WD 456

KT-140-643

OXFORD MEDICAL PUBLICATIONS

A Resuscitation Room Guide

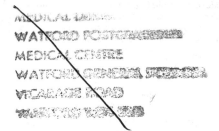

MEDICAL LIBRARY
WATFORD POSTGRADUATE
MEDICAL CENTRE
WATFORD GENERAL HOSPITAL
VICARAGE ROAD
WATFORD WD1 8HB

A Resuscitation Room Guide

Ashis Banerjee

Consultant in Emergency Medicine,
Barnet and Chase Farm Hospitals NHS Trust,
London, UK

and

Chris Hargreaves

Consultant in Intensive Care Medicine
and Anaesthesia, Director of ICU,
The Whittington Hospital NHS Trust,
London, UK

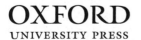
OXFORD
UNIVERSITY PRESS

OXFORD
UNIVERSITY PRESS

Great Clarendon Street, Oxford OX2 6DP

Oxford University Press is a department of the University of Oxford.
It furthers the University's objective of excellence in research, scholarship,
and education by publishing worldwide in

Oxford New York

Auckland Cape Town Dar es Salaam Hong Kong Karachi
Kuala Lumpur Madrid Melbourne Mexico City Nairobi
New Delhi Shanghai Taipei Toronto

With offices in

Argentina Austria Brazil Chile Czech Republic France Greece
Guatemala Hungary Italy Japan Poland Portugal Singapore
South Korea Switzerland Thailand Turkey Ukraine Vietnam

Oxford is a registered trade mark of Oxford University Press
in the UK and in certain other countries

Published in the United States
by Oxford University Press Inc., New York

© Oxford University Press, 2007

The moral rights of the author have been asserted
Database right Oxford University Press (maker)

First published 2007

All rights reserved. No part of this publication may be reproduced,
stored in a retrieval system, or transmitted, in any form or by any means,
without the prior permission in writing of Oxford University Press,
or as expressly permitted by law, or under terms agreed with the appropriate
reprographics rights organization. Enquiries concerning reproduction
outside the scope of the above should be sent to the Rights Department,
Oxford University Press, at the address above

You must not circulate this book in any other binding or cover
and you must impose the same condition on any acquirer

British Library Cataloguing in Publication Data

Data available

Library of Congress Cataloging in Publication Data

Data available

Typeset by Newgen Imaging Systems (P) Ltd., Chennai, India
Printed in Italy
on acid-free paper by Legoprint S.p.A.

ISBN 978–0–19–929807–5 (flexicover: alk.paper)

10 9 8 7 6 5 4 3 2 1

Oxford University Press makes no representation, express or implied, that the drug
dosages in this book are correct. Readers must therefore always check the product
information and clinical procedures with the most up-to-date published product
information and data sheets provided by the manufacturers and the most recent
codes of conduct and safety regulations. The authors and the publishers do not
accept responsibility or legal liability for any errors in the text or for the misuse or
misapplication of material in this work. Except where otherwise stated, drug dosages
and recommendations are for the non-pregnant adult who is not breast-feeding.

Acknowledgements

We wish to express our thanks to our senior adviser on paediatric matters, Dr David Mbamalu, and to Mr Vincent Kika for providing the photographs.

The production of any book requires some support from the proposed audience, and we are grateful to our trainees who have, over the years, identified various clinical questions and the need for a rapid reference text for help in dealing with them. We are indebted to the various individuals who gave up their valuable time to read through and comment on earlier versions of the text

We wish to acknowledge the use of algorithms produced by the Resuscitation Council (UK), the British Thoracic Society, the Intensive Care Society and the Difficult Airway Society, and two algorithms published in the *Postgraduate Medical Journal.*

We have endeavoured to acknowledge all sources of information used in preparation of the text, but would be happy to redress in subsequent editions any inadvertent infringements in the use of information from other sources.

We look forward to receiving any comments and criticisms, which will always be viewed in a constructive spirit

The book would not have taken off had it not been for the vision and support of Catherine Barnes at OUP. We sincerely thank Sara Chare at OUP for patiently and diligently nurturing it through its various gestational stages.

Ashis Banerjee

Chris Hargreaves

Contents

Detailed contents

Preface

The resuscitation room is the hub of intense and focused activity within the emergency department. In most departments, the demands on resuscitation room usage have been steadily increasing, especially linked with the increasing presentation of acutely unwell medical patients to the emergency department.

A wide range of health care professionals contribute to care in this situation. Effective team working hence assumes great importance when working in this environment. The composition and working of teams is thus discussed early in the course of the text.

This book concentrates on important aspects of resuscitation room organization, and emphasizes clinical aspects of management that are of particular importance in this situation. Given the size of the book, it is inevitable that there are alternative views regarding management that may not have been considered or mentioned. Furthermore, the frontiers of evidence-based medicine are rapidly advancing, leading to the potential non-inclusion of some very recent advances. The authors would welcome any suggestions and comments with regard to improving the content of future editions. They, however, sincerely hope that the large majority of users will find it to be a useful adjunct to their clinical practice.

AB
CH

Symbols and abbreviations

+ve	positive
−ve	negative
±	with/without
°	degree
ACE	angiotensin-converting enzyme
ACS	acute coronary syndrome
ACTH	adrenocorticotrophic hormone
AED	automated external defibrillator
AF	atrial fibrillation
aPTT	activated partial thromboplastin time
ARDS	acute respiratory distress syndrome
AV	atrioventricular
bd	bi diem (twice daily)
BiPAP	bilevel positive airway pressure
BP	blood pressure
BSA	body surface area
BTS	British Thoracic Society
CAP	community-acquired pneumonia
CK	creatine kinase
CPAP	continuous positive airway pressure
CPR	cardiopulmonary resuscitation
CSF	cerebrospinal fluid
cm	centimetre
CMV	continuous mandatory ventilation
CNS	central nervous system
COPD	chronic obstructive pulmonary disease
CPAP	continuous positive airway pressure
CPP	cerebral perfusion pressure
CPR	cardiopulmonary resuscitation
CRP	C-reactive protein
CSF	cerebrospinal fluid
CT	computed tomography
CTPA	computed tomographic pulmonary angiography
CVP	central venous pressure
CXR	chest X-ray

DKA	diabetic ketoacidosis
DVT	deep vein thrombosis
ECF	extracellular fluid
ECG	electrocardiograph
ED	emergency department
EEG	electroencephalograph
ELISA	enzyme-linked immunosorbent assay
EPAP	expiratory positive airway pressure
ERCP	endoscopic retrograde cholangio-pancreatography
ESR	erythrocyte sedimentation rate
ETT	endotracheal tube
EVAR	endovascular aortic repair
FBC	full blood count
FFP	frozen fresh plasma
g	gram
GCS	Glasgow Coma Score
GTN	glyceryl trinitrate
h	hour
HCG	human chorionic gonadotrophin
HOCM	hypertrophic obstructive cardiomyopathy
Hct	haematocrit
ICF	intracellular fluid
ICP	intracranial pressure
ICU	intensive care unit
IM	intramuscular
INR	international normalized ratio
IPAP	inspiratory positive airway pressure
IV	intravenous
kg	kilogram
LBBB	left bundle branch block
LFT	liver function test
LMA	laryngeal mask airway
L	litre
LV	left ventricle
LMA	laryngeal mask airway
LVH	left ventricle hypertrophy
MAP	mean arterial pressure
mcg	microgram
MET	Medical Emergency Team
mg	milligram

min	minute
mL	millilitre
MRI	magnetic resonance imaging
MRSA	methicillin-resistant *Staphylococcus aureus*
MSU	midstream urine
NAC	*N*-acetylcysteine
NIV	non-invasive ventilation
NSAID	non-steroidal anti-inflammatory drug
ODP	operating department practitioner
PCI	percutaneous coronary intervention
PCR	polymerase chain reaction
PCWP	pulmonary capillary wedge pressure
PE	pulmonary embolism
PEA	pulseless electrical activity
PEEP	positive end-expiratory pressure
PEFR	peak expiratory flow rate
PO	*per os* (by mouth)
PSV	pressure support ventilation
PT	prothrombin time
PTT	partial thromboplastin time
qds	*quater die sumendus* (4 times a day)
RA	rheumatoid arthritis
RBBB	right bundle branch block
RBC	red blood cell
RSI	rapid sequence intubation
RV	right ventricle
RVH	right ventricle hypertrophy
s	second
SA	sinoatrial
SAH	subarachnoid haemorrhage
SC	subcutaneous
SD	solvent detergent
SIADH	syndrome of inappropriate antidiuretic hormone secretion
SIMV	synchronized intermittent mandatory ventilation
SIRS	systemic inflammatory response syndrome
SLE	systemic lupus erythematosus
STEMI	ST elevation myocardial infarction
tds	*ter die sumendus* (3 times a day)
TIA	transient ischaemic attack
TSS	toxic shock syndrome

TT	thrombin time
U&E	urea and electrolytes
VBG	venous blood gas
VF	ventricular fibrillation
VPC	ventricular premature complex
VT	ventricular tachycardia
vWF	von Willebrand factor
WBC	white blood cell
WPW	Wolff–Parkinson–White

Resuscitation room organization

Introduction

The resuscitation room in the emergency department is set up in a state of immediate readiness to provide staff, equipment, drugs and fluids for actual and potentially life-threatening emergencies. All-round access to the patient permits simultaneous assessment by multiple personnel and practical procedures (in addition to cardiopulmonary resuscitation) to be carried out swiftly and safely. There is usually a designated bay or separate room for children. The equipment may be wall-mounted, or kept in trolleys dedicated to each bay. Whiteboards are useful for documenting key patient details. Ceiling-mounted operating lights are preferably used for illuminating individual bays, which tend to number between two and six. Mobile lead partitions allow for radiation protection of personnel in adjacent bays while X-rays are being taken in a bay. Hand-washing facilities should be available within the room, ideally for each bay.

Some departments have additional equipment such as overhead X-ray gantries and ultrasound machines.

Generally, the resuscitation room is directly accessible from a dedicated ambulance entrance through which thoroughfare is not allowed. The room is placed away from patient circulation areas.

All staff commencing a post in the emergency department will normally attend an induction programme, the content being determined by local policy. It is important as part of induction to the emergency department to become familiarized with the layout of the resuscitation room, resuscitation room procedures and available equipment therein, and to be trained in the use of computer systems, arterial blood gas analysers, automated blood count machines, defibrillators and other devices available. This can be backed up by further familiarization during quiet spells in the department.

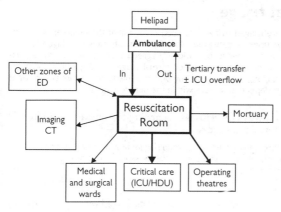

Fig. 1.1 The relationships of the resuscitation room at the 'front end' of the hospital.

Initial triage

Patients are triaged (triage = to sort) on arrival at the emergency department into urgency categories. Priority is usually ranked 1(highest) to 4 (lowest), and is guided by nationally agreed triage scales. Many departments have, however, abandoned formal triage for early decision-making protocols, along with fast tracking of ill patients to the resuscitation room or to high-dependency areas within the department.

> **Care is always prioritized according to clinical need into the following categories:**
>
> 1. Life-threatening emergency requiring immediate resuscitation.
> 2. Very urgent, with strong potential for rapid deterioration or evolution to (1).
> 3. Urgent.
> 4. Standard.
> 5. Non-urgent (but has to be seen and discharged within 4h of arrival!)

To warrant placement in the resuscitation room most patients will be in either category 1 or 2. The general criteria below are used to help in this decision:

- Established or impending cardiac and/or respiratory arrest
- Airway emergencies
- Depressed level of consciousness; coma
- Continuing seizures
- Major trauma and burns
- Major bleeding
- Severe physiological disturbance in any organ system
- Symptoms or signs of serious or potentially serious clinical conditions, e.g. myocardial infarction, left ventricular failure, acute severe asthma, sepsis, etc.

Details of the triage process and recognition of severity of illness are discussed in Chapter 3 'Team approach to resuscitation' p. 48 and p. 50. The major issue is how to identify accurately all very sick patients without false alarms, while not missing patients who appear well but are on the verge of serious deterioration.

For all critically ill patients, prompt recognition of serious problems related to airway, breathing and circulation, and rapid intervention (commonly over minutes at the most) is essential. This requires a combination of adequate clinical skills and experience, appropriate monitoring and rapid access to relevant test results.

Deterioration may quickly progress to cardiorespiratory arrest, which can in many instances be prevented by the provision of optimal care delivered in a timely fashion.

Throughout your time in the emergency department, you will be faced with a broad range of medical and surgical emergencies (particularly trauma) in adults and children.

You should always call for more senior or specialist help if you believe that you do not possess the necessary competence or skills yourself. This may mean activating a 'team call-out', or summoning the assistance of your senior colleagues in the emergency department and/or the duty anaesthetics and/or critical care doctors (see below).

Remember that whatever the circumstances, any patient lacking a patent airway and adequate oxygenation cannot survive for more than a few minutes.

Immediate priorities

Initial care of the critically ill patient, irrespective of the underlying cause, requires a structured approach. This follows the sequence:
- Primary survey with simultaneous resuscitation
- Secondary survey
- Emergency treatment
- Definitive care.

The components of this approach are outlined here.

In general, the order of priority below is adhered to, with vascular access in the form of initial peripheral venous cannulation and blood sampling taking place at the same time.

Standard monitoring of ECG, non-invasive blood pressure and pulse oximetry constitute the essential minimum. The ABCDE approach involves consideration of the following:

1. **A**irway (with cervical spine and **b**reathing) control to deal with airway obstruction with oxygen, intubation and ventilation if needed, as well as dealing with pneumothorax. Immediate drug therapy, e.g. bronchodilators.

   Clinical focus: breathing pattern, respiratory rate and chest excursion, gas exchange as indicated by oximetry and by blood gases.

2. Stabilization of the **c**irculation and haemorrhage control with adequate vascular access, monitoring and fluid therapy. Antiarrhythmics or inotropic support may be needed. External haemorrhage should generally be controllable by local pressure and limb elevation, not by blind clamping of vessels.

   Clinical focus: heart rhythm and rate control, blood pressure and other markers of adequacy of the circulation, e.g. peripheral perfusion, acid–base balance and serum lactate. Direct cardiac output measurement if available.

3. Neurological status (**d**isability assessment): clinical assessment of the level of consciousness and any focal neurological deficit. Intubation to prevent soiling of the lungs if protective reflexes are inadequate. Immediate drug therapy, e.g. anticonvulsants for seizures.

   Clinical focus: Glasgow Coma Score (GCS), focal neurology; remember cerebral perfusion pressure = mean arterial pressure – intracranial pressure.

4. Further **e**xposure and examination to look for diagnostic clues and assess other organ system involvement. In the context of trauma, the secondary survey is done at this stage to exclude other injuries.

   Clinical focus: bladder catheterization and urinary output measurement, and thorough visual inspection of the patient front and back, with log-rolling where necessary.

Other points in immediate care
- Continued or new deterioration in clinical condition warrants repeated and sequential evaluation of airway, breathing and circulation.
- NB: some patients with chronic obstructive pulmonary disease (COPD) and chronic hypercapnia may be sensitive to oxygen, and careful oxygen therapy (commencing with 24 or 28% O_2) is necessary to avoid raising the SpO_2 above 90% in these situations.
  - Excessive inspired oxygen concentration can worsen hypercapnic respiratory failure and may well have been administered in the ambulance.
  - Outside this limited context, it is not appropriate to give low concentrations of oxygen to an acutely unwell patient.
- Non-invasive ventilation (NIV) is increasingly used early in the presentation of respiratory failure in the emergency department in the context of COPD and pulmonary oedema (PE) (see role of NIV p. 188).
  - In the future, NIV is likely to become more commonplace in the acute setting as evidence of its effectiveness accumulates.
  - NIV can avert the need for intubation and invasive ventilation, but has to be used by appropriately trained staff with specialized equipment.

Note keeping/documentation

Due to time pressure and priority of clinical tasks, recording the details of immediate care is often put off until after the patient has been stabilized or notes are sparsely and hurriedly written. Interventions and their timings, especially of which drugs were given and their doses, quantities of fluids and blood products, must be accurately noted as contemporaneously as possible, preferably by a designated 'scribe' (see team approach to resuscitation, p. 46).

Structured documentation should separately outline the state of, and interventions for, airway, breathing, circulation and disability (neurological status). The use of trauma sheets and cardiac arrest proformas where available is recommended.

Remember that early events can have important later repercussions. Medico-legally, written records are far more useful than hazy recollections months afterwards! In general, what has not been written is considered as having not been done, in the absence of proof to the contrary. Electronic monitoring systems with trended data storage are increasingly used to print off the history of all monitored parameters with their timings, and are invaluable in supplementing written records.

Ongoing care

After initial stabilization, a more thorough assessment with meticulous history and examination is required to delineate accurately the diagnosis and extent of the patient's problems.

Further tests can be carried out at this stage as appropriate:
- X-rays and other portable imaging
- ECG
- Blood and tissue fluid specimens for cultures and toxicological screening.

Priorities beyond ABCDE

Although the precise diagnosis is not always immediately important (and indeed, sometimes, many investigations, and many brains put together over several days may be required to recognize the underlying causative condition), treatment must be targeted appropriately.

For example, diuretics will not help pneumonia, antibiotics are of no use in heart failure and bronchodilators are of little value for pulmonary embolus.

Some patients will have a clear single problem, responding to your early care, for which the future management plan will be straightforward and onward transfer to the admitting ward will be appropriate, e.g. asthma or simple pulmonary oedema.

You will also encounter more complex situations where prioritization of interventions will be difficult. The patient could have a simultaneous need for
- More detailed monitoring
- CT imaging
- Major surgery
- Ongoing fluid resuscitation or transfusion
- Transfer to a tertiary centre.

For example, in a patient with septic shock and an acute abdomen, surgery is often briefly delayed until adequate blood pressure and other clinical parameters are achieved. This strategy of 'optimizing' the circulation as part of early goal-directed therapy is thought to improve outcomes in such patients. Time taken has to be traded against the consequences of undue delay with progression of uncontrolled surgical sepsis.

However, with bleeding due to penetrating trauma, immediate surgery is likely to be the only intervention that will salvage the patient, and any delay is detrimental. With major upper gastrointestinal bleeding, urgent endoscopy is usually the most important immediate priority, but this procedure can only be done once the relevant staff and equipment are available.

You need to decide the best order of interventions, balancing the risks and benefits of each procedure against any delay. Competing priorities may make this decision making difficult.

For example in a patient with severe head injury, urgent transfer to a neurosurgical centre may well be needed, but dealing with other life-threatening injuries such as ruptured spleen must take precedence.

Is the patient adequately resuscitated?

Numerical target ranges for physiological parameters in the various organ systems are often used as 'goals' to guide the resuscitation process and monitor response to initial treatment. Some of these can also act as end points to determine when support is optimal. They are also used as part of the early warning scoring systems to activate team call-out.

Goals

Respiration

Some patients may already be commenced on NIV or continuous positive airway pressure (CPAP) and improving.

Circulation

- Heart rate 60–120bpm (adult). Sinus tachycardia above this rate may be inevitable in sepsis, trauma or with high doses of inotropes and after cardiac arrest.
- Capillary refill time: <2s following 5s of pressure on the digit
- Skin perfusion: warm peripheries
- Blood pressure: Systolic >100mmHg
                      MAP ≥70mmHg (adult without co-morbidities)
                      ≥90mmHg (elderly or known hypertension)
                      ≥100mmHg [for adequate cerebral perfusion
                      pressure (CPP) with raised intracranial
                      pressure (ICP).
- Serum lactate <4mmol/l: the level correlates well with the degree of hypovolaemic shock.
- Urine output >0.5ml/kg/h.

The above are indirect markers of cardiac output which can be measured directly (see cardiovascular monitoring techniques p. 260). However, certain methods are only possible in intubated patients and equipment is not widely available outside critical care at present.

Table 1.1

	Awake, spontaneous breathing	Intubated and ventilated
Adequate gas exchange	PaO_2 ≥10kPa with FiO_2 ≤0.5 $PaCO_2$ usually normal or low in hypoxaemic respiratory failure. In improving hypercapnic respiratory failure, pH >7.30 when $PaCO_2$ raised.	PaO_2 ≥10kPa on minimum necessary FiO_2; $PaCO_2$ 5kPa. In hypercapnic states, aim for pH >7.25 ('permissive hypercapnia')
Respiratory rate	>10 and below 25/min	Ventilator set to maintain normocapnia
Protective airway reflexes	Present (if GCS <10 assess need for intubation)	Intubated

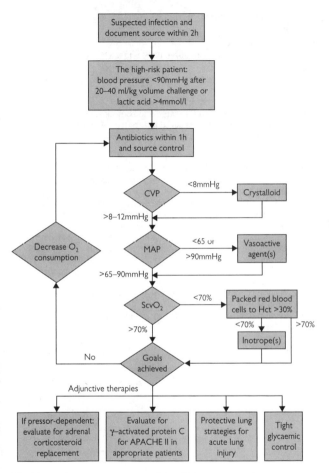

Fig. 1.2 Treatment options in sepsis. CVP = MAP = mean arterial pressure, Scvo$_2$ = central venous oxygen saturation, Hct = haematocrit. Early and innovative interventions for severe sepsis and septic shock: taking advantage of a window of opportunity. Rivers EP, McIntyre L, Morro DC, Rivers KK. *Canadian Medical Association Journal.* 2005; **173**: 1054–1065.
(After Rivers E, *et al.* Early goal-directed therapy in the treatment of severe sepsis and septic shock. *New England Journal of Medicine* 2001; **345**: 1368–1377.)

The algorithmic process in Fig. 1.2 may be extrapolated to other critically ill patients

Level of consciousness

- Ideally, awake and unsedated with GCS >12. GCS <10—requires assessment by critical care-or anaesthetics-trained staff. Some emergency departments have such individuals as members of their own staff.
- All obtunded patients should be nursed on their side.
- Intubated patients are often sedated and sometimes paralysed with muscle relaxants as well as sedated for control of ventilation. Thus GCS assessment is not valid. The GCS prior to intubation is used as a significant baseline measure.

In addition, there should be, with ongoing resuscitation

1. Temperature control. Normothermia should generally be the aim; however, following resuscitation from cardiac arrest mild therapeutic hypothermia is being used for cerebral protection. 'Unconscious adult patients with return of spontaneous circulation after out-of-hospital VF cardiac arrest should be cooled to 32–34°C. Cooling should be started as soon as possible and continued for at least 12–24 hours. Induced hypothermia might also benefit unconscious adult patients with spontaneous circulation after out-of-hospital cardiac arrest from a non-shockable rhythm, or cardiac arrest in hospital' (European Resuscitation Council Guidelines 2005).
2. Correction of metabolic and electrolyte abnormalities (hyperkalaemia, glycaemic control).
3. Correction of anaemia (target Hb 8) and coagulation disturbance (INR <1.5).

Is the patient ready to leave the resuscitation room?

- Whatever the problem, it is dangerous to move a patient who has not been adequately stabilized (or with the potential for rapid deterioration), without necessary monitoring and appropriate escort personnel and back-up equipment.
- Compliance with time limits can only be justified when in the patient's best interest. (for example the 'golden hour' in trauma care). Even in these days of emergency department 98% targets, clinical exceptions are allowed for stabilizing seriously ill patients. Patients should only be moved for clinical reasons and only when it is safe to do so.
- Transport even over short distances within the hospital can present hazards, especially where it is difficult to maintain immediate skilled assistance and when a patient is being moved from the trolley (e.g. in a CT scanner) (refer to patient transfer and transport p. 27).

Key checks before transport even on short journeys in the hospital:
- Oxygen supply
- Drugs and fluids
- Drips and lines secure and working
- Sufficient battery life for infusion pumps and portable monitors
- Working lift available
- Body temperature able to be maintained and patient adequately covered in winter
- Notes, observation charts and test results collated.

Referral and onward external transfer to a specialist centre requires detailed communication and forward planning. Hand-over documentation is crucial. Many such transfers are of ventilated patients with an anaesthetist escort (see section on transfers p. 26).

Where is the appropriate place for the patient to go to from the resuscitation room?

The complexity of care requirements and staffing input are graded by level from 0 (standard ward care) to 3 (intensive care) (*Comprehensive critical care*. Department of Health, 2000)

General ward (level 0, ±1)

- *Admissions ward* (level 0, 1 ± 2)
- *Coronary care unit* (level 1 ± 2)
  - Patients with cardiac problems especially myocardial infarction.
- *Critical care*
  - Level 2 *High dependency* More detailed monitoring than can be provided at the ward level. Basic support of one failing organ system including CPAP for respiratory failure and inotropes for circulatory support.
  - Level 3 *Intensive care* Multiple organ support, i.e. ventilation, renal replacement, etc.

  Local admission arrangements do vary considerably and are dependent on

- Ward capability and expertise (specialty based or generic acute admissions unit)
- Equipment and monitoring provision in a given area
- Staffing levels and availability of cover
- Availability and extent of critical care outreach service (p. 50).

  Decisions about placement are based on the individual factors below as well as the overall clinical picture and circumstances.

- Severity of derangement of physiological parameters and response to initial treatment
- Clinical diagnosis (propensity for deterioration and need for surgery)
- Monitoring requirements
- Complexity of treatment and need for organ system support
- Need for tertiary specialist care not available locally
- Co-morbidities and pre-existing functional reserve*
- 'Treatability' and prospects for recovery, especially with advanced or end-stage disease
- The patient's wishes, any advance directive and DNAR (do not attempt resuscitation) status.

  Bed availability should not be a factor in these decisions. At all times but especially during periods of peak activity and occupancy, safety must be maintained.

---

* This is particularly relevant to surgical patients for whom a lower threshold for post-operative critical care admission is often warranted.

It may be necessary to transfer a patient to a different hospital where the appropriate level of support is available rather than compromise on standards of care when there is no empty bed locally. This is particularly the case for critically ill level 2 and 3 patients. Delayed and suboptimal care has a serious adverse impact on later outcomes.

Care of the critically ill—the essentials

Critical illness often precedes cardio-respiratory arrest, which should in many instances be prevented by the provision of optimal care delivered in a timely fashion.

Caring for the critically ill patient, irrespective of the underlying cause, requires a structured approach, consisting of:
- Primary survey, with simultaneous resuscitation
- Secondary survey
- Emergency treatment
- Definitive care.

Of the above, the component with which the resuscitation room is primarily concerned is the primary survey, along with ongoing resuscitation. The precise diagnosis is not immediately important and indeed this may only be arrived at after extensive investigation.

The primary survey comprises evaluation of:
- Airway (and cervical spine control in the presence of trauma): to prevent upper airway obstruction and/or soiling of the lungs
- Breathing: to ensure adequate ventilation
- Circulation (and haemorrhage control): to ensure adequate vital organ perfusion
- Disability (neurological function), along with:
- Exposure
- Repeated assessments of the above.

Resuscitation involves attention to correction of abnormalities in:
- Airway
- Breathing
- Circulation

Continued or new deterioration in clinical condition warrants repeated and sequential evaluation of airway, breathing and circulation.

Structured documentation should separately outline the state of, and interventions for, airway, breathing, circulation and disability (neurological status).

Universal precautions

Protective measures against diseases spread by blood and other body fluids should be maintained for all patients at all times in the resuscitation room:

- For invasive procedures, the use of gloves and of eye protection (ideally with a visor) are mandatory.
- All open skin lesions, particularly on the hands, should be covered with water-proof adhesive plasters before commencing clinical duties.
- Needles and scalpel blades should be placed into a designated sharps container. Needles must not be re-sheathed prior to disposal. Sharps containers must not be over-filled. Consider the use of safe disposal devices.
- On completion of a procedure, needles and other sharps you have used must be disposed of immediately in a sharps bin. It is dangerous to leave these for others to tidy up.
- All bodily fluids should be immediately disposed of in sealed suction bottles.
- Do not pass or receive sharps from hand to hand—the giver should lay them on a tray or other flat surface and the receiver should pick them up.
- Disposables and clinical waste should be placed in yellow clinical waste bags for incineration.
- Spillages must be dealt with using recommended cleaning fluids and procedures.
- Standard hospital procedures should be followed in the event of a needlestick injury.
- In addition, all staff involved in clinical procedures should be screened for hepatitis B and C, and immunized against hepatitis B.

Body substances requiring the same handling precautions as blood:
- Cerebrospinal fluid (CSF)
- Peritoneal fluid
- Pleural fluid
- Pericardial fluid
- Synovial fluid
- Amniotic fluid
- Semen
- Vaginal secretions
- Breast milk
- Any other body fluid containing visible blood
- Unfixed tissues and organs.

Infection control procedures

These are intended to prevent cross-infection between patients and to reduce hospital acquired infections, especially with resistant organisms such as MRSA.

- Transient carriage of bacteria on the hands of staff is the most common mechanism of spread of MRSA between patients
- Local hospital guidelines should be followed. Remember basic hand hygiene measures, such as washing in water or using alcohol hand scrubs between patients. See clean your hands campaign (www.npsa.uk/cleanyourhands)
- Aseptic precautions should be used for invasive procedures, including wearing sterile gown and gloves and creating an aseptic field by adequate skin cleaning and the application of sterile drapes. The introduction of infection through vascular lines, drains and catheters is a major source of later morbidity
- The patient trolley and reusable equipment in direct patient contact must be cleaned thoroughly between cases
- Most items in potential contact with body fluids and secretions (e.g. oxygen face masks) are now disposable single-use and must not be reused.

Do not attempt resuscitation policy

In general, in the resuscitation room, one should commence resuscitation where indicated, and ask questions later. Selection of patients not to be resuscitated involves the consideration of the following information:

- The patient's own wishes (which may include **an advance directive or written statement made when the individual had capacity**)
- The views of relatives or close friends, especially those holding lasting power of attorney, who may be reporting the known wishes of a patient who cannot communicate
- The patient's prognosis in the intermediate and long term, determined by the presence of incurable and terminal illness
- Objective knowledge of the patient's previous quality of life and previous health
- The expected quality of life in terms of medical and social well-being should resuscitation be 'successful'
- The patient's perceived ability to cope with disability in the environment for which he or she is destined.

Decisions Relating to Cardiopulmonary Resuscitation. A joint statement from the British Medical Association, the Resuscitation Council (UK) and the Royal College of Nursing, London: Resuscitation Council, March 2001.
Resuscitation policy (HSC 2000/028). NHS Executive London, Department of Health, September 2000.

Safe inter-hospital transfer

Inter-hospital transfer is potentially hazardous for the critically ill patient, and requires effective communication between suitably senior members of the medical staff at both ends. Departments need to ensure that they have adequate insurance cover for staff involved in inter-hospital transfers. Individual membership of certain professional bodies, e.g. the Intensive Care Society or the Association of Anaesthetists, includes such cover. In reality, many hospitals provide inadequate or no cover for this purpose. It is important to ensure that the following aspects are taken care of:

Administrative aspects of the preparation for transfer: communication between transferring and receiving units; documentation; X-rays; blood and other investigation reports; copy of all notes; referral letter. Critical care network transfer forms are now comonly available to record and audit transfers.

Preparation of equipment, drugs and personnel
- Equipment: portable mechanical ventilator with airway pressure and tidal volume display, and disconnect alarm
- Adequate supply of oxygen for the journey: spare portable cylinder
- Portable battery-powered multifunction monitor
- Other equipment: suction; battery-powered syringe pumps; battery-powered IV volumetric pumps; intubation equipment; self-inflating bag, valve and mask; venous access equipment; defibrillator; spare batteries; warming blanket
- Drugs: sedative-hypnotic (propofol or midazolam); muscle relaxants; analgesics; anticonvulsants; 20% mannitol; vasoactive drugs; drugs used for CPR
- Cross-matched blood
- Personnel trained in resuscitation.

Preparation of the patient
- Airway: patent and secured, with tracheal intubation as indicated, and tracheal tube position confirmed on chest X-ray (CXR)
- Cervical spine protected where appropriate
- Breathing: adequate spontaneous breathing or assisted ventilation of lungs on transport ventilator; secured chest drains; chest drain placement or thoracostomy in patients requiring helicopter transport if there is a pneumothorax or the potential for developing one—chest drains should not be clamped for transfer; adequate gas exchange confirmed by arterial blood gas estimation
- Circulation: secured venous access with a minimum of two routes of access; adequate control of sources of ongoing bleeding; appropriate fluid replacement in progress
- Disability: appropriate pain relief; seizures controlled; appropriate management of raised intracranial pressure
- Fractures (long bone and pelvic) splinted
- Minimum appropriate monitoring: ECG, transduced invasive blood pressure from arterial line, non-invasive BP cuff back-up, SpO_2; end-tidal CO_2; temperature.

Check list 2: are you ready for departure?
Patient
- Stable on transport trolley
- Appropriately monitored
- All infusions running and lines adequately secured
- Adequately sedated and paralysed
- Adequately secured to trolley
- Adequately wrapped to prevent heat loss.

Staff
- Adequately trained and experienced
- Received appropriate handover
- Adequately clothed and insured.

Equipment
- Appropriately equipped ambulance
- Appropriate equipment and drugs
- Batteries checked (spare batteries available)
- Sufficient oxygen supplies
- Portable phone charged and available
- Money/credit cards for emergencies

Organization
- Case notes, X-rays, results, blood collected
- Transfer documentation prepared
- Location of bed and receiving doctor known
- Receiving unit advised of departure time and estimated time of arrival
- Telephone numbers of referring and receiving units available
- Relatives informed
- Return travel arrangements in place
- Ambulance crew briefed
- Police escort arranged if appropriate.

Departure
- Patient trolley secured
- Electrical equipment plugged into ambulance power supply where available
- Ventilator transferred to ambulance oxygen supply
- All equipment safely mounted or stowed
- Staff seated and wearing seat belts.

Reproduced with permission from the Intensive Care Society.

Transport documentation

The following information should be recorded on transport documentation.

Transfer details

- Patient's name, address, date of birth
- Next of kin, what information they have been given and by whom
- Referring hospital, ward/unit and contact telephone number
- Name of referring doctor and contact telephone number
- Receiving hospital, ward/unit and contact telephone number
- Name of receiving doctor and contact telephone number
- Names and status of the escorting personnel

A medical summary

- Primary reason for admission to the referring unit
- History and past history
- Dates of operations and procedures
- Number of days on intensive care
- Intubation history, ventilatory support and blood gases
- Cardiovascular status including inotrope and vasopressor requirements
- Other medication and fluids
- Type of lines inserted and dates of insertion
- Recent results and MRSA status

A nursing summary

- Nursing care required with reference to the following:

Respiration, cardiovascular parameters, communication methods, nutrition, pain and sedation, sleep patterns, elimination, skin condition, hygiene and social needs.

Patient status during transfer

- Vital signs including ECG, blood pressure SaO_2, $EtCO_2$, temperature, respiratory rate, peak inspiratory pressure, PEEP
- Drugs given during transfer including infusions
- Fluids given during transfer
- Summary of patient's condition during transfer signed by escorting doctor.

Audit data including

- Reason for the transfer
- Whether the transfer was within or outside the local network
- The urgency of the transfer
- Time taken for transfer from time of ambulance request to completion
- Adverse events/critical incidents

(*Guidelines for Transport of the Critically Ill Adult*. Intensive care society, London, 2002).

Breaking bad news

The emergency department can prove to be a challenging atmosphere in which to break bad news, when the staff involved in a failed attempt at resuscitation may themselves be under considerable stress. The death, illness or injury is nearly always sudden and unexpected.

Some ground rules must, however, be followed even in this charged atmosphere in order to do this in an optimal fashion:

- Get your facts right by going through the clinical information and ensure that the relevant documents are available to consult if required
- Ensure a private, quiet and comfortable location, often provided by a designated bereaved relatives' room in proximity to the resuscitation room
- Mobile phones should be switched off and pagers kept on silent mode
- A notice saying 'Do not disturb' affixed to the door is also helpful. This allows for protected time for the encounter.
- All individuals present should be seated at the same level, allowing for eye contact
- Introduce yourself and ensure that you identify who is present and what their relationship to the deceased or seriously ill patient is
- Check what is already known and understood.
- Tissues should be available if required, as should access to tea-and coffee-making facilities
- Clear and unambiguous words should be used, e.g. 'he/she has died', not 'passed away', 'just left us' or 'gone to a better place', which can easily be misconstrued
- No medical jargon should be used
- Attempts at inappropriate humour are best reserved for another occasion
- Allow for a range of emotional responses, ranging from tears, silence, anger, self-pity and a sense of helplessness
- Allow time for questions
- Proceed at the relative's pace
- Write things down or draw diagrams if appropriate and necessary
- Check for understanding as the encounter comes to its natural conclusion
- Offer support, including pastoral and contact with relevant support groups.
- Ensure that the need for notifying the Coroner (or Procurator Fiscal in Scotland) is made known.
- At all times show compassion and understanding.

Care of the dying

For some patients arriving in the resuscitation room, vigorous treatment measures are commenced without the background facts and details of underlying conditions being known. It can later transpire that a patient has advanced malignancy or another untreatable or terminal condition.

At this stage, a decision to discontinue medical intervention can be made. This may be at the request of the patient or their family, or may be arrived at after a full assessment of the clinical picture in conjunction with discussion with relatives.

The emphasis of care is then shifted to comfort measures and preparation for a dignified death.

Many hospitals have now introduced an 'End of Life Care Pathway' to guide the overall care needs. This is based on the Liverpool Care Pathway (www.lcp-mariecurie.org.uk). Further advice may also be available from the local palliative care team or hospice.

The main aims are as below
1. Communication
* Family members are made aware of the diagnosis and imminent death
* Contact details and preferred method for contact are documented
* Religious or psychological support is obtained if requested.
2. Interventions
* Inappropriate monitoring and therapy is discontinued.
3. Drug therapy
* Analgesia, sedation and anti-emetics are prescribed for symptom relief
* Inappropriate medication is discontinued.
  The patient is moved from the resuscitation room to a quiet area.

Referral of a death to the coroner

* A patient who has died in the resuscitation room will nearly always have newly arrived at the hospital and had a rapidly downhill clinical course.
* Detail of the circumstances leading up to the immediate presentation as well as background information on existing medical conditions is often lacking.
* Many cases will involve major injury, drugs and alcohol or other suspicious circumstances, and the identity of the victim may not be known.

The coroner should be notified of any death in the following categories
* Cause of death unknown or unclear
* Accidents, trauma and violence
* Death in or following release from police or prison custody
* Suicide or other poisoning
* Drug and alcohol abuse
* Death during a surgical operation or before recovery from anaesthesia
* Death following non-therapeutic abortion

- Still births where it is thought that the baby was born alive
- Self-neglect or neglect by others
- Industrial or occupational disease
- Any other suspicious or unnatural death.

The coroner's officer (a police officer) will usually gather the necessary details. A post-mortem may well be ordered by the coroner. In cases of suspected manslaughter or murder, the investigation is handed over to the police. A coroner's inquest is deferred until after a Crown Prosecution Service decision and any prosecution is complete.

In Scotland, the Procurator Fiscal handles investigations into deaths in a Fatal Accident Inquiry—this process differs from the coronial system in England.

The function and organization of coroners is currently under review and will be the subject of new legislation.

(Coroner Reform: The Government's Draft Bill Improving Death Investigation in England and Wales www.dca.gov.uk/legist/coroners_draft.pdf)

Basic principles of resuscitation

Airway management

Assess the airway for patency. If the airway is not patent, it should be cleared.

- Clear the airway: head tilt; chin lift; jaw thrust; suction with Yankauer sucker. Keep well-fitting dentures in place wherever possible. Once the airway is cleared, it needs to be maintained patent
- Maintain the airway: oropharyngeal or nasopharyngeal airway initially
- Consider a definitive airway: tracheal tube; laryngeal mask airway; surgical airway.

Assessment of airway patency can lead to one of the following conclusions

- Patent airway: awake subject with coherent speech
- Partial airway obstruction
- Complete airway obstruction
- Airway at risk from obstruction
- Unable to protect airway against aspiration owing to loss of airway reflexes: any patient who accepts an oropharyngeal airway without a gag reflex has an airway at risk from obstruction and from aspiration.

The triple manoeuvre is a combination of

- Head tilt: gentle pressure to the forehead to achieve extension of the upper neck
- Chin lift: gentle lifting of the chin with the tips of the index and middle fingers
- Jaw thrust: lifting forward the mandible using the fingers of both hands behind the angles of the mandible.

The aim of these manoeuvres is to lift the mandible and the hyoid bones anteriorly.

Contraindications to head tilt and chin lift

- Suspected cervical spine injury; however, the risk of not opening the airway needs to be balanced against the presence of potential cervical spine injury
- Previous cervical fusion
- Known cervical spine pathology, including rheumatoid arthritis
- Down's syndrome (atlanto-axial instability).

Assessment of airway patency

- LOOK for chest expansion with inspiration
- LISTEN for airflow at the mouth and nose
- FEEL for airflow at the mouth and nose, using the dorsum
  of the hand

Partial airway obstruction is associated with noisy breathing, and complete airway obstruction with silent breathing and absent breath sounds.

Breathing (ventilation)

Assess adequacy:
- Observe ventilatory activity: look for chest and abdominal movements; listen and feel for airflow at the mouth and nose; count respiratory rate; note respiratory depth and pattern; evaluate for work or effort of breathing
- Continuous auscultation of breath sounds using a monaural precordial stethoscope or a standard stethoscope
- Capnography: normal end-tidal carbon dioxide is 4–5%
- Decompress tension pneumothorax.

Circulation

Venous access.

Fluid bolus: 20mL/kg; 5mL/kg if heart failure is likely; assess the effect on the circulatory status.

Consider inotropic and vasoactive agents (see p. 270)

Table 2.1 Potential sources of blood loss and their recognition

External	Visible
Limbs	Visible
Chest	Chest X-ray
Pelvis	Pelvis X-ray
Abdomen	Ultrasound FAST scan/diagnostic peritoneal lavage

Dysfunction of the CNS

- Ascertain level of consciousness—AVPU scheme (alert, voice, pain, unresponsive)
- Document pupil size, symmetry and light reactions
- Check capillary blood glucose.

Exposure, with environment control

A head-to-toe survey of all aspects of the body, not forgetting the posterior torso, is carried out, all the while ensuring that the patient does not become hypothermic.

Team approach to resuscitation

Introduction

The management of the acutely ill patient in the resuscitation room setting requires a coordinated team approach in order to obtain optimal results. The important elements of the team approach include:
- A pre-assembled team
- Assignment of specific roles
- An identified leader who remains hands-off and maintains overall control
- Horizontal integration of activities
- Observance of universal precautions.

Patients in triage categories 1 and 2 have a huge potential range of disorders that require rapid assessment with simultaneous intervention. Drugs and equipment need to be rapidly deployed in a coordinated way. Smooth and well rehearsed clinical activity along with the essential backup of laboratory, imaging, clerical and portering staff all contribute to the successful team.

The teams called upon to deal with patients in the resuscitation room are:
- Cardiac arrest team
- Trauma team
- Paediatric team
- Medical emergency or critical care outreach team
- Less commonly, obstetrics team
- Major incident response team.

Who should be in the team?
- Emergency medicine doctor
- Emergency department nurse
- Anaesthetics doctor (usually specialist registrar-SpR level)
- Operating department practitioner (ODP)
- Surgical
- Orthopaedic ⎫ doctors usually SpR level, as required
- Medical ⎬
- Paediatric. ⎭

What does each team member do?
Roles relate to the specific expertise of each team member, but all must be competent to deal with the situation in hand. Familiarity with what needs to be done is also crucial. For example, intubation of a trauma patient with suspected cervical spine injury needs in-line stabilization of the neck, application of cricoid pressure and pre-oxygenation all at the same time, requiring close teamwork. Laminated action cards are usefully read by team members while waiting, especially locum members of the staff.

The team leader should be responsible for coordinating the handover from the ambulance crew, who should be questioned for as much detail as may be required to deal with the clinical situation. The patient report form also provides useful information about pre-hospital vital signs and treatments given.

The cardiac arrest team

The remit of the cardiac arrest team is being widely reconsidered. A broader role in attending all very sick patients has been proposed—as the Medical Emergency or Patient at Risk Team. The emphasis is on proactive intervention to deal with problems at an early stage[1].

Aims of an anticipatory team approach
- Early recognition of sick patients and alert of appropriate staff by scoring of abnormal physiological parameters
- Intervene before cardio-respiratory arrest occurs
- Reduce the risk of unexpected death
- Minimize unplanned intensive care unit admissions.

In some hospitals in the UK, critical care outreach teams may cover the emergency department to fulfill this function. In others, the equivalent may be the duty medical registrar and/or critical care or anaesthetics doctors.

The European Resuscitation Council Guideline 2005 Section 4a Prevention of cardiac arrest, states:

> The hospital should have a clearly identified response to critical illness. This may include a designated outreach service or resuscitation team (e.g. MET) capable of responding to acute clinical crises identified by clinical triggers or other indicators. This service must be available 24h per day

The NCEPOD report 2005 'An acute problem?' states
- More attention should be paid to patients exhibiting physiological abnormalities. This is a marker of increased mortality risk.
- Robust track and trigger systems should be in place to cover all inpatients. These should be linked to a response team that is appropriately skilled to assess and manage the clinical problems.

(Reference www.ncepod.org.uk)

The criteria for activating a team call can be derived from the criteria used for medical emergency team activation. These criteria have not been validated (MERIT study) but make physiological sense and can be used to guide the diversion of resources to the most seriously ill patient in the resuscitation room.

Medical Emergency Team (MET) activation criteria

Airway: obstructed or threatened
Breathing: all respiratory arrests
         Respiratory rate <5 or >36/min
Circulation: all cardiac arrests
        Heart rate <40 or >140/min
        Systolic blood pressure <90mmHg
Disability: Sudden fall in level of consciousness
        (fall in GCS by >2 points)
        Repeated or prolonged seizures
Other: any patient who causes concern but does not fit the above mentioned criteria.

1 MERIT study investigators. Introduction of the medical emergency team (MET) system: a cluster-randomised controlled trial. *Lancet.* 2005; **365**: 2091–2097.

Critical care outreach teams

The outreach service may be nurse-led[2] or multiprofessional and operate for variable periods, usually covering ward in-patients. Depending on local arrangements, these teams may be activated to deal with patients in the resuscitation room in the same way as the MET. Activation is dependent upon early warning triggers (patient at risk triggers):

- Respiratory rate <8 or >25 breaths/min
- Pulse oximetry <90% on 35% fractional inspired oxygen
- Pulse <50 or >125bpm
- Systolic BP <90mmHg, >200mmHg, or >40mmHg less than the patient's normal values
- Urine output <30mL/h for 2h
- Sustained alteration in level of consciousness or fall in GCS of 2 points in the past hour
- Staff concerns about the patient.

2 Ball C, Kirby M, Williams S. Effect of the critical care outreach team on patient survival to discharge from hospital and readmission to critical care: non-randomised population based study. *British Medical Journal*, 2003; **327**: 1014–1016.

Cardiac arrest protocol

Pre assignment of roles is useful in dealing with a cardiac arrest. The procedure listed below is not meant to be prescriptive, and merely outlines a system that we have found useful in personal practice.

Announced on departmental tannoy as cardiac arrest call to resuscitation room

2222 call activated

Team: minimum 4; optimum 6.

6-member working hours team
- Team leader
- Airways doctor: takes charge of airway
- Circulation doctor: obtains venous access + administers drugs + obtains arterial blood gases
- Compressions nurse/doctor: starts chest compressions/defibrillates; alternates with scribe
- Scribe nurse/doctor: starts clock + writes details on whiteboard, documenting time of arrest, time of CPR, defibrillation attempts, drugs administered
- Runner: attaches leads.

4-member out-of-hours team
- Team leader
- Airways doctor
- Circulation doctor: obtains venous access + attaches leads + drugs + scribe
- Compression/defibrillation—alternates with circulation doctor
- Runner.

Trauma team activation criteria

The trauma team is often assembled following an alert from ambulance service paramedics before the patient arrives at the hospital, allowing valuable preparation time. Activation based on historical criteria almost invariably leads to over-triage, but it is always preferable to activate a team response followed by stand-down as appropriate, rather than losing control over a potentially life-threatening situation. In some emergency departments, the initial response may be initiated in-house, with recruitment of support from in-patient specialities as and when required.

Historical circumstances:
- Motor vehicle accident:
  - Impact speed >40mph
  - Death of another occupant in the vehicle
  - Ejection of patient from vehicle
  - Severe damage to vehicle
  - Vehicle roll-over
  - Incident with five or more casualties
- Pedestrian/cyclist
  - Impact speed >30mph
  - Fall from higher than standing height.

Abnormal physiology
- Respiratory distress
- Airway compromise or obstruction
- Respiratory rate <9 or >30/min
- Irregular breathing
- SaO_2 <90%
- Shock
- Systolic blood pressure <90mmHg
- Pulse rate <50 or >120bpm
- Peripheral hypoperfusion
- Neurological dysfunction
- Reduced level of consciousness
- Repeated seizures.

When does the team stand down?

- Although a patient has been stabilized and is ready to move out of the resuscitation room, responsibility for the patient continues until care is formally handed over. This may be to theatres, the critical care unit or an acute ward
- The sickest patients, especially when ventilated, will need a trained medical escort (almost always the anaesthetist) as well as nursing presence
- Remember that the patient is leaving a safe, controlled environment and may still have outstanding problems needing definitive intervention (especially with major trauma)
- Detailed monitoring with frequent recording of observations needs to be continued

- The team's activity and interventions need to be documented thoroughly in the records, and events communicated to the patient's family
- After an unsuccessful or complex case, particularly if problems are encountered pertaining to delivery of optimal care, time needs to be set aside for staff debriefing and, if need be, completion of an incident report.

Chapter 4

Cardiac arrest and peri-arrest management

Introduction

Cardiac arrest is the cessation of effective circulation, manifested by loss of responsiveness and the absence of respiratory effort, which may be accompanied by impalpable central pulses. All medical and nursing staff involved in cardiac arrest management in the resuscitation room should be trained to at least intermediate life support standard, and preferably to advanced life support standard. The Resuscitation Guidelines 2005 have considerably simplified the procedures involved in advanced life support. While the basic life support algorithm has been incorporated in the text, it applies mainly to lay rescuers. In the hospital situation, it is customary to proceed to advanced life support.

Causes of cardiac arrest

Cardiac disease
- Ischaemic heart disease
- Cardiomyopathy
- Myocarditis
- Cardiac trauma and tamponade.

Respiratory
- Hypoxia
- Hypercapnia.

Circulatory
- Hypovolaemia
- Tension pneumothorax
- Air/pulmonary embolism
- Vagal reflex activation.

Metabolic
- Potassium disorders
- Acute hypercalcaemia
- Circulating catecholamines
- Hypothermia.

Drug effects

Miscellaneous
- Electrocution
- Drowning.

Cardiac arrest management

Cardiac arrest team activation is achieved by ringing a universal internal activation number in the UK: 2222. A stop clock or wall clock should be activated with commencement of active resuscitation. Apart from the presence of team members, some emergency departments may give family members the option to be present at the resuscitation of a close relative, especially if this is a child.

The information that should be obtained from the ambulance crew includes time of collapse, time of arrival on the scene, timing of shocks and of medications delivered, and whether bystander CPR was given. Any available relevant past medical history should also be received.

Chest compression

- The patient should be on a firm surface
- Stand, on a platform if necessary, to the patient's side
- Place the heel of one hand on the middle of the lower half of the sternum, and the other on top. Avoid pressing on the xiphoid, which can lead to liver laceration.
- Keep both arms straight and lock both elbows in extension
- Depress the sternum 4–5cm in adults.
- In children, a site is chosen in the lower one-third of the sternum, one fingerbreadth above the xiphisternum. The sternum is depressed by one-third of the depth of the chest. Two fingers are employed in infants, and either one or both hands in children over 1yr of age
- A rate of 100 compressions per min is indicated in adults, and at least 100 compressions per min in children and babies
- The duration of compression should be 50% of the compression–relaxation cycle. Unless otherwise stated, the duration of compression should equal that of relaxation
- A 30:2 compression:ventilation ratio is employed
- Interruptions to chest compression should be minimized, being kept under a maximum of 10s
- Adequate compression produces about 25–30% of the usual cardiac output, and generates a systolic blood pressure between 60 and 80mmHg, and cerebral blood flow of 10–15% of normal. It must be remembered that coronary perfusion pressure is predominantly determined by diastolic blood pressure, being equivalent to diastolic blood pressure minus central venous pressure. Palpation of a central pulse (carotid or femoral) is not a reliable way of assessing the adequacy of compressions.
- Change over regularly to avoid fatigue.

Alternative experimental closed chest CPR methods

- Mechanical piston-driven CPR
- Simultaneous compression and ventilation: SCV CPR
- Interposed abdominal compression: IAC CPR
- CPR with abdominal binding
- CPR with medical anti-shock trousers
- High-impulse CPR
- Circumferential thoracic vest CPR
- Active compression–decompression: ACD CRP: Ambu CardioPump
- Phased chest and abdominal compression–decompression: lifestick.

CPR techniques and devices. *Circulation* 2005; **112**: IV47–IV50.

Precordial thump

- Witnessed and monitored cardiac arrest; defibrillator leads not attached; administration should not delay application of defibrillator pads.
- Can convert ventricular fibrillation or ventricular tachycardia to sinus rhythm.
- Usually best performed within 15–30s of the occurrence of arrest; in most successful cases, within 10s.
- Delivered with the ulnar border of the tightly clenched fist, which delivers a sharp impact to the lower half of the sternum from a height of 20cm, followed by immediate retraction of the fist.
- For witnessed monitored VF, however, immediate defibrillation is the treatment of choice.

Cardiac arrest rhythms

- Non-VF/VT: asystole; pulseless electrical activity
- VF or pulseless VT.

Effective CPR

- The presence of a palpable central pulse is an unreliable guide to assess the adequacy of chest compressions. Absence of a central pulse implies very little forward flow
- Increase in end-tidal CO_2 is probably the most reliable indicator. This indicates delivery of CO_2 to the lungs and reflects cardiac output. A rise to normal or high levels implies effective CPR. Persistently low CO_2 means a poor cardiac output from either poor technique or an underlying cause such as massive pulmonary embolism. Absent endotracheal CO_2 may indicate inadvertent oesophageal intubation, which should be checked by immediate laryngoscopy.
- Improving acid–base status, as measured by rising venous or arterial blood pH. Central or mixed venous pH is more meaningful than arterial pH.
- Metabolic acidosis is invariably present after all but the briefest cardiac arrest, with raised base deficit and plasma lactate.

Indications for the termination of CPR

- Prolonged attempt of 20–30min without return of spontaneous circulation
- Adequate advanced life support procedures during the resuscitation attempt: airway, drugs and electricity
- Core temperature restored to 30–32°C
- A terminal rhythm, e.g. asystole, agonal rhythm
- Bedside trans-thoracic echocardiography allows evaluation of cardiac wall motion. If motion is detected, this suggests that continued resuscitation in the presence of pulseless electrical activity may be beneficial.

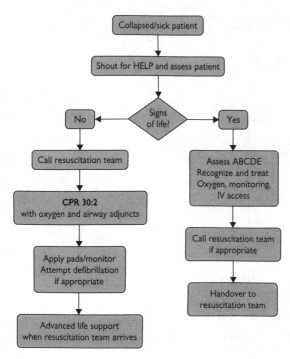

6

Fig. 4.1 In-hospital resuscitation. Reproduced with permission by the Resuscitation Council (UK).

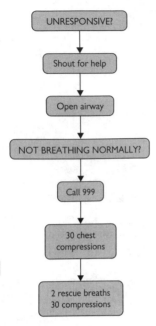

Fig. 4.2 Adult basic life support. Reproduced with permission by the Resuscitation Council (UK).

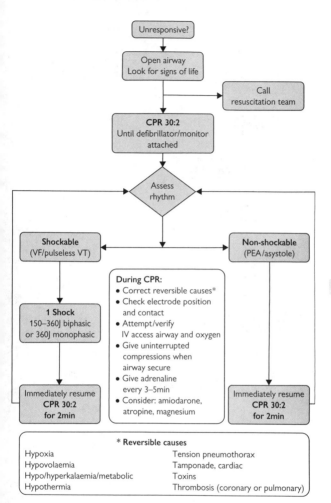

Fig. 4.3 Adult advanced life support algorithm. Reproduced with permission by the Resuscitation Council (UK).

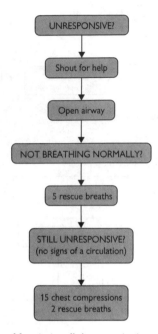

After 1min call the resuscitation team then continue CPR

Fig. 4.4 Paediatric basic life support (health care professionals with a duty to respond). Reproduced with permission by the Resuscitation Council (UK).

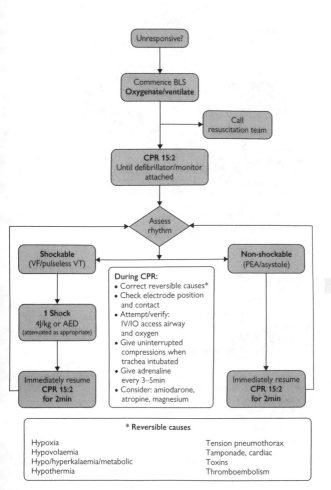

Fig. 4.5 Paediatric advanced life support. Reproduced with permission by the Resuscitation Council (UK).

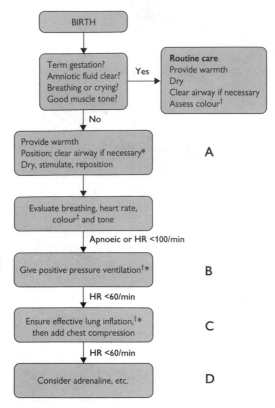

Fig. 4.6 Newborn life support. Reproduced with permission by the Resuscitation Council (UK).

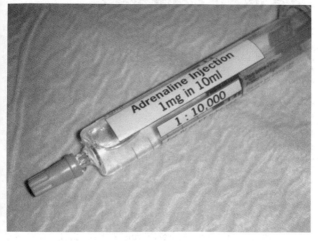

7

Fig. 4.7 Pre-loaded adrenaline (epinephrine).

Drugs used in cardiac arrest

There is no robust evidence to support the use of drugs in cardiac arrest management. Drug administration must not lead to interruptions in CPR or delay the delivery of shocks.

The aims of administered medication include:
• Improved myocardial perfusion
• Improved myocardial contractility
• Reduction of afterload
• Suppression of abnormal cardiac rhythms
• Correction of acidosis.

Mode of administration

• Usually by IV injection, preferably through a central vein.
• Peripheral venous administration should be followed by a 20mL flush with normal saline and limb elevation for 10–20s.
• Alternatives when venous access has not been established:
1. Via the tracheal tube:
    • Drugs are absorbed via the mucosa of the bronchial tree
    • Two to three times the IV dose is diluted in 10mL of sterile water or, alternatively, the contents of a pre-filled syringe are used
    • The drug can be placed directly into the tracheal tube but is preferably injected down a sterile suction catheter passed beyond the tracheal tube tip
    • Administration is followed by five ventilations to allow dispersal of the drug in the bronchial tree.
    • Epinephrine/adrenaline, atropine, lidocaine and naloxone can be given by this route.
2. Via the intraosseous route: although mainly used in paediatric practice, this route is also effective in adults.

Epinephrine (adrenaline)

• 1mg (10mL of 1:10000 or 1mL of 1:1000) or 2–3mg diluted into 10mL sterile water via the tracheal tube
• In children: 10mcg/kg (0.1mL/kg 1 in 10000) IV 100mcg/kg via the tracheal tube (1mL/kg 1 in 10000 or 0.1mL/kg 1 in 1000); best avoided as it may have a paradoxical effect
• Repeated after every 3–5min of CPR
• It is thus given immediately before alternate shocks
• The dosage may need to be reduced where the patient is on sympathomimetic drugs, therapeutic or recreational drugs.

Effects

• Improved coronary perfusion (increased aortic diastolic pressure): alpha-adrenergic effect
• Reduced perfusion to non-vital organs: alpha-adrenergic effect
• Increased intensity of ventricular fibrillation: beta-adrenergic effect
• Stimulates cardiac stimulation: beta-adrenergic effect.

Atropine

- 3mg single dose for asystole or PEA with bradycardia (<40/min or <60/min if poor cardiac reserve)
- 6mg via tracheal tube
- 20mcg/kg or 30mcg/kg via the tracheal tube.

Amiodarone

300mg diluted in 5% dextrose to a volume of 20ml (or from a pre-filled syringe); if VF/VT persists after more than three shocks, this precedes the fourth shock. In children, the dose is 5mg/kg in 5% dextrose.

A further 150mg bolus is given for recurrent/refractory VT/VF, followed by an infusion of 900mg over 24h if return of spontaneous circulation occurs.

Magnesium sulphate

- 8mmol or 2g(4mL of 50% magnesium sulphate) over 1–2min; can be repeated after 10–15min
- 1mL 50% magnesium sulphate = 2mmol = 500mg.
- In children: 25–50mg/kg to a maximum of 2g (equating to 0.05–0.10mmol/kg).
- Two concentrations exist in ampoule form:
  - 20mL of 20% (= 16mmol = 4g)
  - 2mL of 50% (= 4mmol = 2g)
- 4, 5 and 10mL pre-filled syringes of 50% solution are also available.

  Magnesium is indicated for refractory VF/VT if there are any of the following:
- A suspicion of hypomagnesaemia(e.g. potassium-losing diuretic therapy)
- Torsade de pointes on the ECG
- Digoxin toxicity.

Lidocaine

- 100mg(1–1.5mg/kg)
- Additional bolus of 50mg if necessary
- Not more than 3mg/kg during the first hour
- This is used if amiodarone is not available and not if amiodarone has already been used.

Sodium bicarbonate

- 50mL of 8.4% solution: 50mmol
- In children: 1–2mL/kg of 8.4% solution
- Profound and life-threatening acidosis (pH <7.1; base deficit >10)
- Cardiac arrest associated with hyperkalaemia or with tricyclic antidepressant overdose; prolonged cardiac arrest(based on arterial blood gases).

Vasopressin

- 40U
- Half-life: 20min
- Effect: absence of beta-adrenergic activity leads to lower myocardial oxygen consumption
- Currently it is believed to have no advantage as a vasopressor over adrenaline.

Calcium
- 10mL 10% calcium chloride: 6.8mmol
- In children: 0.2mL/kg slow IV

This is indicated for pulseless electrical activity due to one of the following:
- Hyperkalemia
- Hypocalcemia
- Hypermagnesemia
- Calcium channel blocker overdose.

Endobronchial route for drug administration
- Adrenaline, atropine, lignocaine and naloxone can be given by this route
- The recommended dose is twice the IV dose
- The drug should be diluted to a total volume of 10mL with sterile water or isotonic saline
- It is injected through a catheter passed beyond the tip of the tracheal tube.

Antiarrhythmic drugs in peri-arrest situations

Adenosine
- 6mg rapid bolus, followed by saline flush
- Three further doses of 12mg every 1–2min as required.

Atropine
- 0.5 (500mcg)–1.0mg IV, repeated after 3–5min as required to a maximum of 3mg.

Amiodarone
- 150mg diluted in 5% dextrose to a volume of 20mL over 10min; a further 150mg may be given
- or 300mg (5mg/kg) in 250ml 5% dextrose over 1hour, followed by 900mg (15mg/kg) over 24h.

Digoxin
- 500mcg in 50mL 5% dextrose over 30min IV; depending on response, up to a further 500mcg can be given in two divided doses of 250mcg.

Lidocaine
- 50mg IV; repeat every 5min to a maximum of 200mg.

Verapamil
5–10mg over 2min IV; repeat 5mg 5min later if necessary

Flecainide
100–150mg (2mg/kg) over 30min IV.

Esmolol
40mg (500mcg/kg) over 1min, followed by an infusion of 4mg/min (50mcg/kg/min).

Procainamide
20–30mg/min to a maximum of 1g.

If appropriate, give oxygen, cannulate a vein, and record a 12-Lead ECG

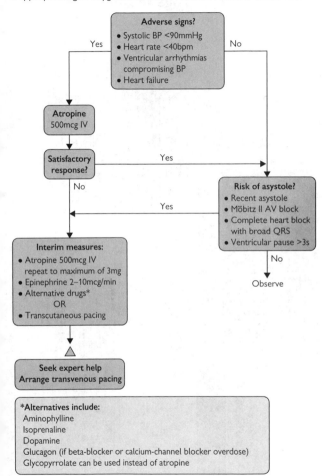

Fig. 4.8 Bradycardia algorithm (includes rates inappropriately slow for the haemodynamic state). Reproduced with permission by the Resuscitation Council (UK).

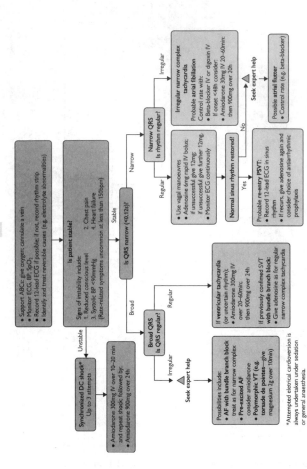

Fig. 4.9 Tachycardia algorithm (with pulse). Reproduced with permission by the Resuscitation Council (UK).

Potentially reversible causes of cardiac arrest

Four Hs
- Hypoxia
- Hypovolaemia
- Hyperkalaemia; hypocalcaemia; acidaemia
- Hypothermia.

Four Ts
- Tension pneumothorax
- Tamponade
- Therapeutic or toxic substance ingestion
- Thrombo-embolic circulatory obstruction.

Defibrillation

- Early defibrillation in sudden cardiac arrest is a key part of the 'chain of survival'
- Avoiding delay in shock delivery is paramount; however, after prolonged VF arrests, a preliminary phase of cardiac compressions is recommended prior to attempted defibrillation ('blue hearts do not start')
- The charge energy for successful defibrillation is lower with moden biphasic waveform machines
- There is widespread use of automated external defibrilators in the pre-hospital setting.

Components of a defibrillator
- Power source
- AC/DC converter to provide a direct current
- Capacitor to store direct current
- A switch to charge the capacitor
- Discharge switches to complete the circuit from the capacitor to the paddle electrodes
- Paddles or pads
  - Electrode paddles which allow ECG monitoring; paddle size (cross-sectional area) 12–20cm^2 for infants and children <10kg in body weight; 50–80cm^2 for adults). They deliver the shock via conducting gel pads placed on the chest wall
  - Pre-connected adhesive gel pads (these are preferred) allow hands-free operation and are associated with less delay in delivering shocks (along with shorter interruptions to compressions).

Procedure for defibrillation
- Confirm cardiac arrest: unresponsive and apnoeic
- Switch on ECG (connect red leads to right shoulder, yellow to left shoulder, and green anywhere): check rhythm on lead II
- **Switch on** defibrillator
- Confirm VF from ECG monitor or defibrillator paddles—**rhythm check**
- Apply gel pads to right clavicle and over the cardiac apex (apico-anterior configuration)
- Apply paddles firmly onto water-based gel pads
- Remove nitrate patches or ointments in order to prevent explosions
- Avoid placement on ECG electrodes and on implanted pacemaker or defibrillator casing
- **Select required energy level: for biphasic defibrillators 150J at least or if unsure of effective energy range of device use 200J; for monophasic defibrillators 360J**
- Stop high flow oxygen
- Ensure that the synchronization switch is OFF
- **Charge paddles** by pressing charge buttons on handles; do not charge paddles in the air or wave charged paddles in the air (only charge paddles when on the patient)—**Charging! verbal warning**

- Warn to stand clear along with visual check around the bed or trolley to ensure that no one is making contact with anything touching the patient—**stand clear!**
- Check monitor and **discharge** by depressing both discharge buttons on the handles simultaneously—**SHOCKING!**
- The paddle force should be 8kg in an adult and 5kg in children aged 1–8yrs when using adult paddles
- Follow the shock by 2min of CPR before performing a rhythm check. A single shock replaces the three-stacked shocks of the 2000 Resuscitation Guidelines
- If a shock is not required, the charged paddles should be replaced in the defibrillator, and the charge is dumped by either turning off the monitor–defibrillator or by changing the selected energy level
- In pre-hospital situations, with more than a 5min delay to defibrillation, preliminary CPR is recommended.

Shock sequence

360J (4J/kg)—monophasic
360J thereafter
150–200J—biphasic
150–200J thereafter

Optimum paddle diameter

Adult: 8–13cm
Child: 8–10cm
Infant: 4.5–5cm

If defibrillation is unsuccessful:
- Check paddle position and skin contact
- Improve myocardial metabolism: intubate; ventilate with 100% oxygen; maximize external cardiac compression.

Factors that lower the VF threshold
- Hypoxia
- Hypercapnia
- Metabolic acidosis
- Myocardial ischaemia
- Hypothermia
- Electrolyte abnormalities: Na, K, Ca, Mg.

Reduction of trans-thoracic impedance
- Larger paddle diameter: 10–13cm in adults
- Conductive electrode paste or gel pads
- Pressure on paddles (8kg) improves paddle–skin contact
- Delivery of shock during the expiratory phase. Air is a poor electrical conductor. Hence the impedance is slightly reduced when the lung volume is lower.
- Repeated counter-shocks with a short interval in between: stacked shocks have, however, been abandoned in the Resuscitation 2005 Guidelines as they interrupt chest compression.

Avoid placement of paddles on
- ECG electrodes
- Breast tissue
- Medicated (nitrate) patches
- Implanted pacemaker module or pulse generator of implantable cardioverter–defibrillator: paddles should be 12–15cm away.

Waveforms employed for defibrillation
All new defibrillators and AEDs use biphasic defibrillation. Older defibrillators use a monophasic discharge where current flows in one direction only between the paddles. In newer biphasic machines, the current flow is reversed during the shock. The advantage of a biphasic shock is that defibrillation is achieved with lower energy delivery, resulting in less myocardial damage.

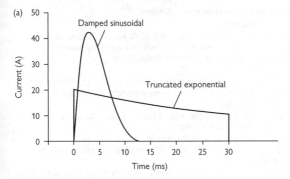

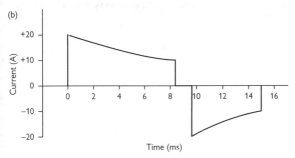

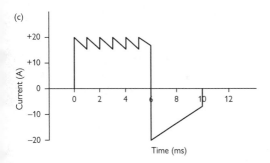

Fig. 4.10 (a) Monophasic: damped sinusoidal (sine wave) (gradual return to zero current flow or truncated with exponential decay (abrupt return to zero current flow): current in the positive direction only.
(b) Biphasic (bi-directional) sinusoidal: reversal of the current polarity midway through the discharge gives both positive and negative current.
(c) Biphasic truncated: positive truncated exponential waveform followed immediately by a negative truncated exponential waveform.

Automated external defibrillator—features
- Compact and portable
- Utilizes disposable adhesive electrode pads with pre-connected leads
- Gives visual and voice prompts and instructions to lay operators to turn the machine on, and to attach defibrillation electrode pads to the chest wall
- Reads ECG, recognizes VF (or other shockable rhythm) and delivers a counter-shock automatically or semi-automatically according to a pre-programmed algorithm
- Provides a programmed print-out of critical ECG data; stores ECG rhythms and shocks with timing
- Manual over-ride is not always possible
- These devices should not be used on wet patients, who should be dried off prior to use
- AED devices nowadays have paediatric attenuation pads, which reduce the energy delivered to children aged from 1 to 8yrs. Currently these devices are not used on infants.

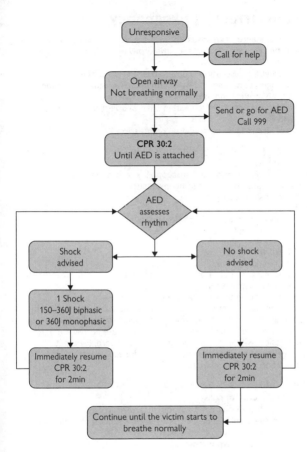

Fig. 4.11 AED algorithm.

Cardiac arrest in pregnancy

Ensure the presence of an anaesthetist and an obstetrician. A paediatrician may also be required if emergency hysterotomy or Caesarean section is performed.

- Below 24wks, resuscitation is directed at survival of the mother
- Above a gestational age of 24wks, attempts are made to save the life of both mother and infant
- The infant must be delivered within 5min of arrest for the best chance of survival
- Delivery also relieves aorto-caval compression.

Important physiological differences in the pregnant woman

Airway and breathing:
- More rapid desaturation and susceptibility to hypoxaemia
- Lower oesophageal sphincter incompetence
- Increased risk of aspiration.

Circulation:
- Aorto-caval compression by the enlarged uterus
- Venous return and cardiac output are reduced in the supine position.

Management

- Airway: continuous cricoid pressure prior to tracheal intubation; an endotracheal tube (ETT) of internal diameter 0.5–1.0mm smaller than in a non-pregnant woman
- Breathing: capnography to confirm tracheal tube position
- Circulation: placement in the left lateral decubitus position, aided by a wedge under the right flank, while performing cardiac compressions. Uterine pressure in the supine position may cause aortocaval compression, with impaired venous return and cardiac output
- Remove foetal monitoring leads while performing electrical defibrillation to prevent arcing.

Sudden collapse in pregnancy and reversible causes of cardiac arrest

Remember the 4 Hs and 4 Ts as for all cardiac arrests
- Haemorrhage: ruptured ectopic pregnancy, antepartum haemorrhage; ruptured aneurysm (e.g. splenic artery)
- Seizure: eclampsia; hyponatraemia
- Unrecognized or decompensated cardiac disease (remember rheumatic valve disease in recent immigrants)
- Thromboembolism
- Aortic dissection
- Septic shock.

Anaphylaxis

This is a type I allergic reaction (immediate hypersensitivity), mediated by specific IgE antibodies to an allergen. The onset of the reaction is usually within 5–10min of exposure, evolving to the full-blown reaction within 10–30min, and it may lead to death. However, delayed onset and biphasic responses have also been described. Anaphylactoid reactions are clinically similar or indistinguishable, but do not depend on IgE release—the distinction is of little value and the term anaphylactoid is being gradually abandoned. The mediators of anaphylactic reactions include pre-formed mediators (e.g. histamine), *de novo* mediators (e.g. leukotrienes, prostaglandin D$_2$, and platelet-activating factor) and cytokines (e.g. tumour necrosis factor and interleukin-4). Beta blocker therapy increases the severity of the reaction and anatagonizes the therapeutic effect of adrenaline.

Common causes
- Foods: peanuts; tree nuts; strawberries; fish; shellfish; eggs; milk
- Insect stings: bees; wasps
- Drugs: antibiotics (penicillin); aspirin; non-steroidal anti-inflammatory drugs (NSAIDs); intravenous anaesthetics and muscle relaxants; opioid analgesics; radiographic contrast media
- Vaccines
- Latex rubber.

Features
- A rapid onset of symptoms
- Laryngeal oedema, laryngospasm and bronchospasm; stridor (upper and/or lower airway obstruction)
- Cardiovascular collapse: profound hypotension and marked tachycardia
- Skin signs: redness, intense itching, urticaria, angioedema of the face and oral mucosa
- Nausea, vomiting, diarrhoea and abdominal pain
- Reduced level of consciousness
- Diagnostic problems arise from a lack of consistent clinical manifestations, and varying combinations of the listed features can occur.

Management
- Discontinue exposure to the causative agent: e.g. remove the sting.

Airway
- Oxygen 10–15L/min via a face mask with an oxygen reservoir bag.

Breathing
- Salbutamol 5mg nebulized in oxygen for bronchospasm
- Bag and mask ventilation
- Tracheal intubation and ventilation if:
  - Cardio-respiratory collapse
  - Airway obstruction
  - Stridor.

If stridor is present, awake fibreoptic intubation may become necessary, and skilled anaesthetic help should be urgently summoned.

Circulation

- **Epinephrine/adrenaline** 0.5mL (0.01mL/kg) of 1:1000 (1mg/mL) solution (500mcg) IM; repeat after 5min if there is no clinical improvement.

Age	Dose
6–12yrs	0.25mL (250mcg)
6 months to 6yrs	0.12mL (120mcg)
<6 months	0.05mL (50mcg)

- In extreme cases, 0.1mL/kg of 1:10 000 (1mg/10mL) solution can be given slowly IV with continuous ECG monitoring. The maximum initial intravenous dose is 100mcg (i.e. 1mL of 1:10 000 solution).
- The IV route is limited to immediately life-threatening shock with profound circulatory failure, or with anaphylaxis occurring during general anaesthesia. Multiple boluses may be needed or, preferably, an infusion can be used, commencing at 0.05mcg/kg/min.
- Fluid infusion: 1–2L (20mL/kg) as a bolus if there is evidence of shock.

Adjunctive measure

- Chlorphenamine 10–20mg slow IV over 1min; continued for 48h to prevent relapse; the dose is 5–10mg for children aged 6–12yrs, and 2.5–5mg for children aged 1–6yrs.
- Ranitidine (H_2 receptor antagonist) 50mg IV to complete the histamine blockade
- Hydrocortisone 200mg IV and repeated 6 hourly
- Inhaled beta-2 agonist for bronchospasm, e.g. salbutamol
- Provide with self-administered adrenaline/epinephrine syringes (EpiPen or EpiPen Junior). These provide a fixed dose of 0.3mL of 1 in 1000 solution (300mcg) for adults and 0.3mL of 1 in 2,000 solution (150mcg) for children.
- Recommend obtaining a Medic Alert bracelet or necklace (www.medicalert.co.uk) or a wallet card
- Serum sample for mast cell tryptase may be useful in obscure anaphylactic reactions to confirm the diagnosis retrospectively; this is an investigation only available in tertiary referral centres. Ten mL of clotted blood is sent to the reference laboratory. The normal level ranges from 0.8 to 1.5ng/mL
- Avoid non-cardiac-selective beta-blockers, which may impair the effectiveness of epinephrine by antagonizing its beta-agonist activity
- Consider notifying the Medicines and Health Care Products Regulatory Agency (MHRA)
- Consider follow-up by a specialist in allergy/clinical immunology.

Differential diagnosis of anaphylaxis

- Other types of angioedema: hereditary angioedema (C1 esterase deficiency); angiotensin–converting enzyme (ACE) inhibitors
- Upper airway swelling with skin changes and tachycardia: severe cellulitis of the throat and neck; erythema multiforme from streptococcal tonsillitis
- Bronchospasm with tachycardia: acute severe asthma.

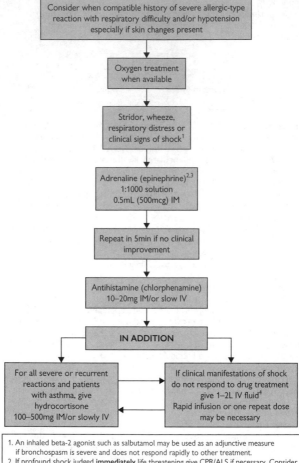

Consider when compatible history of severe allergic-type reaction with respiratory difficulty and/or hypotension especially if skin changes present

Oxygen treatment when available

Stridor, wheeze, respiratory distress or clinical signs of shock[1]

Adrenaline (epinephrine)[2,3] 1:1000 solution 0.5mL (500mcg) IM

Repeat in 5min if no clinical improvement

Antihistamine (chlorphenamine) 10–20mg IM/or slow IV

IN ADDITION

For all severe or recurrent reactions and patients with asthma, give hydrocortisone 100–500mg IM/or slowly IV

If clinical manifestations of shock do not respond to drug treatment give 1–2L IV fluid[4] Rapid infusion or one repeat dose may be necessary

1. An inhaled beta-2 agonist such as salbutamol may be used as an adjunctive measure if bronchospasm is severe and does not respond rapidly to other treatment.
2. If profound shock judged **immediately** life threatening give CPR/ALS if necessary. Consider **slow** IV adrenaline (epinephrine) 1:10 000 solution. This is **hazardous** and is recommended only for an experienced practitioner who can also obtain IV access without delay. Note the different strength of adrenaline (epinephrine) that may be required for IV use.
3. If adults are treated with an adrenaline autoinjector, the 300mcg will usually be sufficient. A second dose may be required. Half doses of adrenaline (epinephrine) may be safer for patients on amitriptyline, imipramine or beta-blocker.
4. A crystalloid may be safer than a colloid.

Fig. 4.12 Anaphylactic reactions: treatment algorithm for adults by first medical responders. Reproduced with permission by the Resuscitation Council (UK).

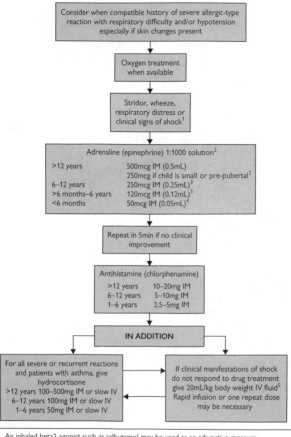

Consider when compatible history of severe allergic-type reaction with respiratory difficulty and/or hypotension especially if skin changes present

↓

Oxygen treatment when available

↓

Stridor, wheeze, respiratory distress or clinical signs of shock[1]

↓

Adrenaline (epinephrine) 1:1000 solution[2]

>12 years	500mcg IM (0.5mL)
	250mcg if child is small or pre-pubertal[3]
6–12 years	250mcg IM (0.25mL)[3]
>6 months–6 years	120mcg IM (0.12mL)[3]
<6 months	50mcg IM (0.05mL)[4]

↓

Repeat in 5min if no clinical improvement

↓

Antihistamine (chlorphenamine)

>12 years	10–20mg IM
6–12 years	5–10mg IM
1–6 years	2.5–5mg IM

↓

IN ADDITION

For all severe or recurrent reactions and patients with asthma, give hydrocortisone
>12 years 100–500mg IM or slow IV
6–12 years 100mg IM or slow IV
1–6 years 50mg IM or slow IV

If clinical manifestations of shock do not respond to drug treatment give 20mL/kg body weight IV fluid[5] Rapid infusion or one repeat dose may be necessary

1. An inhaled beta2-agonist such as salbutamol may be used as an adjunctive measure if bronchospasm is severe and does not respond rapidly to other treatment.
2. If profound shock judged **immediately** life threatening give CPR/ALS if necessary. Consider **slow** IV adrenaline (epinephrine) 1:10 000 solution. This is **hazardous** and is recommended only for an experienced practitioner who can also obtain IV access without delay. Note the different strength of adrenaline (epinephrine) that may be required for IV use.
3. For children who have been prescribed an adrenaline autoinjector, 150mcg can be given instead of 120mcg, and 300mcg can be given instead of 250mcg or 500mcg.
4. Absolute accuracy of the small dose is not essential.
5. A crystalloid may be safer than a colloid.

Fig. 4.13 Anaphylactic reactions: treatment algorithm for children by first medical responders. Reproduced with permission by the Resuscitation Council (UK).

Airway and breathing management

Introduction

- Early airway assessment and control are essential components of the respiratory management of all acutely ill patients—for whom oxygenation is always a crucial priority
- Apart from witnessed primary cardiac arrest—where defibrillation takes precedence—ensuring a patent airway and delivering oxygen into the lungs is the immediate aim, fundamental to successful patient care by preventing hypoxaemia
- The clear airway may be threatened by many widely different disease processes and at different levels from the front of the face down to the bronchi
- Tracheal intubation is the definitive way of securing the airway to by-pass any obstruction, permit positive pressure ventilation and regulate gas exchange with high oxygen concentrations if needed. It also provides access for tracheal suction
- Recognition of the difficult airway and predicting the occasions when intubation will be complicated and will need highly specialized intervention is important but not easy. It is important always to have a clear back-up plan of action in the anticipation of failure
- Patients arriving in the resuscitation room can present some of the most challenging airway problems requiring urgent skilled anaesthetic and even surgical intervention

For patients in respiratory failure, intubation and ventilation is the tried and tested method of respiratory support and still essential in most circumstances

- As well as ensuring gas exchange, airway control by intubation is also the definitive way to safeguard the unconscious patient against aspiration pneumonitis when protective reflexes have been lost
- In severe head injury and other situations where ICP may be raised, intubation and ventilation assists in ICP control
- Monitoring of oxygen saturation by pulse oximetry indicates whether or not oxygenation is being achieved far more reliably than visual appearances of skin colour. Oximetry must be immediately available at all times. An additional minimum monitoring standard is capnography which must also be available wherever intubation is undertaken, both to confirm tracheal tube placement and to demonstrate effectiveness of ventilation breath by breath.

Indications for emergency airway management

- Cardiac arrest
- Major head injury
- Multiple trauma
- Burns with inhalational injury
- Respiratory failure
- Drug overdose
- Neurological problems: stroke; status epilepticus
- Anaphylaxis
- Foreign body in the airway.

Signs indicative of inadequate air exchange
- Increased difficulty in breathing
- Increased work of breathing
- Inefficient cough
- Noisy breathing: stridor (inspiratory with extra-thoracic airway obstruction; expiratory with intra-thoracic airway obstruction); gurgling (secretions); crowing (laryngeal spasm); snoring (oropharyngeal obstruction).

Features of increased work of breathing

- Tachypnoea
- Flaring of alae nasi
- Intercostal, subcostal, suprasternal and supraclavicular recession or retraction
- Use of accessory muscles of respiration: sternomastoids; strap muscles; trapezius muscles
- Expiratory grunt: exhalation against a partially closed glottis
- Inspiratory descent of thyroid cartilage (tracheal tug)
- Altered inspiratory: expiratory ratio (normally 1:2)
- Paradoxical breathing: abdominal see–saw movement, with chest expansion and abdominal expansion being desynchronized (sinking chest with rising abdomen, and vice versa). Thus inward chest movement and outward abdominal movement occur simultaneously on inspiration, producing a rocking-boat respiratory pattern.

With fatigue, these signs tend to subside, indicating imminent respiratory arrest, while simultaneously often lulling the inexperienced into a false sense of security.

Table 5.1 Respiratory rate by age

Age (years)	Respiratory rate (breaths/min)
<1	30–40
1–2	25–35
2–5	25–30
5–12	20–25
>12	15–20

Patterns of altered breathing

These mainly occur when there has been an extensive brain injury and in the presence of raised intracranial pressure. The patient will normally be deeply unconscious with a low GCS. They are usually an indicator of the need for intubation to control gas exchange and intracranial pressure, as well as protecting the airway.

- Cheyne–Stokes breathing: periodic and rhythmic waxing and waning in rate and depth followed by apnoea; seen with bilateral lesions involving the basal ganglia and thalamus
- Central neurogenic hyperventilation: increased rate and depth; seen with lesions in the midbrain and upper pons
- Apneustic breathing: 2–3s pauses after full or prolonged inspiration; seen with lesions in the lower pons
- Cluster breathing: clusters of irregular breathing and periods of apnoea at irregular intervals; seen with lesions in the lower pons and upper medulla
- Ataxic breathing: irregular and unpredictable pattern of breathing; seen with lesions in the medulla.

Features of paediatric upper airway

- Relatively large head size with small mouth and short neck; more prominent occiput. The neck tends to be flexed in the supine position, with distortion of the airway leading to obstruction. This can be overcome by placement of a small folded towel under the shoulders
- Narrow nares and choanae, leading to greater dependence on nasopharyngeal patency; infants under 6 months of age are obligate nose breathers
- Large relatively short tongue, which increases airway resistance
- Relatively smaller oral cavity and mandible
- Larger tonsils and adenoids
- Increased angulation of the base of the tongue and the glottic aperture
- High glottis and larynx (C3–4)
- Long and floppy U-shaped epiglottis with axis angled 45° posteriorly to that of the trachea
- Slanting vocal cords with high attachment (C4)
- Narrow cricoid ring, which is the narrowest part of the airway
- Short and posteriorly angulated trachea

Special measures for the paediatric airway

- Slight neck extension; neutral position in infant
- Straight laryngoscope blade to directly lift the epiglottis for vocal cord visualization
- Un-cuffed ETT in children up to the age of 10yrs.

Elective airway evaluation

Mouth opening

Mouth opening should be 6–8cm (3–4 finger breadths). The thyromental distance should be 6–8cm (3–4 finger breadths). This is the straight line distance between the thyroid notch and the lower border of the mentum (chin) with the head extended.

Mallampati score

This is evaluated while sitting up with head in neutral position and maximal opening of mouth with maximal tongue protrusion. Visible pharyngeal structures are used in the process of scoring. The scoring system does carry the disadvantage of noticeable interobserver variability.

- Class 1: soft palate, uvula, fauces and anterior and posterior tonsillar pillars seen
- Class 2: as above, but view of the tonsillar pillars is prevented by tongue
- Class 3: only soft palate and base of uvula seen
- Class 4: soft palate not seen at all; only hard palate visible.

Cormack and Lehane classification

- Laryngoscopic view
- Grade I: all or most of the glottis visible
- Grade II: only the posterior part of the glottis visible
- Grade III: whole of the glottis not visible
- Grade IV: epiglottis not visible.

Predictors of difficult airway

- History of snoring
- Large tongue
- Inability to see soft palate, uvula or faucial pillars
- Limited mouth opening, i.e. trismus
- Micrognathia, or a small and receding mandible
- Short neck
- Cervical spine abnormalities/immobility
- High arched palate
- Upper airway obstruction from bleeding, trauma, burns, inhalation injury, cranio-facial abnormality, or infection
- Morbid obesity
- Pregnancy.

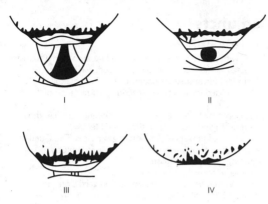

Fig. 5.1 Classification of laryngoscopy views. (Cormack and Lehane).

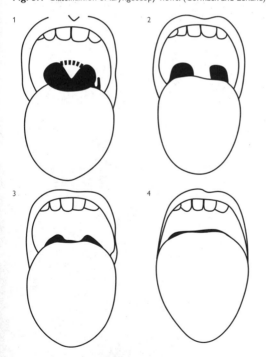

Fig. 5.2 View during the Mallampati Test Score.

Airway adjuncts

Oropharyngeal (Guedel) airway

- S-shaped airway with a large flange, a reinforced bite area, and a tubular lumen for increased air flow and insertion of a suction catheter
- Sizes range from 000 for premature babies to 4 for large adults. Sizes 3, 4 and 5 are used for adults, representing a size range of 80–100mm
- Size can be measured by the distance between the incisors (i.e. the midline of the mouth) and the angle of the mandible
- Should not be placed in presence of an intact gag reflex. The Guedel airway can elicit a gag reflex if inserted in a conscious subject, provoking vomiting or laryngeal spasm.

The two methods for placement:

- Insertion in the inverted position, concave side upwards, on the hard palate and rotated 180°, followed by continued insertion into the oropharynx
- Insertion in the unrotated position under direct vision with the aid of a tongue depressor blade or of a laryngoscope blade.

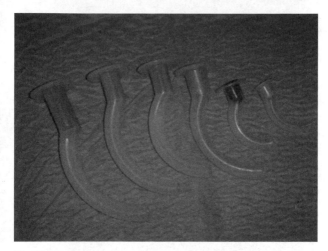

Fig. 5.3 Guedel airways.

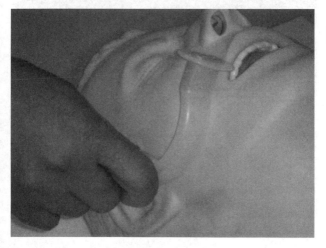

Fig. 5.4 Insertion of an oropharyngeal airway.

Nasopharyngeal airway

- Soft tube made of rubber or pliable plastic with a bevel and a flange at the opposite ends (flange prevents overinsertion)
- Sizes: 6–8mm internal diameter (adult female: 6–7mm; adult male: 7–8mm). The desired length is from the tragus of ear to the tip of the nose.
- These airways are of a fixed length. Selection of the appropriate diameter airway will usually also give the right length. Shortened ETTs can be used in children as small size nasopharyngeal tubes are not available
- In the patient with a clamped jaw or when insertion of an oropharyngeal airway has failed, nasopharyngeal airway insertion can rapidly provide a clear airway and access for suctioning to the pharynx. Some unconscious patients with a partial gag reflex will tolerate this better than an oral airway
- Should not be placed in the presence of facial fractures, base of skull fractures and CSF leak, and when coagulopathy is present
- Insert lubricated into the most patent airway, horizontal to the palate, advancing with a twisting motion until maximal airflow is heard.

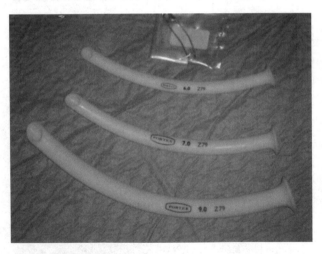

Fig. 5.5 Nasopharyngeal airways.

Face mask application

- Single operator ventilation is difficult and requires considerable practice.
- Use the thumb and index finger to hold the mask down on to the face, covering the nose and mouth, to provide an air-tight seal
- Use the other three fingers to support the angle of the mandible to prevent airway obstruction. The little, ring and middle fingers lift the chin and thrust the jaw forwards
- The other hand is used to compress the bag
- With two person ventilation, one person can use both hands to maintain an air-tight seal
- If the patient has dentures, they are best retained to ensure a better fit.

Although described separately here, assessment of breathing and respiratory adequacy is often made alongside airway assessment as the two are closely interrelated. The priority is to ensure adequate oxygenation with saturation of 90–95%.

If this cannot be quickly achieved or if the patient is in severe respiratory failure, intubation needs to be considered early, and appropriate staff summoned.

Table 5.2 Size of the oropharyngeal airway

Age	Size	Length (cm)
Pre-term	000,00	3.5, 4.5
Neonate to 3 months	0	5.5
Three months to 1 year	1	6.0
2–5 years	2	7.0
>5 years	3	8.0

Bag and mask ventilation

A self-inflating bag (Ambu or Laerdal) with an attached reservoir and a high flow of oxygen (10–15L/min) can deliver 85–90% inspired oxygen via a face mask. A unidirectional valve on either side of the mask permits venting of the exhaled tidal volume (eliminating exhaled CO_2 from the inspired gas system) and prevents the inspiration of room air.

The bag must be continually inflated throughout the ventilatory cycle to ensure the highest FiO_2 and adequate CO_2 evacuation.

The bags are available in three sizes: 240mL, 500mL, and 1600mL. Self-inflating bags should be fitted with a pressure release valve (30–45cm H_2O pressure), protecting the lungs from barotrauma, that can be over-ridden if necessary.

Ventilation can be further improved by using the oral or nasal airway. Chest movement must be produced with each ventilation delivered.

Predictors of difficult bag and mask ventilation
• Excessive facial hair (beards)
• Obesity
• Advanced age
• Snoring.

To improve mask seal:
• Apply water-soluble lubricant to the facial hair in the presence of beards and moustaches
• Replace dentures in edentulous patients
• Fluff and compress gauze sponges (4 × 4) and insert into the cheeks to create an improved mask seal. There is, however, a potential for losing or causing airway obstruction.

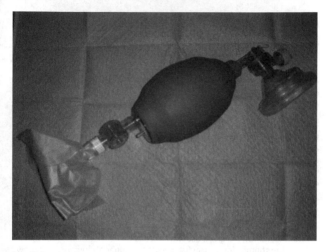

Fig. 5.6 Bag and face mask.

Adult and paediatric choking

Mild obstruction, with the preservation of the ability to breathe, speak and cough: encourage continued coughing only.

Severe obstruction, with inability to breathe, speak or cough:
• Up to five back blows
• Followed by five abdominal thrusts
• Followed by alternating five back blows with five abdominal thrusts.

Features associated with foreign body airway obstruction in children
• Sudden onset of respiratory distress
• Coughing, choking or stridor
• Playing with or ingesting small objects, e.g. peanuts, beads
• Can present with either effective or ineffective coughing.

Heimlich manoeuvre (subdiaphragmatic abdominal thrust)
• Wrap arms around the victim's waist
• Interlock hands, making a fist with one hand
• Place the thumb side of the fist against the upper abdomen, just below the xiphoid
• Press into the upper abdomen with quick upward thrusts.

Foreign body removal
• A blind finger sweep can be used for a conscious adult in extremis, but not in children. A hooking manoeuvre may be used to remove the impacted foreign body
• Direct vision removal using a laryngoscope and Magill forceps should be considered.

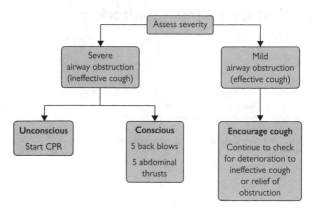

Fig. 5.7 Adult choking treatment.

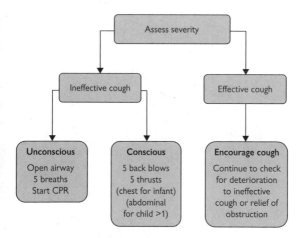

Fig. 5.8 Paediatric foreign body airway obstruction treatment.

Figures 5.7 and 5.8 are reproduced with permission by the Resuscitation Council (UK).

Respiratory system monitoring techniques

Gas exchange
- Pulse oximetry
- Arterial blood gases
- Trans-cutaneous blood gases.

Pulmonary mechanics
- End-tidal carbon dioxide capnography
- Airway resistance
- Airway pressure measurements and waveforms
- Compliance.

Pulse oximetry

- The oximeter probe is usually applied to a finger or to an ear lobe. Care needs to be taken to avoid pressure necrosis with prolonged use by relocation of the probe to other digits
- The technique involves a combination of dual wavelength spectro-photometry and photoplethysmography
- The probe contains two light-emitting diodes producing beams at red (660nm) and infrared (940nm) frequencies, and a photo-detector. The difference in absorbance between oxyhaemoglobin and deoxyhaemoglobin is greatest at 625nm. The isobestic point of oxyhaemoglobin and deoxyhaemoglobin, where the molecular absorption coefficient is identical for both molecules, is 805nm
- The signal is analysed by a microprocessor, programmed to analyse mathematically both the DC and AC components at 660 and 940nm
- A display is provided of oxygen saturation, pulse rate and a plethysmographic waveform of the pulse. The monitored heart rate should normally coincide with the oximetric pulse rate. Any discrepancies may indicate failure to detect arterial pulsation, thereby compromising the reliability of the readings obtained
- It is not an indicator of the adequacy of alvelolar ventilation, for which arterial blood gases are required
- A variable pitch bleep provides an audible signal of changes in saturation; alarm limits can be set for a low saturation value and for both high and low pulse rates.
- Accurate to within ±2% in the 70–100% range. Errors can occur at lower saturations as the relationship of red/infrared absorption to saturation is non-linear. Within the 95–100% range, arterial blood gas analysis is required to provide an accurate estimation of arterial pO_2

The accuracy of pulse oximetric readings may be affected by the following conditions:

Underestimation of SpO_2
- Low flow states, associated with low pulse pressure. This is related to vasoconstriction, associated with hypovolaemia, peripheral arterial disease or cold exposure
- Motion artefact
- Ambient light: overhead fluorescent light; infrared heat lamp
- Pigmentation: vital dyes (methylene blue); dark skin; bilirubin (jaundice); dark-coloured nail polish/synthetic fingernails (usually not a problem with current devices)
- Very low haemoglobin concentration (<5g/dL)
- Altered PaO_2: SpO_2 relationship (shift of oxyhaemoglobin dissociation curve)
- Low PaO_2.

Overestimation of SpO_2
- Dysfunctional haemoglobins: carboxyhaemoglobin; methaemoglobin (>10%). In methaemoglobinaemia, the SpO_2 tends to be 85% irrespective of the actual SaO_2 or PaO_2.

Monitoring of tissue oxygenation
Derived variables
- Oxygen delivery
- Oxygen consumption
- Blood biochemistry: lactate; pyruvate

Measurements using specific devices or techniques
- Pulse oximetry
- Tissue oximetry:
  - Transcutaneous PO_2
  - Conjunctival PO_2.

Key points in the use of pulse oximeters in emergency medicine
- Pulse oximeters are calibrated for adult haemoglobin
- When used in suspected carbon monoxide poisoning, the attending health care professional needs to be aware of the possibility of falsely high SpO_2 readings
- Must not be used with patients suspected of having other abnormal haemoglobins
- Oximetry does not indicate the adequacy of alveolar ventilation. Severe hypercapnia may be present without hypoxaemia, especially when supplementary oxygen is being given
- There is a non-linear relationship between SpO_2 and oxygen partial pressure, which depends on the oxyhaemoglobin dissociation curve.

Capnography

Capnography involves the continuous monitoring of exhaled and inhaled carbon dioxide concentrations (partial pressures) in order to produce a recording of the carbon dioxide concentration over time. Infrared absorption spectrographic analysis is used to determine the end-tidal partial pressure of carbon dioxide. Carbon dioxide sensors can be mainstream (in-line and incorporated in the breathing system) or side-stream (with continuous sampling from the breathing system via a side connector at a rate of 150mL/min). Side-stream analysers have a slower response time of 1–2s, and may underestimate the measured value of carbon dioxide owing to gas mixing. The analysing unit is usually a modular component of a multifunction patient monitor and this may be wall-mounted or portable. Small, portable, battery-operated individual capnographs are also available.

The capnogram is a continuous wave trace of carbon dioxide concentration over time, characterized by a sharp rise in carbon dioxide concentration followed by a plateau.

- Ascending limb: carbon dioxide in the gas from rapidly emptying alveoli: steep EXPIRATORY UPSTROKE
- Alveolar plateau: carbon dioxide concentration in uniformly ventilated alveoli: EXPIRATORY PLATEAU
- Descending limb: from the end-tidal point (highest end-tidal carbon dioxide), corresponds to inspired fresh gas with clearing of carbon dioxide from the previous expiration. The end-tidal carbon dioxide approximates the true alveolar pCO_2: steep INSPIRATORY DOWNSTROKE
- Zero baseline: carbon dioxide concentration of inspired gas.

The end-tidal CO_2 is displayed as a number next to the trace. It is usually given in kPa but can sometimes be in % or in mmHg. 1kPa is approximately 1% and = 7.5mmHg.

A disposable end-tidal carbon dioxide detector uses a chemical pH indicator (metacresol) for CO_2 detection. In the presence of endotracheal intubation, cyclical colour changes are observed.

Clinical use of capnography in the acute setting

- Mandatory for all intubated, ventilated patients (see ventilation p. 176)
  - Acts as disconnection and apnoea alarm
  - Permits adjustment of ventilation to normocapnia without need for frequent blood gas analysis
  - Indicates presence of re-breathing (if inspired CO_2 concentration is >0)
- The CO_2 waveform can indicate bronchospasm (sloping plateau—see Fig 5.10 below)
- In a patient breathing spontaneously via a tight fitting mask, end-tidal CO_2 reflects the $PaCO_2$ non-invasively (but this can be an under-estimate)
- Hypoxaemia refers to a relative deficiency of oxygen in the arterial blood as measured by arterial oxygen tension

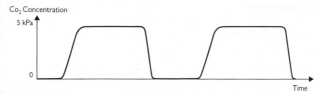

Fig. 5.9 A normal end-tidal CO_2 waveform.

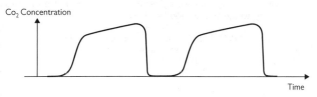

Fig. 5.10 A rising plateau indicating a small airway obstruction in COPD or asthma.

- Hypoxia refers to inadequate oxygen delivery at a cellular level, and cannot be directly measured. This can be due to inadequate tissue perfusion, with or without hypoxaemia
- Hypoxia can be present without hypoxaemia. Sustained severe hypoxaemia inevitably leads to hypoxia.

Mechanisms of hypoxaemia

Broadly speaking, defects arise from defects in ventilation or in gas exchange.
- Low inspired partial pressure of oxygen
- High altitudes
- Hypoxic gas mixture administration. On an anaesthetic machine, safety features prevent this—it is not possible to give nitrous oxide without oxygen due to interlocking of the rotameters and mandatory use of oxygen analysers.

Alveolar hypoventilation
- Central neurological causes: coma; head injury; status epilepticus; narcotic overdose
- Peripheral neurological causes: spinal cord injury; neuromuscular disease.

Ventilation–perfusion mismatch
- Impaired ventilation: reduced FiO_2; atelectasis; pneumothorax; bronchospasm
- Impaired perfusion: pulmonary embolism; congenital cardiac lesions with shunt.

Diffusion defects
- Acute respiratory distress syndrome (ARDS)
- Pulmonary oedema
- Pneumonia
- Interstitial fibrosis.

Air contains 21% oxygen (the remainder being mainly nitrogen).
- Oxygen tension or partial pressure is usually expressed in kilopascals (kPa), the non-metric unit being mmHg (conversion 1kPa = 7.5mmHg).
- One atmosphere pressure is 101kPa at sea level. Thus, each 1% is 1kPa. In theory, blood could have a maximum PaO_2 of 21kPa when breathing air. However, the oxygen partial pressure falls in a series of downward steps from air to the arterial blood as shown Fig. 5.11.

In health, normal PaO_2 breathing air also falls with increasing age.

30yrs	13–14kPa (approximate values)
50yrs	12kPa
70yrs	11kPa
90yrs	9.5kPa

Relationship between oxygen partial pressure and oxygen saturation
- PaO_2 and SaO_2 are not related in a linear fashion but follow a sigmoid curve as shown in Fig. 5.12.
- Oxygen binds extensively to haemoglobin at the lungs where PaO_2 is 13kPa. However, even a substantial fall in PaO_2 to 7kPa results in only a small drop in SaO_2 from 99 to 90%
- Pulse oximetry will detect this change in SaO_2, but it is important to appreciate that a further small drop in PaO_2 will result in a large and dangerous fall in SaO_2
- Conversely, when PaO_2 is 10kPa, SaO_2 is 95%, and further increases in inspired oxygen concentration will bring about only a marginal rise in SaO_2.

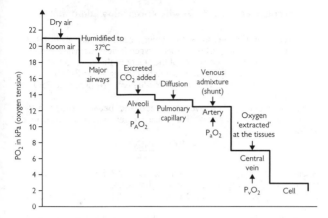

Fig. 5.11 Diagram showing the stepwise fall in oxygen tension from inspired air to the tissues. In health, the difference between alveolar and arterial PO_2 (i.e. A–a gradient) is small.

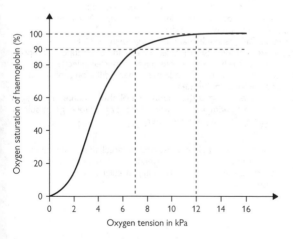

Fig. 5.12 An oxygen–haemoglobin dissociation curve showing the relationship between PaO_2 (X-axis) and SaO_2 (Y-axis).

Estimating predicted PaO_2 when breathing additional oxygen

- Oxygen saturation measured by oximetry remains relatively high over a wide range of PaO_2 values. When oxygen is being administered, this can mask a serious impairment of the ability of the lungs to transfer oxygen. This can only be appreciated by looking at the PaO_2 on a blood gas sample and comparing the value with the predicted PaO_2 as shown below

The alveolar gas equation gives the relationship between FiO_2 and PaO_2 where P_AO_2 is the theoretical or ideal oxygen partial pressure in the alveoli.

$$P_AO_2 = PiO_2 - \frac{PaCO_2}{R} + F$$

where R is the respiratory quotient, normally 0.8. F is a small correction factor and PiO_2 is inspired oxygen partial pressure

- Arterial oxygen tension (PaO_2) should be 1–2kPa lower than P_AO_2 in health
- Thus, for a given $PaCO_2$ (say 5 kPa) the predicted alveolar PO_2 will be 7kPa less than the inspired oxygen tension (PiO_2) in kPa.

Alveolar–arterial PO_2 difference (A–a gradient or PAO_2–PaO_2 gradient)

- The difference between the predicted PaO_2 and the measured arterial PaO_2 is an indication of the severity of impairment of oxygenation
- For example, in a patient breathing 50% oxygen, PiO_2 will be 50kPa.
- The predicted PAO_2 will be 43kPa.
- If the actual PaO_2 is say 10kPa, then the gradient is 33kPa. It is essential to recognize that even though arterial PaO_2 and SaO_2 appear acceptable, there is actually a very serious oxygen transfer defect
- In this case, the drop in PaO_2 indicates either a diffusion problem, a shunt or a combination of the two.

This example also highlights the importance of always noting the oxygen concentration being administered when recording a blood gas result or saturation reading from a pulse oximeter.

Shunt

- Intracardiac: abnormal pulmonary–systemic circulation connections
- Intra-pulmonary: pulmonary arterio-venous malformations; hepato-pulmonary syndrome (dilated pulmonary vascular bed with chronic liver disease).

Mechanisms of hypoxaemia

- Low ambient oxygen
- Alveolar hypoventilation: CO_2 retention: type II respiratory failure
- Impaired alveolar–capillary diffusion: type I respiratory failure
- Ventilation–perfusion mismatch: type I respiratory failure
- Venous admixture shunt (perfusion without ventilation)
- Ventilation without perfusion: dead space.

Table 5.3 Arterial hypoxaemia.

	Response to 100% O_2	$PaCO_2$	Alv-art gradient
Hypoventilation	Yes	R	N
Diffusion defect	Yes	L	R
Shunt	No	R/N	R
V–P mismatch	Yes	L/R/N	R

R = raised; N = normal; L = low.

Oxygen therapy

Hypoxia not only leads to organ dysfunction but also, if severe and prolonged, predisposes to permanent organ damage. The primary role of oxygen therapy is to increase the oxygen delivery to the tissues in states of tissue hypoxia. Oxygen delivery also depends on an adequate cardiac output, haemoglobin concentration and haemoglobin/oxygen saturation, which should be optimized in the hypoxic patient.

Oxygen has both physiological and pharmacological actions, a dose–response relationship and the potential for adverse effects. Oxygen should be prescribed as any other drug, in writing, specifying the mode of delivery, flow rate and concentration.

The maintenance of cellular respiration requires adequate alveolar ventilation, a functioning gas exchange surface, the capacity to transport oxygen to the tissues and intact tissue respiration (reliant on the mitochondrial cytochrome oxidase system). Cellular hypoxia results in cell membrane ion pump dysfunction, intracellular oedema, leakage of intracellular content into the extracellular space and inadequate regulation of intracellular pH.

The goal of oxygen therapy is to correct hypoxaemia by achieving an arterial oxygen saturation greater than 92% in the presence of normally functioning haemoglobin. In patients with COPD and chronic CO_2 retention, a target oxygen saturation of around 88–90% may be acceptable as higher inspired oxygen concentrations suppress the hypoxic drive. A higher target oxygen saturation is required for patients with abnormal haemoglobins that do not effectively bind oxygen.

Period of tolerance for anoxia	
Brain	<3min
Kidneys and liver	15–20min
Skeletal muscle	60–90min
Vascular smooth muscle	24–72h

Organ viability depends on both flow of blood and blood oxygen content. These figures are approximate and depend on metabolic rate, body temperature and adequacy of perfusion (or severity of ischaemia).

Recommendations for instituting oxygen therapy (American College of Chest Physicians and National Heart, Lung and Blood Institute)

- Cardiac and respiratory arrest
- Hypoxaemia: paO_2 <8kPa; SaO_2 <90%
- Hypotension: systolic blood pressure <100mmHg
- Low cardiac output and metabolic acidosis (HCO_3 <18mmol/L)
- Respiratory distress: respiratory rate >24/min.

Sources of oxygen

Room air contains 21% oxygen, and expired air contains 16% oxygen. Medical gas sources for oxygen therapy are of two types: wall oxygen and gas cylinders. Medical gas sources require administration devices that reduce the system working pressure between the gas source and the patient.

$$DO_2 \text{ (delivery)} = \text{cardiac index} \times SaO_2 \times Hb = 400mL/min/m^2$$
$$VO_2 \text{ (consumption)} = \text{cardiac index} \times (SaO_2 - SvO_2) \times$$
$$Hb = 170mL/min/m^2.$$

Safe use of oxygen

- FiO_2 should be selected to target an appropriate SaO_2, and an excessively high FiO_2 is both unnecessary and wasteful. The FiO_2 must be increased until a safe SaO_2 is maintained
- Prolonged high FiO_2 (>0.6) can lead to alveolar collapse and absorption atelectasis, and to free oxygen radical-induced tissue toxicity. These concerns should not preclude the use of appropriately high inspired oxygen concentrations for patients in the resuscitation room. The only exceptions to this provision are in the presence of COPD with chronic CO_2 retention and with paraquat poisoning
- In the context of severe respiratory disease with reliance on the hypoxic drive, graduated oxygen therapy with $PaCO_2$ measurement is necessary to avoid worsening hypercapnia
  - NB: these patients may be given excess oxygen during ambulance transport
  - NB: nebulizers should be driven by air rather than oxygen
- Oxygen is a fire and explosion hazard as it strongly supports combustion. Smoking in the presence of oxygen can lead to flash burns
- Oxygen should be prescribed on the drug chart: delivery device, flow rate and target SpO_2 should be specified.

Practical oxygen therapy in dyspnoeic states

Acute severe dyspnoea

- High flow oxygen: 60% via a venturi mask
- Aim to keep SpO_2 >90%, equivalent to a PaO_2 of 8kPa.

Chronic type 2 respiratory failure

- 24 or 28% oxygen via a venturi mask initially; titrate to SpO_2 and arterial blood gases
- Nebulized bronchodilators: drive by air at >8L/min; supplement
- FiO_2 by oxygen through nasal cannulae for the duration of nebulized therapy
- Aim to keep SpO_2 at 80–90%.

Risks of oxygen

Fire hazard
Pulmonary oxygen toxicity: with delivery of high concentrations (>60%) over a prolonged period (>48h)

Oxygen delivery devices

Oxygen delivery devices can be divided into fixed and variable performance systems

Fixed performance systems

These provide predictable and consistent FiO_2 independent of fluctuations in the pattern of breathing (minute ventilation and peak inspiratory flow rate).

- Continuous positive airway pressure: mask with tight seal
- High flow masks: Venturi masks entrain a known amount of room air via Bernoulli's principle and constant pressure-jet mixing, depending on the rapid velocity of oxygen passing through a restricted orifice. High oxygen flow velocity results in air entrainment through side ports in the device, distal to the jet orifice. The masks utilize colour-coded interchangeable components, with varying bore, which are marked with the recommended oxygen flow rate. The inspired gas flow is higher than the peak inspiratory flow rate. The expired gases are rapidly flushed away, with no rebreathing and no increase in dead space.

Variable performance systems

These depend on oxygen flow rate, room air entrainment, ventilation and device function (capacity and the presence of leaks). The FiO_2 may vary with the size of the oxygen reservoir, oxygen flow rate and the ventilatory pattern of the patient e.g. tidal volume, peak inspiratory flow rate, respiratory rate and minute ventilation. These systems are more economical and enhance patient comfort.

- Nasal catheter: foam-padded catheter inserted into one nostril, the other end being connected to an oxygen source
- Nasal prongs: plastic tubing with two prongs or cannulae, one for each nostril
- Low flow masks: Hudson, MC, Edinburgh, Harris: two side ports allow room air entrainment and exit for exhaled gases; no valves
- Low flow masks with unidirectional expiratory valves and reservoir bags
- T pieces
- Face tents
- Head box
- Tracheostomy collars.

Low flow devices provide flows at less than the inspiratory flow rate, and high flow devices provide flows that are higher than the inspiratory flow rate. The provision of low or high flow does not reflect the FiO_2 potential (oxygen concentration) of the inspired gas. For a given flow rate of oxygen, the greater the ventilation rate of the patient, the lower the FiO_2 as the patient inspires more room air.

Oxygen delivery systems

Low flow:
- Nasal cannula
- Simple mask
- Masks with reservoirs
- Partial rebreathing
- Non-rebreathing

High flow:
- Venturi masks
- Mechanical aerosol systems

Oxygen delivery—general principles

- Simple face masks can deliver 40–60% of oxygen at 10–12L/min. They tend to migrate to the forehead, around the neck, and to bedsheets or the floor
- Partial rebreathing masks can deliver 70–90% of oxygen at 6–15L/min. The flow rate must be high enough to keep the reservoir bag two-thirds full during inspiration
- Non-rebreathing bags have an attached reservoir bag and multiple one-way flaps on the mask vent ports. They can deliver 90–100% oxygen at 15L/min.

Nasal cannula

Nasal cannulae can be used if the desired oxygen concentration is under 50%. The FiO_2 delivered varies between 0.25 and 0.50, with oxygen flow rates between 1 and 6L/min. Flow rates above 6L/min do not convey any added benefit.

The cannulae require prongs, delivery tubing, adjustable restraining headband, oxygen flowmeter and occasionally a humidifier (for high flow rates >4L/min; rarely employed). The prongs protrude 1cm into the nostril. A rough rule of thumb for the inspired oxygen concentration provided is an increment of 3%/L/min of oxygen flow. High flow rates (5–6L/min) are uncomfortable and produce mucosal drying, hence requiring humidification of inspired gas. The cannulae, however, are well tolerated and permit eating, drinking and the administration of oral medication while in place.

Flow through nasal cannulae depends on multiple factors including:
- Oxygen flow rate
- Nasal resistance
- Oropharyngeal resistance
- Mouth breathing
- Inspiratory flow rate
- Tidal volume of the patient.

In general, the nasal cannula is not useful where high and pre-determined inspired oxygen concentrations are required.

Ventimask	Colour code
2L/min: 24%	Blue
4L/min: 28%	White
8L/min: 35%	Yellow
10L/min: 40%	Red
15L/min: 60%	Green

Functions of reservoir or rebreathing bag
- Provision of a supply of gases for inspiration
- A pressure-limiting device for breathing systems
- Can be used to manually ventilate the lungs

Reservoir bag and mask systems

With non-rebreathing masks, exhaled gases are prevented from entering the fresh gas reservoir by a uni-directional valve added to the inlet port between the mask and the reservoir bag. The valve vents exhaled gases while preventing the inhalation of room air. The patient can inhale only from the reservoir bag and can exhale through separate one-way valves on the sides of the mask.

With partial rebreathing masks, there is no uni-directional valve between the mask and the reservoir bag. Open vents allow the escape of exhaled gas into the ambient air. Some exhaled dead space gas with a high FiO_2 enters the reservoir bag and is inhaled by the patient. The remaining two-thirds of the exhaled gas is vented through exhalation ports in the mask.

Supplemental oxygen device	Achievable FiO_2
Nasal cannula	0.21–0.30
Mask	
Simple	0.6
Partial rebreathing	0.6
Non-rebreathing	0.9–1.0
Venturi mask	0.24–0.6

Heliox
- Consists of 80:20 helium: oxygen mixture
- Can be used with a non-rebreathing mask in situations where a high FiO_2 is not required
- It reduces the density of delivered gas, thereby reducing the work of breathing. This may be especially beneficial in the presence of airway obstruction, although postulated benefits remain unproven.

Arterial blood gases

The arterial pO_2 reflects arterial oxygenation.
The arterial pCO_2 reflects alveolar ventilation.

Capillary blood from the earlobe, fingertip or heel can be substituted for arterial blood, particularly in infants and children, but has the disadvantage of requiring the area of sampling to be heated for 10–15min.

Air bubbles must be expelled, the needle sealed promptly and the syringe capped air tight. The syringe should be rolled between the hands and the sample repeatedly inverted to allow adequate mixing of the sample.

The arterial blood sample must be processed promptly (within 20min), or cooled to 4°C on ice if a delay is anticipated-this maintains the blood gas values stable for 1–2h.

Pitfalls in sample collection
- Excess sodium heparin in the collection syringe can lead to a dilutional effect, reducing the $PaCO_2$ and HCO_3. Syringes pre-packaged with dry lyophilized heparin are preferable
- Air bubbles in the blood sample can increase the PaO_2
- Arterial catheter dead space filled with flush solution can lead to misrepresentation of blood gas values.

Analysis of blood gas results

pH
Acidosis: pH <7.35; H+ >44nmol/L
Alkalosis: pH >7.45; H+ <35nmol/L
Strictly speaking, the terms acidaemia and alkalaemia may be used in the above situation, acidosis and alkalosis referring to the excess production of acid or base, respectively.

Acidosis
Respiratory: $PaCO_2$ >6kPa (45mmHg)
Metabolic: HCO_3 <22mmol/L.

Alkalosis
Respiratory: $PaCO_2$ <4.7kPa (35mmHg)
Metabolic: HCO_3 >26mmol/L.

Normal values

pH	7.35–7.45
PaO$_2$	12.5–13.0kPa (95–100mmHg) on room air (young adult)
PaCO$_2$	4.7–6.0kPa (35–45mmHg)
Standard HCO$_3$	22–26mmol/L
Base excess	+ 2 to –2mmol/L
Alveolar–arterial oxygen gradient	0.5–3.0kPa
Anion gap	8–15mmol/L

Anion gap

$(Na^+ + K^+) - (Cl^- + HCO_3^-)$

8–12mmol/L

A high anion gap indicates unmeasured anions contributing to metabolic acidosis, such as lactate, ketoacids and salicylates.

Acidosis correction

(Base deficit × body weight in kg)/3 = mL of 8.4% sodium bicarbonate (1mL = 1mmol). It is preferable to use 1.26% sodium bicarbonate which is less irritant to veins.

Acidosis correction with a base is only indicated for severe and life-threatening acidosis, in the presence of tricyclic antidepressant overdose or after prolonged cardiac arrest.

Deleterious effects of acidosis

Cardiac
- Impaired sinus node function
- Depressed myocardial contractility
- Depressed diastolic depolarization
- Depressed ventricular fibrillation threshold
- Depressed catecholamine responsiveness.

Vascular
- Depressed systemic vascular resistance
- Increased pulmonary vascular resistance
- Depressed systemic vascular responsiveness to catecholamines.

Key point

Recheck arterial blood gases 20–30min following a change in the oxygen prescription for an acutely unwell patient

Arterial blood gases—an approach to interpretation

Decreased pH

Raised $paCO_2$	Respiratory acidosis
Compensation	Proportionate increase in HCO_3
Greater than expected increase in HCO_3	Respiratory acidosis + metabolic alkalosis
Less than expected increase in HCO_3	Respiratory acidosis + metabolic acidosis
Decreased HCO_3	Metabolic acidosis
Proportionate reduction in $paCO_2$	Compensation
Greater than expected reduction in $paCO_2$	Metabolic acidosis + respiratory alkalosis
Less than expected reduction in $paCO_2$	Metabolic acidosis + respiratory acidosis

Raised pH

Decreased $paCO_2$	Respiratory alkalosis
Proportionate reduction in HCO_3	Compensation
Greater than expected reduction in HCO_3	Respiratory alkalosis + metabolic acidosis
Less than expected reduction in HCO_3	Respiratory alkalosis + metabolic alkalosis
Raised HCO_3	Metabolic alkalosis
Proportionate increase in $paCO_2$	Compensation
Greater than expected increase in $paCO_2$	Metabolic alkalosis + respiratory acidosis
Less than expected increase in $paCO_2$	Metabolic alkalosis + respiratory alkalosis

Peripheral venous blood gases

PvO_2 5–5.6kPa (37–42mmHg)
$PvCO_2$ 5.6–6.7kPa (42–50mmHg)
pH 7.34–7.42

In general, there is a good correlation between pH and PCO_2 values obtained by venous and arterial sampling

Tracheal intubation

- One should always have a back-up protocol for dealing with failed intubation, with not more than three attempts being made at a given time
- Pre-oxygenation with 100% oxygen for a minimum of 15s, preferably for up to 3min
- Check ETT cuff for leaks by inflation and deflation of the balloon with 10mL of air
- Check the blade and handle of the laryngoscope to ensure that the light is functioning
- Position (align axes of oral cavity, pharynx and trachea): head extended at atlanto-occipital junction + lower neck flexed with a small pillow under the occiput. This sniffing the morning air position tenses the soft palate, lifts the tongue off the posterior pharyngeal wall and lifts the epiglottis from the laryngeal opening. In trauma victims, the forehead straps and sandbags are preferably removed, along with the front por- tion of the hard collar. An assistant provides manual in-line stabilization of the cervical spine by holding each side of the patient's head with the fingertips on the mastoid processes and the thumbs on the occiput. In infants, a neutral position should be used
- The laryngoscope is held in the left hand and the curved Macintosh number 3 or 4 blade introduced into the mouth along the right side of the tongue, displacing it to the left
- The blade is advanced till the tip is positioned in the gap between the base of the tongue and the epiglottis—the vallecula
- The vocal cords are exposed by lifting the jaw and tongue base forward with the laryngoscope, in the direction the laryngoscope handle is pointing. The axis of the laryngoscope handle is lifted at a 45° angle, pulling the tongue away from the upper incisors. The laryngoscope blade and handle should not be used in a levering motion, and pressure should not be placed directly on the teeth, lips or gums
- The tracheal tube is introduced into the right mouth and advanced through the cords under direct vision until the cuff disappears below the cords
- The procedure should last <30s

A gum elastic bougie (Eschmann tracheal tube introducer or stylet), 60cm long, can be used to intubate the trachea when the cords are not visible, with the rail-roading of an ETT over it. This is particularly useful in situa- tions requiring advanced airway control in the presence of suspected cervical spine trauma.

Laryngoscopes comprise a handle, a blade (consisting of a spatula, flange and tip) and light. Blades can differ in length, width and curvature. The spatula is used to depress the tongue, the side flange holds the tongue out of the field of view and the tip is used to elevate the epiglottis. The handle contains batteries and the light source. Standard laryngoscope blades are single use disposable, with a fibreoptic light channel, and a light source in the handle.

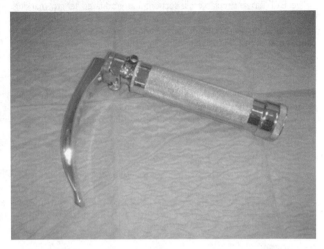

Fig. 5.13 A Laryngoscope.

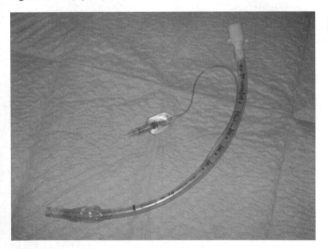

Fig. 5.14 An Endotracheal tube.

The ETT has a circular cross-section, and graduated length markings mark the distance in centimetres to the bevelled end of the tube. A high-volume, low-pressure cuff is connected to an external pilot balloon, which has a self-sealing valve to allow injection and removal of air from a syringe. The balloon monitors the state of inflation of the cuff and is used to allow inflation and deflation of the cuff. Air is injected until there is no longer a leak of air on inflation of the lungs. The Murphy eye is a hole on the left side just before the tip and allows some ventilation of the left lung if the tip of the tube enters the right main bronchus.

In emergencies, size 8.0 tracheal tubes for adult males and 7.0 for adult females are usually appropriate.

Table 5.4 Endotracheal tube size

	Internal diameter (mm)
Neonate	
<2kg	2.5
2–3.5kg	3.0
6 months	3.5
2yrs	4.5
4yrs	5.0
6yrs	5.5
8yrs	6.0 cuffed
12yrs	7.0 cuffed
Adult	7.0–8.0 cuffed

Guides to tube size
• Size of little finger
• (Age in years/4) + 4 = size in mm.

Table 5.5 Optimal endotracheal tube length

Size (mm)	Length (cm)
2.5	11
3.0	11
3.5	11.5
4.0	13
4.5	14
5.0	15
5.5	17
6.0	18
6.5	19
7.0	20
7.5	21
8.0	22
9.0	23

Guides to tube length
• Oral tube: length in cm = (age/2) + 12
• Nasal tube: length in cm = (age/2) + 15
Depth of insertion(cm) = internal diameter of tube (mm) × 3.

Confirmation of tracheal tube placement

Clinical methods

- Observation of passage of the tube through the vocal cords during intubation
- Mist in the ETT from condensation; water vapour in the breathing system during expiration
- Auscultation of bilaterally equal breath sounds in the axillae
- Absence of air sounds on auscultation over the epigastrium during ventilation
- Observation of symmetrical chest expansion during ventilation
- Absence of gastric contents within the tube
- A normal, and somewhat subjective, reservoir bag compliance
- Maintenance of oxygenation
- None of these methods is completely reliable.

Technical methods

- Detection of expired carbon dioxide with a capnograph (displays realtime carbon dioxide waveforms) or a mass spectrometer for at least six breaths
- Oesophageal detector device (negative pressure test): application of suction to a tube within the trachea allows free aspiration of gas as the tracheal walls are rigid. Application of suction to an oesophageal tube does not allow aspiration of gas
- Fibreoptic bronchoscope: visualization of tracheal rings and bifurcation (carina).

If there is doubt about the correct placement of an ETT, it should be removed and re-inserted.

Correct length of tube

- It is the length of the tube in the trachea that is critical
- Ideally the tip of the tube should be 1cm above the carina in an adult
- Stimulation of the carina can cause bronchospasm, and severe coughing if the patient is unparalysed
- Accidental endo-bronchial intubation leads to de-aeration and collapse of the left lung
- A tube that is too short allows tip position changes with flexion and extension of the neck. Neck flexion can lead to accidental extubation.
- Tracheal tubes are supplied at a standard uncut length with a separate 15mm connector. The connector is pushed firmly into the proximal end of the tube either at full length or after cutting the tube to a shorter length
- In UK practice, tubes are traditionally cut to give 1–2cm of tube protruding beyond the teeth when the tube tip is correctly placed in the lower trachea. The tube's end connector is then attached to a catheter mount (see Table 5.5).

- Tube lengths are often quoted in centimetres from the tip to the teeth as a guide. These lengths are imprecise. It is always necessary to confirm correct tube placement at laryngoscopy.

Securing the tube after placement

- The tracheal tube can be tied or taped in position. Until it has been securely fastened, it should be held by hand
- The tube should be fixed so that the length marking at the teeth does not move in or out
- Placement of a Guedel airway adjacent to a tracheal tube prevents the patient biting down on the tube, protecting against obstruction.

Potential for dislodgement/malposition of the tracheal tube

- Turning or moving the patient on the trolley or on transfer to bed or CT scanner or operating table
- Procedures around the head and neck: insertion of a nasogastric tube; insertion of a central venous line
- Staff moving around the head end of the trolley can accidentally pull on the ventilation tubing, thereby displacing the tracheal tube.

Recognition of tension pneumothorax

- Progressive respiratory distress
- Progressive cardiovascular failure
- Absent breath sounds in association with hyper-resonant percussion note
- Progressive tracheal deviation
- Distended neck veins
- Subcutaneous air leak.

Management

X-ray confirmation of diagnosis is not required, the diagnosis being a clinical one. There is some indication that tension pneumothorax is over-diagnosed resulting in iatrogenic morbidity. Tension is not synonymous with a large pneumothorax, and must be accompanied by signs of shock consequent on impaired venous return due to mediastinal compression. Immediate decompression is necessary via the anterior second intercostal space, followed by intercostal tube drainage.

Peri-intubation problems

Stiff lungs
Blood, secretions or foreign bodies in the airway
Obstructed ETT
Right main stem bronchus intubation
Pneumothorax
Air space disease

Hypoxia
Oesophageal intubation
Dislodged ETT
Obstructed ETT
Tension pneumothorax

Hypotension
Hypovolaemia
Tension pneumothorax

Principles of tracheal suction
- Always pre-oxygenate
- Use a sterile catheter and gloves
- Suction with withdrawal, over a 5–10s period
- Insert with suction off, and withdraw with suction on
- Consider instillation of sterile isotonic saline if secretions are thick.

Suction devices
The pipeline vacuum unit consists of:
- A suction hose inserted into a wall terminal outlet
- A controller (to adjust the vacuum pressure)
- A reservoir jar
- Suction tubing
- A suitable sucker nozzle or catheter: the Yankauer sucker is available in adult and paediatric sizes. The paediatric size has a side hole which can be occluded by a finger.
- Portable suction devices, commonly operated by a hand or foot pump.

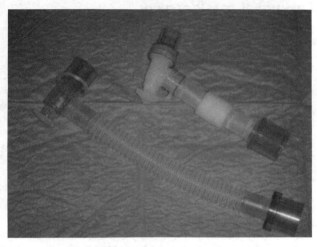

Fig. 5.15 Catheter mounts.

Laryngeal mask airway

Features of the classic laryngeal mask airway

- An elliptical inflatable latex-free mask is attached at a 30° angle to a curved breathing tube, which opens into the concavity of the cuff ellipse through a fenestrated aperture. The mask has an inflatable outer cuff attached to a pilot tube with a pilot balloon and self-sealing valve
- The cuff forms a high-volume, low-pressure seal over the laryngeal inlet
- A longitudinal black line along the back of the tube aids in orientation during placement. With correct placement, the line is dorsal and in the midline, facing the upper incisors
- The proximal end of the tube is fitted with a standard 15mm male connector for attachment to the breathing system. A barred aperture prevents the epiglottis from obstructing the tube
- The laryngeal mask airway can be used as a route for ventilation and oxygenation, or as a conduit for the passage of an ETT, flexible bronchoscope, airway catheter, light wand or other equipment to facilitate tracheal intubation
- The Fastrach intubating LMA allows blind passage of a soft-tipped flexible reinforced tracheal tube through the lumen. It consists of a rigid curved tube with a metal-guided handle and a distal silicone laryngeal cuff. The cuff aperture contains an epiglottis elevating bar and guiding ramp permitting the passage of a specially designed tracheal tube by the use of the Chandy manoeuvre to be directed toward the glottis. This allows blind tracheal intubation.

Technique of passage

- The head extended and neck flexed (sniffing) position is optimal but not mandatory
- The cuff should be checked for leaks when fully inflated, and then fully deflated prior to insertion
- The posterior surface of the mask is lubricated with a water-soluble gel
- The deflated laryngeal mask airway is passed backward and upward along the hard and soft palates, being guided by the gloved dominant index finger. It is advanced gently into the hypopharynx until the resistance of the upper oesophageal sphincter is encountered. The size and shape prevent further passage into the oesophagus
- Inflation of the cuff without holding the tube allows optimal seating of the mask. With cuff inflation, the laryngeal mask airway advances 1–2cm out of the oropharynx
- A correctly placed laryngeal mask airway lies in the hypopharynx, bordered superiorly by the base of the tongue, laterally by the piriform fossae, and inferiorly by the cricopharyngeus or upper oesophageal sphincter

Contraindications to the LMA

- Pharyngeal pathology, e.g. retropharyngeal abscess
- Obstructive lesions below the glottis
- Limited mouth opening.

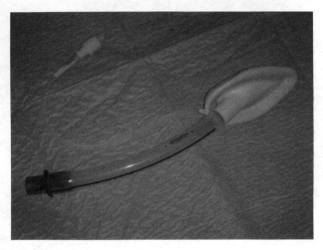

Fig. 5.16 Laryngeal mask airway.

Table 5.6 Laryngeal mask airway

Size	Weight (kg)	Internal diameter (mm)	Cuff volume (ml)
1	<6.5	5.25	2–5
2	6.5–20	7.0	7–10
2.5	20–30	8.4	12–14
3	30–70	10.0	15–20
4	70–90	10.0	25–30
5	>90	11.5	30–40

Airway trolley contents

- Facemasks of various sizes
- Oral and nasopharyngeal airways of various sizes
- Self-inflating resuscitating bag with reservoir and oxygen tubing
- Working laryngoscopes: Macintosh; Magill; McCoy; short handle laryngoscope
- Laryngeal masks of various sizes; intubating laryngeal mask if available
- ETTs: cuffed and non-cuffed of all sizes
- Syringes of all sizes
- Intubation aids: stylets; gum elastic bougies; Magill's forceps; airway exchange catheter (Aintree catheter)
- Large IV cannulae; scalpel
- Needle cricothyroidotomy set
- Retrograde tracheal intubation equipment
- Fibreoptic laryngoscope.

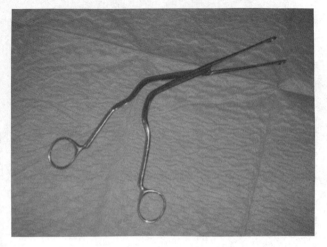

Fig. 5.17 Magill's forceps.

Aids to intubation

- Gum elastic bougie: a semi-rigid flexible stylet that is 60cm long and 15F in diameter. There is an angled distal tip to allow anterior placement. It is passed in the midline, being kept well anterior to avoid oesophageal entry. A 90° counter-clockwise rotation of the tube aids successful railroading of the ETT with the bougie in place.
- McCoy's laryngoscope: modification of Macintosh blade with a hinged tip at the distal end which is elevated by a lever at the proximal end
- Airway exchange device
- BURP technique: backward, upward and rightward pressure on the thyroid cartilage
- Awake intubation
- Fibreoptic endoscopy
- Light wand/illuminated stylet: an intubating stylet with a handle and a malleable, fibreoptic light source at its tip.

Failed intubation carries the risks of tissue hypoxia, aspiration of gastric contents and trauma to the upper airway. Many of the devices listed below require special anaesthetic expertise, but may still have a place in emergency room practice.

Options with failed intubation
Special airway devices
- Laryngeal mask airway
- Lighted stylet (light wand)
- Oesophageal–tracheal combitube
- Pharyngotracheal lumen airway.

Retrograde intubation.

Needle cricothyroidotomy with trans-tracheal jet ventilation.

Fibreoptic intubation with fibreoptic laryngoscope or bronchoscope.

Tracheostomy: surgical; percutaneous dilatational.

The Difficult Airway Society website at www.das.uk.com provides algorithmic flowcharts for difficult intubation, failed rapid sequence induction and failed ventilation.

Flexible fibreoptic intubating laryngoscope components
- Control unit: tip deflection control knob; eye piece; dioptre adjustment ring (focusing); suction channel
- Flexible insertion cord
- Light-transmitting cable
- Other: bite block; oral airway; endoscopic face mask; defogging agent.

Oesophageal–tracheal combitube
- The multilumen oesophageal airway device constitutes an improvement over the oesophageal obturator airway device
- Two lumens: oesophageal with an open proximal end and an occluded distal end with perforations at the pharyngeal level; tracheal with open proximal and distal ends

- Two inflatable cuffs: a large proximal white cuff (85mL) inflated in the pharynx; a smaller distal blue cuff (10mL) to seal off the proximal oesophagus or trachea
- Ventilation is allowed between the cuffs
- The tube is lubricated and passed blindly over the tongue until the upper incisors are between the two black lines
- One lumen will always provide access to the trachea. Ventilation is usually achieved through the oesophageal lumen, and less frequently through the tracheal lumen.

Cricothyroidotomy

This is an emergency procedure to gain access to the airway in order to oxygenate the lungs when intubation via the vocal cords is not possible and all attempts at oxygenation are failing, usually in the context of supraglottic airway obstruction.

The cricothyroid membrane covers the front of the larynx between the cricoid and thyroid cartilages. These cartilages give the larynx its rigid structure but the membrane can be punctured in the midline to gain access to the airway at this level. (the trachea commences below the level of the cricoid cartilage).

It has the following advantages:
• It is thin
• The area is relatively avascular and away from the thyroid gland which lies lower down
• The landmarks are consistent and easily palpable
• The crico-thyroid space can be stretched and dilated to accommodate a tube of sufficient diameter to permit oxygenation and ventilation in an emergency
• The trachea has a softer wall which is more flexible and lies deeper and is less reliably accessible by needle puncture.

Potential hazards of cricothyroidotomy
• Bleeding: puncture away from the midline can injure major blood vessels in the neck
• Pneumomediastinum, pneumothorax and surgical emphysema: with placement outside the airway, positive pressure ventilation will inflate the tissues around the airway
• Perforation of the oesophagus—by passing through the back wall of the larynx or upper trachea
• Failure of insertion: in some older subjects, the membrane is calcified and very tough.

Commercial cricothyroidotomy kits are available that use:
• Cannula over needle: oxygenation is through the cannula
• Guidewire through the needle (Seldinger) with dilator to introduce a wider tube: connected to breathing circuit
• Verress needle, trocar and tube kit (Portex PCK—Smiths industries) It can also be done surgically.

Check local policies and airway protocols and familiarize yourself with equipment and its location.

Needle cricothyroidotomy
• Attach a 10mL syringe to a 12 or 14G Venflon, with 1mL of air in the syringe
• Identify the cricothyroid membrane
• Stabilize the trachea with finger and thumb
• Insert the Venflon in the midline through the cricothyroid membrane at 45°, aiming caudally into the trachea
• If air is ejected from the syringe and aspirated back, the cannula is in the trachea

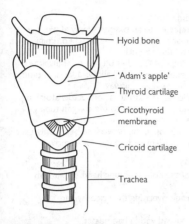

Fig. 5.18 Cricothyroidotomy.

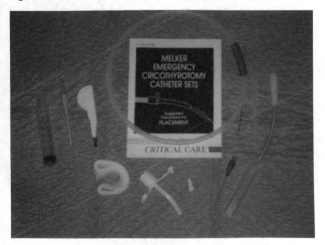

Fig. 5.19 Cricothyroidotomy set.

- The syringe and trocar are removed
- The hub of the cannula is connected to an oxygen supply at 15L/min via tubing with a Y connector or a side hole in the attached tubing between the oxygen supply and the cannula
- Jet insufflation, with 1s occluding the Y, and 4s off (i.e. a 1:4 inspiration:expiration ratio). The 4s expiratory period allows adequate time for expiration through the patient's upper airway
- Alternatively, use a 2mL plastic syringe barrel as connector, attaching the Luer tip to the cannula and the wide end to the oxygen tubing
- Carbon dioxide elimination is via the upper airway as normal
- Prepare for surgical cricothyroidotomy, the procedure being only used for up to 30–45min owing to inefficient carbon dioxide removal.

Surgical cricothyroidotomy

- The thumb and index finger of the non-operating hand stabilize the thyroid cartilage
- A 3–4cm vertical incision is made overlying the cricothyroid membrane
- The edges of the incision are spread with a haemostat
- The tracheal level is identified
- A small tracheostomy tube (internal diameter 4–6mm) is inserted through the cricothyroid membrane and secured.

Tracheostomy

Principles of tracheostomy

- This requires considerable surgical expertise and should never be attempted by the untrained. It is best performed once temporary airway control has been achieved, and preferably in the operating theatre.
- A transverse incision is made midway between the suprasternal notch and the cricoid cartilage
- The incision is deepened through the skin, subcutaneous tissue and platysma
- The strap muscles are separated by blunt dissection
- The thyroid isthmus is transected vertically in the midline. The cut ends are suture-ligated
- A cricoid hook is placed between the cricoid cartilage and the first tracheal ring to pull the trachea superiorly
- The tracheal incision is made.

Rapid sequence intubation

Rapid sequence intubation

This is the use of pharmacological adjuncts to facilitate, and to prevent adverse effects of tracheal intubation, in particular the aspiration of gastric contents. RSI provides amnesia, sedation, muscle relaxation, and minimizes the haemodynamic responses to intubation. This leads to optimal conditions for emergency intubation. Potent IV anaesthetic agents should only be used by those with appropriate competence and training in airway management and the ability to deal safely with an anaesthetized patient. The dose required in the acutely unwell, especially the elderly and those with medical co-morbidities, is often considerably less than for a fit and healthy adult.

The basic steps include:
• Preparation
• Pre-oxygenation
• Sedation
• Application of cricoid pressure
• Muscle relaxation
• Tracheal intubation.

Personnel

• Intubation is carried out by an anaesthetist or other competent and proficient operator
• Trained assistance: in the resuscitation room, A&E nursing staff may assist with application of cricoid pressure. if not appropriately trained, an (ODP) or anaesthetics nurse is necessary.

Equipment checklist

• Tipping trolley (to tilt the head down in the event of regurgitation)
• Guedel airways
• Breathing circuits
Minimum: self-inflating bag with mask and reservoir
In addition: single use, disposable anaesthetic breathing circuit
• HME bacterial filter
• Catheter mount
• Appropriate sizes of ETT usually cut to length
• Syringe for inflating cuff
• Laryngoscope with appropriate blades (sizes 3 and 4 for adults)
• + at least one working spare laryngoscope
• Working suction with Yankauer sucker
• Aids for difficult intubation
    • Bougie
    • Introducing stylet
    • McCoy laryngoscope.

Minimum monitoring standard

• ECG
• Non-invasive (cuff) blood pressure
• Pulse oximetry
• Capnography (to measure expired CO_2 after intubation, essential for confirmation of correct tube placement) with waveform display.

Pre-intubation preparation and checks

All equipment must be checked prior to use
- Suction turned on and tucked under pillow
- Endotracheal tube cuff checked for integrity
- Two laryngoscopes working
- Drugs drawn up
- Adequate access behind top of trolley which is at the correct height
- Assistant ready to apply cricoid pressure
- One other 'circulating' helper available
- Patient optimally positioned with sufficient pillows
- Monitoring attached and display clearly visible
- Patent venous access with flush or running drip.
- Attention to the circulation if unstable.

Directed AMPLE history
- Allergies
- Medicines, drugs of abuse
- Past medical history; previous anaesthesia
- Last oral intake
- Events, including pre-hospital course.

Technique
- Check availability of equipment and drugs before commencing
- Ensure a skilled assistant is present, who normally stands on the right side
- Pre-oxygenation with a close-fitting non-rebreathing face mask: 100% oxygen for 3–5min of normal tidal volume ventilation; avoid positive pressure ventilation. This allows the washout of nitrogen from the functional residual capacity of the lungs, leaving a substantial oxygen reservoir. This reservoir makes more time available for intubation in the presence of a difficult airway
- A combative patient may require the administration of haloperidol 5–10mg IM
- IV induction agent (rapid onset sedative–hypnotic)
- IV muscle relaxant (suxamethonium), which follows on immediately after the induction agent

Cricoid pressure should be applied (to compress the oesophagus between the posterior aspect of the complete cricoid ring and the body of C6 vertebra, preventing passive regurgitation of gastric contents) at the time of injection of the induction agent, until the tracheal cuff is inflated and tube position confirmed. Hold the cricoid cartilage ring between the thumb and middle finger and exert direct backward pressure, mainly with the index finger. The recommended pressure to be applied is at least 30 Newtons, approximately 6.7 pounds of force. The manoeuvre should not be employed in the presence of vomiting. If vomiting occurs, the pressure should be released and the patient turned into a lateral decubitus position.

Laryngoscopy and intubation should be performed after suxamethonium fasciculation is observed to have stopped.

Verify tube position by auscultation over both sides of the chest and over the stomach, along with end-tidal carbon dioxide monitoring.

Special considerations for a full stomach include:
- Passage of a nasogastric tube
- Prokinetic agents
- H_2 receptor antagonists
- Antacids.

Table 5.7 Rapid sequence intubation (emergency airway course scheme) (RM Walls)

Time	Action (seven Ps)
0–10min	Preparation: assemble all necessary equipment, drugs, etc.
0–5min	Pre-oxygenation
0–3min	Pre-treatment
0	Paralysis with induction: administer induction agent by IV push, followed immediately by paralytic agent by IV push
0 + 20–30s	Protection: apply Sellick's manoeuvre; position patient for optimal laryngoscopy
0 + 45s	Placement: assess mandible for flaccidity, perform intubation; confirm placement
0 + 1min	Post-intubation management

Walls RM, Editor-in-Chief. Manual of Emergency Airway Management, 2nd edn Philadelphia, Lippincott, Williams & Wilkins, 2004.

Rapid onset sedative–hypnotics

Propofol
6 months–8years: 2.5–4mg/kg
8–12years: 2.5mg/kg
12–18years: 1–2.5mg/kg
>18years: 1.5–2.5mg.
Typically, in adults, a dose of 2mg/kg is employed.
- Ultra-short-acting agent
- In 20mL ampoules, 10mg/mL (1% solution in lipid emulsion)
- Onset of action: 30–60s (one arm–brain circulation)
- Duration of action: 3–5min
- Elimination half-life: 1–3h
- Water insoluble and highly lipid soluble
- Reduces intracranial pressure, by reducing cerebral blood flow
- Causes dose-dependent respiratory depression and reduction in blood pressure; in the presence of shock the dose should be reduced to about 0.2–3mg/kg
- There are minimal residual central nervous system depressant effects
- Pain on injection, especially if injected into small veins on the dorsum of the hand.

Etomidate
6 months–8yrs   300mcg/kg
>8y: 100–300mcg/kg (2mg/mL)
- Short-acting agent; imidazole derivative
- In 10mg ampoules, 2mg/mL (0.2%), ready for use
- Onset of action: 30–60s
- Duration of action: 6–10min
- Elimination half-life: 2–4h
- Can cause pain on injection
- Little accumulation with repeated administration
- No myocardial depression, allowing greater cardiovascular stability; minimal effects on heart rate and blood pressure. This makes it ideal for use for most trauma patients.
- Reduces intracranial pressure, cerebral blood flow and cerebral metabolic rate
- High incidence of extraneous muscle movement, minimized by opiate analgesia or short-acting benzodiazepines
- Causes transient, reversible, dose-dependent adrenal cortical suppression; the effects on outcome are not clear.

Thiopentone
6–8mg/kg in infants
5–6mg/kg in children
3–5mg/kg in adults
25mg/mL (2.5% solution)
- Onset of action: 10–20s
- Duration of action: 7min
- Reduces cerebral blood flow, cerebral metabolic rate for oxygen and intracranial pressure

- Some effects may persist for 24h
- Can cause morbidity from accidental intra-arterial injection or from tissue extravasation.

Ketamine

- 6 months–12years: 1–2mg/kg
- 6 months–18years: 1–4.5mg/kg (usually 2mg/kg)
- 1–2mg/kg over 1min, 10 or 50mg/mL

(analgesic effect); onset of action within 1min; duration of action: 5–10min; full recovery within 60min

- 4.0mg/kg for complete dissociative anaesthesia
- Dose-related CNS depression is characterized by profound amnesia and analgesia associated with open eyes (apparent wakefulness), a slow nystagmic gaze and EEG dissociation between the thalamo-cortical and limbic systems (dissociative anaesthesia) reflected as sensory–cognitive dissociation
- Dose-related sympathomimetic agent, producing increased blood pressure, heart rate, cardiac output and myocardial oxygen demand, along with increased cerebral metabolic rate for oxygen; and bronchodilatation. It is the only induction agent with bronchial smooth muscle relaxant properties
- A potent cerebral vasodilator; raises intracranial pressure
- Increases muscle tone; associated with purposeless motor activity and random eye movements
- Can induce copious secretions. Secretions may be prevented by the administration of glycopyrrolate 0.2mg IV
- Maintains laryngeal protective airway reflexes. Loud breathing is common and can be corrected by optimizing airway opening. This is usually not related to laryngospasm
- No significant ventilatory depression or hypotension
- Emergence reactions: high incidence of hallucinations and other transient psychotic sequelae
- Slower recovery time

Fentanyl 1–5mcg/kg

- High potency synthetic opioid causing profound respiratory depression
- Minimal histamine release and consequent adverse cardiovascular effects
- Rapid serum clearance
- Rapid onset of action: 90s
- Duration of action: 30–40min after a bolus dose but cumulative in repeat doses or with infusion.

Alfentanil 3–8mcg/kg
Midazolam 0.1–0.3mg/kg

- Highly water-soluble benzodiazepine
- Lipid solubility at physiological pH allows rapid redistribution from the brain to non-active sites
- Onset of sedation within 3–5min, with peak action at 10min
- High first-pass metabolism in the liver
- Short elimination half-life of 1–4h.

Properties of the ideal sedative agent
- High lipid solubility
- Water-soluble formulation
- No post-injection pain, venous irritation or propensity to produce tissue damage on extravasation
- Rapid and smooth onset of action (<90s)
- Predictable dose response
- Short clinical and elimination half-life; rapid metabolism to pharmacologically inactive metabolites
- Analgesic properties
- Pharmacological effects independent of electrolyte, acid–base and protein-binding abnormalities
- No adverse effects
  - No respiratory depression
  - No histamine release
  - No excitatory phenomena
- No hypersensitivity reactions
- No drug interactions
- No deleterious haemodynamic effects
- Clearance independent of organ function
- Predictable recovery to pre-administration mental status
- No extubation or emergence phenomena
- Reversible with antagonist.

Neuromuscular relaxants

These drugs are used as a component of general anaesthesia to produce muscle paralysis for intubation and the control of ventilation. In a rapid sequence intubation (see p. 156) suxamethonium is the relaxant used. After successful intubation, a non-depolarizing relaxant is used to maintain paralysis.

Depolarizing agent: non-competitive antagonist of acetylcholine

- Suxamethonium 1.0–2.0mg/kg (onset 30–45s; duration 3–5min—the action is terminated by hydrolysis by plasma cholinesterase activity)
- 2mL ampoules containing 50mg/mL
- Causes transient and generalized fasciculations after 10–15s following injection, associated with transient rises in intracranial and intraocular pressures.

Non-depolarizing agents: competitive antagonists of acetylcholine

- Vecuronium 0.1–0.4mg/kg
- Rocuronium 0.6–1.2mg/kg
- Pancuronium 0.05–0.20mg/kg (0.10mg/kg)
- Atracurium 0.4–0.6mg/kg
- Cisatracurium 0.15–0.20mg/kg.

Duration of action of neuromuscular blocking agents

- Cisatracurium 30–40min
- Suxamethonium 3–5min
- Atracurium 30–40min
- Vecuronium 30–40min
- Rocuronium 30–40min
- Pancuronium 60–120min.

Adjuncts

- Lidocaine 1–2mg/kg depresses the cough reflex and reduces bronchospasm (its role is controversial; there is no evidence that pre-treatment in RSI for head injury reduces intracranial pressure)
- Fentanyl 1–5mcg/kg (rapid acting analgesic)
- Atropine 10–20mcg/kg.

Properties of the ideal neuromuscular blocking agent for the critically ill

- Rapid onset of action
- Non-depolarizing
- No autonomic side effects
- No histamine release
- Not dependent on liver or kidney function for metabolism or elimination
- Metabolites inactive at the neuromuscular junction.

Adverse effects of suxamethonium
- Increased ICP
- Increased intraocular pressure
- Increased intragastric pressure
- Release of intracellular potassium: hyperkalaemia
- Myalgia
- Masseter spasm
- Trigger for malignant hyperthermia
- Stimulation of muscarinic acetylcholine receptors of the sinoatrial (SA) node
- Bradycardia
- Prolonged apnoea in the presence of plasma cholinesterase deficiency.

Reversal of non-depolarizing neuromuscular blockade
Anticholinesterase drugs:
- Neostigmine 0.07mg/kg (maximum 5mg)
- Pyridostigmine 0.2mg/kg(maximum 10mg)
- Anticholinergic agent to prevent the muscarinic effects of anticholinesterase agents
- Atropine 0.02mg/kg (maximum 1mg) + glycopyrrolate 0.01mg/kg.

Signs of adequate reversal
Ability to lift the head for 5s
Flexion of arms and legs
Inspiratory force > -25cm H_2O.

Ongoing sedation
- Midazolam 0.1mg/kg boluses or 1–4mcg/kg/min infusion
- Morphine 0.1mg/kg boluses or 10–40mcg/kg/h.

Ongoing paralysis
- Atracurium 0.25mg/kg boluses
- Vecuronium 0.05mg/kg boluses or 1–10mcg/kg/min infusion
- Pancuronium 0.02mg/kg boluses
- Rocuronium 0.2mg/kg boluses.

Management after uneventful intubation

1. Pass nasogastric or orogastric tube size 16 or 18Fr. This may require Magill's forceps (refer to procedures section for method of confirming correct placement p. 140)
2. Ongoing sedation and muscle relaxation. Sedative drugs will need to be administered once the initial bolus of anaesthetic agent is wearing off:
- Midazolam boluses (usually 1–2mg initially or an infusion of 2–10mg/h)
- Propofol infusion (25 up to 200mg/h)

A non-depolarizing muscle relaxant is also needed,e.g.
- Vecuronium initially 10mg
- Atracurium initially 30–50mg

Depending on the circumstances, opiate analgesics are also often used, e.g. fentanyl or morphine.

3. Ongoing mechanical ventilation and appropriate monitoring (see p. 176).
4. CXR to confirm ETT and nasogastric tube positions (may wait till central venous catheter is also placed).

Failed intubation

Even if there is no anticipated difficulty before starting, it may not be possible to get the tube in because of a poor view of the larynx:
- Blood, vomit or secretions obstructing the view
- Poor positioning of the head and neck
- Poor laryngoscopy technique or incorrect size blade
- Badly applied cricoid pressure
- Equipment failure
- Genuine anatomical difficulty.

Try
- Optimizing patient position
- Manually manipulating the larynx over the front of the neck to bring larynx into view (see BURP technique p. 172)
- A different laryngoscope with a bigger or smaller blade
- Use of a bougie to get behind the epiglottis into the trachea. The ETT tube is then passed over the bougie.

There should be a maximum of three attempts at intubation (fewer if hypoxaemia develops)

It is dangerous to persist if the patient is beginning to desaturate, and mask ventilation with 100% oxygen should be commenced whilst cricoid pressure is maintained.

Senior help should be summoned.

Options with failed intubation
- If oxygenation with a bag and mask is possible, insertion of a laryngeal mask can be attempted. Then ventilate with 100% O_2 via the LMA until senior help arrives
- If LMA ventilation fails and the patient cannot be oxygenated, use of an oral airway with facemask and maximal jaw thrust is tried—cricoid pressure can be reduced to see if this helps
- If hypoxaemia develops, this becomes a 'can't intubate can't ventilate' scenario which may require urgent cricothyrotomy or retrograde intubation (see below can't intubate, can't ventilate p. 174)
- It is possible that before this stage, the dose of suxamethonium given initially will be wearing off and spontaneous breathing may resume. It is safer to maintain the airway with a mask and oxygen in this situation until senior help arrives.

Anticipated difficult intubation

- In the patient with features of an abnormal upper airway (see airway assessment above), special techniques are often needed to intubate the patient safely. The degree of urgency and severity of airway obstruction will determine how to proceed. It is essential that experienced anaesthetics help is summoned quickly and in some situations an ENT surgeon will also need to be standing by
- Nebulized adrenaline (epinephrine) may help whilst preparations for intubation are made. Dose of adrenine: 2mg in 5ml normal saline for adult (2ml 1:1,000).
- In a completely stable, awake and cooperative patient, there may be time for imaging and fibreoptic nasendoscopy to delineate the exact diagnosis before proceeding. Remember that such patients can deteriorate quickly, and moving a patient away from a safe area can be very risky. This is the case with stridor due to upper airway swelling especially where infection is the cause
- In more urgent situations, intubation may have to be completed within minutes.
- The technique used depends on local circumstances, preferences and the expertise of the team involved. No one method is always right or appropriate for all situations.

The choice is between

1. Standard intubation after IV anaesthesia with extra intubation aids available—this may result in failed intubation as described earlier.
2. Awake fibreoptic intubation (usually via the nose with topical local anaesthesia).
3. Gas induction of anaesthesia, 'breathing the patient down' until deeply anaesthetized with a volatile anaesthetic agent then attempting laryngoscopy—this has the advantage that oxygenation and spontaneous breathing are maintained.
4. Surgical tracheostomy under local anaesthesia or after gas induction of facemask general anaesthesia.

These methods are outlined below

Aids to intubation with a laryngoscope when difficulty is anticipated

BURP technique

Backward, upward and rightward pressure on the thyroid cartilage—this can help bring the vocal cords into better view at laryngoscopy when there is an anterior larynx or short mandible and only a grade 3 view (see earlier Cormack and Lehane classification). See p. 104–105.

Gum elastic bougie

- Semi-rigid flexible stylet that is 60cm long and 15 F in diameter
- Angled distal tip to allow anterior placement
- It is passed in the midline under the epiglottis, being kept well anterior to avoid oesophageal entry
- As it passes down the trachea, the tip can often be felt 'bumping' over the tracheal rings

- A 90° counter-clockwise rotation of the tube aids successful railroading of the endotracheal tube with the bougie in place. This is particularly useful in situations requiring advanced airway control in the presence of suspected cervical spine trauma.

Tracheal tube introducer or stylet

- This is a malleable, plastic-coated metal introducer that is placed (lubricated) inside the ETT before intubation to stiffen and provide curvature to the lower end of the ETT
- After intubation it is carefully withdrawn without pulling the ETT back out.

McCoy's laryngoscope

A modification of Macintosh blade with a hinged tip at the distal end which is elevated by a lever alongside the handle. It is useful to lift the epiglottis and improve a grade 3 view.

Light wand/illuminated stylet

This is an intubating stylet with a handle and a malleable, fibreoptic light source at its tip. Transillumination of the upper trachea indicates correct placement in the airway. The ETT is then advanced into place.

Retrograde intubation

A needle is passed through the cricothyroid membrane and a guidewire is passed upwards into the larynx. It should appear in the pharynx and an ETT can then be inserted over it.

Awake fibreoptic intubation

- The fibreoptic bronchoscope is threaded with a lubricated ETT of small size
- The nose and upper airway are anaesthetized with local anaesthetic
- The bronchoscope is passed through the nasopharynx with the ETT.
- When the vocal cords are seen, local anaesthetic is sprayed via the suction channel of the 'scope
- The scope is then advanced through the larynx into the trachea and the ETT slid forwards over the 'scope
- Correct position of the tube is confirmed (ie above the carina) and the scope withdrawn
- The lungs are ventilated with oxygen via a breathing circuit
- The patient can then be sedated.

Gas induction of anaesthesia maintaining spontaneous breathing

- Anaesthetic (Boyle's) machine and skilled anaesthetics input are required.
- May be used if fibreoptic intubation is not available
- It may be safer if time permits (and according to local protocols) to move the patient to the operating theatres, as surgical airway access may need to follow.
  In outline,
- 100% oxygen is given via a facemask and breathing circuit

- A volatile agent (usually sevoflurane) is gradually introduced in increasing concentration
- Maintaining the airway may be difficult, and early introduction of an oral airway can cause laryngeal spasm
- Once deeply anaesthetized, laryngoscopy is attempted
- Provided the airway is maintained and the lungs can be gently inflated manually with a bag and mask, other methods such as an intubating LMA can also then be deployed
- Surgical tracheostomy can also be done in this situation if intubation appears impossible—providing a patent airway and spontaneous breathing can be maintained

Surgical tracheostomy

In the rare situation with a stable awake patient where intubation appears impossible, tracheostomy can be performed under local anaesthesia.

As described above, the airway should be maintained under gaseous anaesthesia whilst the tracheostomy is performed—this can be the best option with some types of airway swelling affecting the pharynx.

Can't intubate, can't ventilate

A patient may present with such rapid airway obstruction that there is no time for assessment, recognition or preparation. The standard methods for laryngoscopy and intubation are used. If these are unsuccessful—as described under failed intubation, you are faced with a rapidly deteriorating situation with worsening hypoxaemia and, within a short time, the heart will stop.

Rescue techniques to gain rapid access to the airway and provide oxygen via the cricothyroid membrane are the only remaining option (see cricothyroidotomy p. 150).

Failed intubation, increasing hypoxaemia and difficult ventilation in the paralysed anaesthetized patient: rescue techniques for the 'can't intubate, can't ventilate' situation

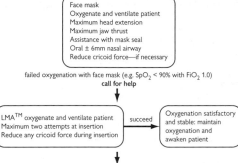

failed intubation and difficult ventilation (other than laryngospasm)

> Face mask
> Oxygenate and ventilate patient
> Maximum head extension
> Maximum jaw thrust
> Assistance with mask seal
> Oral ± 6mm nasal airway
> Reduce cricoid force—if necessary

failed oxygenation with face mask (e.g. SpO$_2$ < 90% with FiO$_2$ 1.0)
call for help

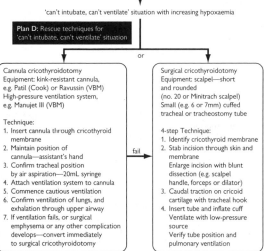

LMA™ oxygenate and ventilate patient
Maximum two attempts at insertion
Reduce any cricoid force during insertion

→ succeed →

Oxygenation satisfactory and stable: maintain oxygenation and awaken patient

'can't intubate, can't ventilate' situation with increasing hypoxaemia

Plan D: Rescue techniques for 'can't intubate, can't ventilate' situation

or

Cannula cricothyroidotomy
Equipment: kink-resistant cannula, e.g. Patil (Cook) or Ravussin (VBM)
High-pressure ventilation system, e.g. Manujet III (VBM)

Technique:
1. Insert cannula through cricothyroid membrane
2. Maintain position of cannula—assistant's hand
3. Confirm tracheal position by air aspiration—20mL syringe
4. Attach ventilation system to cannula
5. Commence cautious ventilation
6. Confirm ventilation of lungs, and exhalation through upper airway
7. If ventilation fails, or surgical emphysema or any other complication develops—convert immediately to surgical cricothyroidotomy

→ fail →

Surgical cricothyroidotomy
Equipment: scalpel—short and rounded (no. 20 or Minitrach scalpel)
Small (e.g. 6 or 7mm) cuffed tracheal or tracheostomy tube

4-step Technique:
1. Identify cricothyroid membrane
2. Stab incision through skin and membrane
   Enlarge incision with blunt dissection (e.g. scalpel handle, forceps or dilator)
3. Caudal traction on cricoid cartilage with tracheal hook
4. Insert tube and inflate cuff
   Ventilate with low-pressure source
   Verify tube position and pulmonary ventilation

Notes:
1. These techniques can have serious complications—use only in life-threatening situations
2. Convert to definitive airway as soon as possible
3. Post-operative management—see other difficult airway guidelines and flow charts
4. 4mm cannula with low-pressure ventilation may be successful in a patient breathing spontaneously

Fig. 5.20 Difficult airway society guidelines flow-chart 2004. Reproduced with permission from the Difficult Airway Society.

Mechanical ventilation

Mechanical ventilation follows on from emergency airway management and intubation and is needed to support the breathing of a patient in the emergency situations below.
1. For impending or established upper airway obstruction.
2. In acute respiratory failure
- for oxygenation
  - pneumonia including aspiration pneumonitis
  - pulmonary oedema
  - asthma
  - chest trauma
- for CO_2 control
  - ICP control in head injury
  - hypercapnic respiratory failure.
3. For airway protection in the unconscious patient
- overdose
- intracranial problems.
4. For provision of anaesthesia before urgent surgery in the multiply injured trauma patient.

Virtually all patients who have been intubated will be ventilated mechanically as unassisted spontaneous breathing through an ETT is not appropriate.

When is ventilation inappropriate?

The decision on suitability for and appropriateness of invasive respiratory support with ventilation and consequent intensive care admission can be difficult. The following groups of patient may be deemed inappropriate for intensive care support:
- Background of chronic severe respiratory disease with very poor exercise tolerance (i.e. end-stage disease)
- Progressive irreversible neuromuscular diseases (e.g. motor neurone disease)
- Underlying advanced or disseminated malignancy
- Extensive stroke or intracranial haemorrhage (some of these patients may be appropriate for consideration of organ donation at a later stage).

The patient's wishes (if known) are taken into account along with background detail including previous admissions to ICU, exercise capacity and pre-existing quality of life.

In practice, for many patients the required information is not immediately available and urgent ventilation is undertaken on empirical clinical appearances.

For some patients, non-invasive ventilation or CPAP may be the first intervention or can be made a 'ceiling' of support. In some hospitals, as part of the 'do not resuscitate' policy there is also a 'do not intubate' decision.

Criteria for starting mechanical ventilation

The need for ventilation is decided on the overall clinical picture as well as objectively measurable parameters and their trends over time.

Indications for mechanical ventilation

Inadequate ventilation and increased work of breathing (impaired CO_2 clearance)

- Respiratory rate >35 breaths/min
- $PaCO_2$ >8kPa and pH <7.25 (i.e. hypercapnia)
- These are objective parameters that can be easily measured. The additional parameters listed below may not be measurable in sick patients. However, the clinical picture of rapid and shallow breathing with a weak cough in combination with hypercapnia is a reliable guide. Hand-held spirometers that measure tidal volume are available.
- Tidal volume < 5mL/kg
- Vital capacity < 15mL/kg
- Negative inspiratory force <25cm H_2O
- VD/VT ratio >0.6.

Inadequate oxygenation (hypoxaemia)

Hypoxaemia is defined as a PaO_2 <11kPa on 40% oxygen or higher (PaO_2 <8kPa on FiO_2 >0.6)

Alveolar–arterial oxygen gradient on FiO_2 of 1.0 >47kPa.

Basic principles of ventilation

The principles of safe ventilation apply in resuscitation room practice, as elsewhere:

- The inspiratory phase is under positive pressure, whereas expiration is passive
- This reversal of intrathoracic pressure can have a major impact on the circulation by reducing venous return and can lead to severe hypotension and cardiac arrest. One needs to be prepared for this possibility
- Excessively high airway pressures should be avoided to minimize the risk of barotrauma and hypotension
- Adjustments to settings after starting ventilation are made gradually in response to adequacy of gas exchange
- Pulse oximetry indicates oxygenation continuously
- Capnography indirectly reflects the arterial CO_2 level and clearance as well as breath by breath monitoring of airway patency and disconnection
- Arterial blood gas sampling more accurately indicates these gas exchange parameters and needs to be done regularly when a patient is first ventilated.

Classification of ventilators

- Method of cycling: volume; time; pressure; flow
- Inspiratory phase gas control: volume; pressure
- Power source: electrical; pneumatic.

Phases of intermittent gas flow with a mechanical ventilator

- Inspiratory phase: pressure generated (constant pressure); flow generated (constant flow rate)
- Inspiratory to expiratory change over or cycling: time, pressure, volume or flow cycled
- Expiratory phase: passive
- Expiratory to inspiratory change over or cycling: patient cycling or patient triggering; time cycling
- The physiological inspiratory: expiratory ratio is 1:2.

Which ventilator?

These vary considerably in sophistication and features.

In the resuscitation room setting, a ventilator may be incorporated into the equipment available on an anaesthetic machine—some machines have a built in ventilator or it may be free-standing.

Alternatively, a portable (transport) ventilator can be used. This has the advantage of allowing ventilation to continue without changing over machine when the patient is moved elsewhere (CT scanner, ICU, theatre).

For complex ventilation requirements, a fully specified intensive care ventilator may need to be obtained. Similarly, for small children, a designated paediatric ventilator may be needed.

Setting up the ventilator

Safety checks

Most machines will be left ready to 'switch on and go' but preliminary checks are always needed before connecting to the patient

Gas source connected?

- Oxygen (and possibly air) hose connected to wall socket outlets or oxygen cylinder with Schrader valve socket.

Mains electricity cable connected?

Battery charged?

Patient breathing circuit connected and leak tested? (some are permanently fitted, others are disposable single use)

Bacterial filter connected to circuit?

Alarms working and correctly set?

Monitoring equipment available and working?

- Capnograph
- Oxygen analyser
- Oximetry and ECG and blood pressure device connected to the patient.

Initial ventilator settings (see Fig. 5.21)

These will depend on the particular ventilator and the mode of ventilation selected. Most machines have an area where settings are adjusted and a display screen for patient parameters.

- IMV/SIMV mode
- Set inspired oxygen concentration at 100% (FiO$_2$: 1.0) initially and reduce to lowest level that maintains an acceptable SaO$_2$
- Set tidal volume at 7–10mL/kg
- Set rate at 10–14 breaths/min

- Set Positive end-expiratory Pressure if required to at least 5cm H_2O
- Set inspiratory: expiratory ratio 1:2 (long expiratory time) to 1:3
- Set inspiratory flow rate at 50–100L/min
- Set volume and pressure alarms
- Set reasonable trigger sensitivity.

Ventilator alarms

- Disconnection
- Pressure development outside the pre-set range
  - Leakage
  - Reducing compliance
  - Partial airway obstruction
- Gas supply failure
- Power failure
- Reduction of FiO_2
- Apnoea.

Connecting the patient to the machine

- Ventilation after intubation will initially be by hand with a breathing circuit or a self-inflating bag (p. 112)
- With appropriate settings, and after confirming correct operation, the ventilator circuit is attached to the catheter mount from the ETT.
- The capnograph must be in the patient circuit
- Watch for chest movement and the appropriate capnograph waveform and end-tidal CO_2 level
- The ventilator should display appropriate exhaled tidal volume and airway pressures.

Ventilator–user interface

Primary controls

- Mode
- Rate
- Tidal volume or pressure
- Flow or inspiratory time
- PEEP
- FiO_2.

Secondary controls

- Pause
- Sigh.

Alarms

Monitored parameters

- Pressure
- Volume
- Waveforms.

STEP 1
Ventilatory mode
Assist control—Initial mode (especially if patient sedated, limited efforts)
SIMV—consider if some respiratory effort, dysynchrony
Pressure support—only if good patient effort, more comfortable

STEP 2
Oxygenation
FiO_2: begin with 100% (FiO_2), reduce according to SaO_2
PEEP: begin with 5cm H_2O, increase according to SaO_2 and haemodynamic effects
Aim for SaO_2 >90%, FiO_2 <60%

STEP 3
Ventilation
Tidal volume: begin with 7–10mL/kg
Rate: begin with 10–14/min, higher if acidotic
Pressure limit: set at 50cm H_2O initially
Aim for less than 35cm H_2O

STEP 4
Fine tuning
Breath parameters can be adjusted to minimize peak airway pressure
Triggering: in spontaneous modes, adjust to minimize effort
Inspiratory flow rate of 40–80L/min: higher if tachypnoeic, lower if high pressure is alarming
I:E ratio: 1:2, either set or as function of flow rate
Flow pattern: decelerating ramp reduces peak pressure

STEP 5
Monitoring
Cardiovascular parameters: blood pressure, ECG (very close attention needed in hypovolaemic or shocked patients)
Ventilator: tidal volume, minute ventilation, airway pressures
Arterial blood gases, pulse oximetry

After
Lapinsky SE, Slutsky AS. Ventilator
Management In: Wachter, RM, Goldman L, Hollander H, eds. *Hospital Medicine.*
Philadelphia: Lippincott Williams and Wilkins, 2000; 105–114.

Fig. 5.21 Algorithm for initiating mechanical ventilation.

Transport ventilator

Ideal features for a transport ventilator in the resuscitation room

- Portable but robust
- Simple operation with clear controls (user interface)
- Adult and paediatric capability
- Securely mountable to prevent patient injury
- Integrated monitoring display and alarm functions with both audible and visible capability
- Visual readout of circuit pressure, volume expired, frequency, inspiratory time, inspiratory waveform
- FiO_2 continuously variable from ambient air to 100% oxygen
- Economical on gas consumption for driving the ventilators (sensible portable cylinder size can be used during transfer)
- Has pressure control as well as volume control capability
- Able to deliver mandatory and spontaneous breathing modes, e.g. SIMV and pressure support
- Capable of providing measurable PEEP.
- Variable I:E ratios.
- Circuit easily sterilized, with minimal dead space, minimal resistance, minimal connections, and low internal compliance
- Internal batteries with at least 4h run time. Mains power supply as well
- Fitted with a demand valve
- Back-up manual ventilation equipment available
- Security label with name of hospital and department

Examples
- Drager Oxylog 2000, 3000
- Pulmonetic Systems LTV1000.

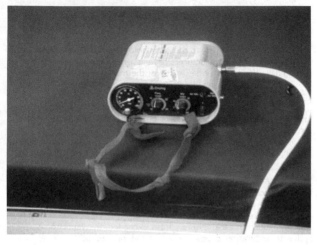

Fig. 5.22 Portable ventilator.

Ventilatory modes

Ventilatory modes

This is a confusing topic as the terminology is somewhat bewildering. Differing ventilator manufacturers have assigned different names to what is essentially the same mode. Many of the modes have been developed for use in the critically ill patient in an intensive care setting to aid weaning from ventilation.

In most situations in the resuscitation room, complex ventilator features are often irrelevant and have potential for inappropriate use and error.

It is essential that a ventilator is only set up by those who have had proper training for the specific machine available and are competent in its safe use.

Volume control ventilation

On inspiration, the preset tidal volume is delivered with whatever inspiratory pressure is required (up to the set high pressure limit)—this normally ensures that the set tidal volume is received.

If the maximum set pressure limit is exceeded, the ventilator normally cycles to expiration prematurely and the pre-set tidal volume is not necessarily delivered.

As the set breath rate is increased, the duration of inspiration may shorten—because the I:E ratio is often held constant (see example in setting the I:E ratio below).

The I:E ratio is adjustable separately on most machines in this mode.

Pressure control ventilation

Here, the inspiratory time and an inspiratory pressure are set. The delivered tidal volume is determined by the compliance of the chest and airways resistance.

A careful watch needs to be kept on tidal volume as it can either go up or down very rapidly. Tidal volume alarms must be set appropriately.

Setting the rate also determines the I:E ratio as the inspiration time has been fixed (see settings and controls above).

The I:E ratio may be set at 1:1 or inversely by at 2:1 if oxygenation is poor.

This cannot be used in situations such as asthma where air trapping is a danger. Here, the I:E ratio is kept at 1:3.

CMV (continuous mandatory ventilation) also called intermittent positive pressure ventilation (IPPV)

- The ventilator delivers the set breath rate
- Most machines give 'volume-controlled' breaths
- Some also have the option of 'pressure control'
- The patient cannot trigger additional breaths.

In the context of emergency ventilation with a sedated and paralysed patient, this mode is perfectly adequate

SIMV (synchronized intermittent mandatory ventilation)
- Mandatory breaths are delivered at the set rate by volume control or pressure control (above)

The ventilator detects the patient's respiratory effort and breaths synchronize with spontaneous breathing

This mode is usually used with pressure support (below).

PSV (pressure support ventilation)
- This is used to support spontaneous breathing
- The ventilator delivers inspiratory flow up to the pre set support pressure level after sensing of a patient inspiratory effort
- Typical support pressure is 10–20cm H_2O. PEEP is also usually set: 5cm H_2O typical
- The breath is terminated when the inspiratory flow drops (usually to 25% of peak). Thus tidal volume is variable and depends on compliance, airway resistance and breathing pattern.

All breaths are patient triggered—if patient breathing is not detected after a set time interval (usually 20–30s), the machine alarms and a back-up apnoea mandatory ventilation kicks in

When used with SIMV (above), the patient receives mandatory breaths but spontaneous breaths in between are augmented by pressure support.

NB: pressure support is measured above PEEP

Peak inspiratory pressure = pressure support + PEEP

On some machines designed for non-invasive use, pressure support ventilation is known as bilevel positive airway pressure or BIPAP (e.g. Respironics Bipap®)

Inspiratory positive airway pressure (IPAP) is the high set pressure.

IPAP = pressure support + PEEP

Expiratory positive airway pressure (EPAP) is the same as PEEP

Matching mode and settings to clinical need
CMV and SIMV
For a paralysed or apnoeic intubated patient, mandatory ventilation is needed, i.e. the machine delivers breaths at a pre-set rate. On many machines, SIMV behaves in the same way as CMV when the patient is not breathing spontaneously

Volume control or pressure control
In volume control, tidal volume is pre-set.

It is appropriate for patients who are intentionally kept sedated (for e.g. ICP control in head injury)
- Standard mode with I:E ratio normally at 1:2 for any patient with relatively normal lungs
- Can lead to excessively high airway pressures with poor lung compliance
- rate and tidal volume will determine CO_2 clearance and are adjusted to maintain normocapnia.

In pressure control, inspiratory time and set inspiratory pressure interact with patient chest compliance to determine tidal volume.

In patients with poorly compliant or 'stiff' lungs, high inflation pressures which would result if using volume control are avoided e.g. pulmonary oedema, pneumonia, lung contusion.

The combination of pressure control ventilation used with an inverse I:E ratio and higher levels of PEEP is also referred to as protective lung ventilation

- Lower tidal volumes (6–8 mL/kg) are often used
- Resulting lower peak and end inspiratory plateau pressures are thought to cause less damage to the lung by avoiding overinflation and excessive stretch
- By holding the lung open at end inspiration with PEEP, end-tidal collapse is avoided
- This also reduces cyclical shear forces on the alveoli.

By 'recruiting' or reopening collapsed parts of the lung, this strategy improves oxygenation especially in the face of alveolar oedema as ventilation–perfusion matching is improved.

NB it is dangerous to use long inspiratory times in asthma, COPD and when a pneumothorax with air leak is present.

What I:E ratio (inspiratory:expiratory ratio)

1:2 typically used in a patient without severe lung problems
1:3–1:4 may be needed in asthma
1:1–2:1 used to aid lung recruitment in severe hypoxaemia.
Safe adjustment of I:E ratio
- Inspiratory time is usually adjustable
- Inspiratory pause time may be added on some machines.

The relationship between inspiratory time and set breath rate can cause the I:E ratio to vary especially when using pressure control.
Example
10 breaths/min each breath is 6s long
I = 2s E = 4s I:E = 1:2
Rate changes to 20 breaths/min each breath is now only 3s
I = 2s E is now only 1s I:E ratio 2:1.

What PEEP

5cm H_2O is typical
10cm H_2O for lung recruitment as described above, can be higher in specialized situations

In asthma and COPD, PEEP is set at zero or worsening air trapping can occur.

Effects of positive end-expiratory pressure

- Increased alveolar recruitment
- Increased functional residual capacity
- Minimizes intrapulmonary shunt
- Redistribution of pulmonary blood flow

- Redistributes lung water from alveoli to interstitium: increased extra-vascular lung water
- Reduced cardiac output
- Pulmonary barotrauma.

> ### Relative contraindications to PEEP
>
> - Hypotension
> - Right heart failure
> - Raised intracranial pressure
> - Right to left intracardiac shunts
> - Asymmetrical or focal lung disease
> - Bronchopleural fistula

Spontaneous breathing modes
- Only available on more sophisticated machines
- Not often used in the emergency setting in an intubated patient but allows the patient to maintain their own respiratory efforts.

Pressure support
- Set typically at 10–20cm H_2O to achieve a tidal volume of 8–10mL/kg
- When used with SIMV, the patient receives the minimum number of set breaths but can breathe 'in between' as well.

CPAP
- In an intubated patient, work of breathing may be too high and $PaCO_2$ may rise
- If spontaneous breathing is excellent with acceptable tidal volume, with well maintained blood gases and no greater level of support is needed, it can be appropriate.

Patient trigger
This is the detection of the patient's inspiratory effort by the machine and results in delivery of a supported breath to the patient which is synchronized to coincide with the onset of the spontaneous breath.

This will either be a mandatory breath or a pressure-supported breath.

Sensitivity can be adjusted and the machine detects a change in either pressure or flow. Flow triggering is faster with a greater sensitivity.

Non-invasive ventilation

Non-invasive ventilation refers to ventilatory support that is provided using a mask and thus does not involve invasion of the trachea. This is easier to set up and allows for intermittent ventilatory support, with eating, drinking, verbal comunication and cooperation with physiotherapy being retained. Lack of tracheal invasion abolishes complications associated with the presence of a tracheal tube, including upper airway trauma and infection, and allows the retention of normal protective and humidification mechanisms. Non-invasive ventilation can be used to avoid invasive ventilation, while other treatments are continued to optimize the patient's condition.

In the last decade, evidence is emerging of the benefits in lower mortality and reduced hospital stay from non-invasive ventilation if this is deployed early in hypercapnic respiratory failure due to COPD, also in cardiogenic pulmonary oedema and possibly a wider range of acute respiratory failure scenarios. For this reason, the technique is becoming more widely available in the resuscitation room setting[1] to avert the need for intubation in these groups of patients.

Caution still needs to be applied to avoid the widespread and indiscriminate use of NIV in situations where clear evidence of benefit has yet to emerge. Inappropriate delay to intubation can be harmful to some patients. Where available, local guidelines should be followed as well the guidance of national bodies such as the British Thoracic Society

Modes

- CPAP provision of positive airway pressure during spontaneous ventilation throughout the respiratory cycle; can be delivered via face or nasal mask or by nasal prong. Technically, this does not constitute ventilation
- Pressure support ventilation: bi-level or biphasic positive airway pressure (inspiratory pressure support and expiratory positive airway pressure): provision of partial ventilatory assistance, the ventilator supporting the patient's inspiration combining inspiratory pressure support and positive end-expiratory pressure; delivered via face or nasal mask
- Pressure- or volume-limited intermittent positive pressure ventilation External jacket ventilator providing constant pressure, oscillation or ventilation.

Equipment

- High gas flow (10–20L/min) from a pressurized gas supply, a gas turbine or a Venturi jet mechanism
- An expiratory resistor capable of maintaining the desired PEEP, yet offering a low resistance to expiratory flow
- Minimal length, wide bore, tubing, usually provide as disposable circuits
- Bacterial/viral filter
- A flow or pressure sensor for identification of inspiratory effort, and triggering positive inspiratory pressure support

1 L'Her E. noninvasive ventilation outside the intensive care unit: A new standard of care? (editorial) *Crit. Care Med.* 2005; **33**: 1642–1643.

- Ability to control and deliver a wide range of FiO_2
- Provision of pressure-relief safety valves.

Indications for NIV (British Thoracic Society)
- Chronic obstructive pulmonary disease with respiratory acidosis (pH 7.25–7.35)
- Hypercapnic respiratory failure secondary to chest wall deformity or neuromuscular disease
- Cardiogenic pulmonary oedema unresponsive to CPAP
- Weaning from tracheal ventilation.

Prior to setting up NIV
- A CXR should be taken to exclude pneumothorax
- Maximal and optimal medical therapy should have been administered
- Arterial blood gases should have been obtained; an arterial line is optimally placed.

Desirable characteristics of masks for NIV
- Low dead space
- Transparent
- Light weight
- Easy to secure; most masks use cloth strips and Velcro to secure the mask
- Adequate seal with low facial pressure; nasal and oro-nasal masks often have an open cushion with an inner lip
- Non-irritating and non-allergenic
- Disposable
- Cheap.

Patient interfaces for NIV
- Nasal mask, which should fit just above the junction of the nasal bone and cartilage, directly at the sides of the nares, and just below the nose above the upper lip
- Oro-nasal mask, which should fit from just above the junction of the nasal bone and cartilage to just below the lower lip.

Selection guidelines for non-invasive ventilation for patients with acute respiratory failure

Identify patients requiring ventilatory assistance
Usually patients with COPD, heart failure and, with caution, in pneumonia

Symptoms and signs of acute respiratory distress: moderate to severe dyspnoea, more than usual; and respiratory rate >24, accessory muscle use, paradoxical breathing in COPD

Gas exchange abnormalities: PaO_2 <6kPa, $PaCO_2$ >6.5kPa, pH <7.35 or PaO_2/FiO_2 <40kPa

Contraindications (exclude those at increased risk with NIV)
• Respiratory arrest
• Medical instability: hypotensive shock; uncontrolled cardiac ischaemia or arrhythmias
• Agitated or uncooperative
• Drowsy or GCS <13
• Facial trauma, burns or surgery, or anatomical abnormalities interfering with mask fit
• Unable to protect airway: impaired cough and swallowing mechanism (impaired bulbar function); vomiting
• Excessive upper airway secretions
• Pneumothorax

Beneficial effects of CPAP

• Recruitment of collapsed alveoli
• Increased end-expiratory lung volume
• Reduced alveolar–arterial gradient
• Improved lung compliance
• Reduced work of breathing

Setting up non-invasive ventilation

In most hospitals, this is commenced by members of the intensive therapy unit, respiratory nurses or by members of critical care outreach teams. In some instances, emergency department staff may be trained for this purpose.

- The procedure is explained to the patient to maximize compliance with use
- The appropriate face mask is applied. The smallest mask to fit the face should be used. Face mask size is usually determined by using a measure gauge (sizer). Padding might need to be applied to the nasal bridge to minimize the effects of prolonged pressure
- The ventilator is turned on
- Oxygen is attached to the patient interface at a flow rate of 2L/min initially
- The mask is strapped in place
- A humidification system is connected
- The lower level of airway pressure support is EPAP and the higher level is IPAP
- EPAP(expiratory positive airway pressure) is set at 2cm H_2O and increased in steps of 1–2cm until the patient triggers the ventilator with all inspirations
- IPAP (inspiratory positive airway pressure) is set at 6cm H_2O and increased in steps of 1–2cm to the maximum the patient can tolerate without a significant air leak
- EPAP is always lower than IPAP to allow expiration.
- If IPAP is set on zero, the patient will receive CPAP
- The respiratory rate should be kept under 25 breaths/min
- The aim is to obtain an SpO_2 of 90% or more.

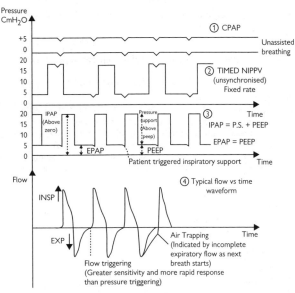

Diagram illustrating modes of non-invasive ventilation
1. CPAP (continuous positive airway pressure)
2. Timed Non-Invasive Positive pressure ventilation)
3. Triggered BIPAP (bilerel positive airway pressure)

IPAP inspiratory positive airway pressure
EPAP expiratory positive airway pressure

Fig. 5.23 Diagram illustrating modes of non-invasive ventilation.

When to use non-invasive ventilation

Patients
- COPD
- Chest wall deformity, neuromuscular disorder, decompensated
- OSA
- Cardiogenic pulmonary oedema, unresponsive to CPAP.

Blood gases
- Respiratory acidosis (Pa_{CO_2} >6.0 kPa, pH <7.35 or H^+ >45 nmol/L) which persists despite maximal medical treatment and appropriate controlled oxygen therapy (patients with pH <7.25 or H^+ >56 nmol/L respond less well and should be managed in an HDU/ICU)
- Low A–a oxygen gradient (patients with severe life-threatening hypoxaemia are more appropriately managed by tracheal intubation).

Clinical state
- Sick but not moribund
- Able to protect airway
- Conscious and cooperative
- Haemodynamically stable
- No excessive respiratory secretions
- Few co-morbidities.

Contraindications excluded
- Facial burns/trauma/recent facial or upper airway surgery
- Vomiting
- Fixed upper airway obstruction
- Undrained pneumothorax.

Pre-morbid state
- Potential for recovery to quality of life acceptable to the patient
- Patient's wishes considered.

How to set up non-invasive ventilation

1. Decide about management plan if trial of NIV fails, after discussion with senior medical staff, and document in the notes.
2. Decide where trial of NIV should take place (ICU, HDU or respiratory ward).
3. Consider informing ICU.
4. Explain NIV to the patient.
5. Select a mask to fit the patient and hold it in place to familiarize the patient.
6. Set up the ventilator.
7. Attach the pulse oximeter to the patient.
8. Commence NIV, holding the mask in place for the first few minutes.
9. Secure the mask in place with straps/headgear.
10. Reassess after a few minutes.
11. Adjust settings if necessary.
12. Add oxygen if SpO$_2$ <85%.
13. Instruct the patient how to remove the mask and how to summon help.
14. Clinical assessment and check arterial blood gases at 1–2h.
15. Adjust settings/oxygen if necessary.
16. Institute alternative management plan if PaCO$_2$ and pH have deteriorated after 1–2h of NIV on optimal settings. If no improvement, consider continuing with NIV and reassess with repeat arterial blood gas analysis after 4–6h. If no improvement in PaCO$_2$ and pH by 4–6h, institute alternative management plan.

Components of an anaesthetic machine

Anaesthetic machines may be available in resuscitation areas. They should only be used by individuals with appropriate anaesthetic experience. The main components are as follows:

- Compressed gas supplies: supply pipe from a central source, with reserve cylinders on the trolley
- Pressure gauges
- Reducing valves or pressure regulators, which control gas release from a high pressure system
- Flow meters, consisting of tapered glass tubes with spinning aluminium bobbins
- Vaporizers for volatile anaesthetic agents
- A common gas outlet for delivery of gases and vapours to the patient
- Magill attachment of corrugated rubber or plastic tube, reservoir bag and spill valve
- T-piece system: this consists of an inspiratory limb connected to the patient, and an expiratory limb, which serves as a reservoir for fresh gas.

There are no unidirectional or overflow valves, and no breathing bag. The open (expiratory) limb conveys expired gas to the atmosphere; continuous flow from the fresh gas limb flushes expired gas from the expiratory limb. Performance therefore depends on the role of fresh gas flow and on the ventilatory pattern of the patient.

Safety features

- Colour-coded pressure gauges
- Colour-coded flow meters
- An oxygen flow meter controlled by a single touch-coded knob
- An oxygen concentration monitor or analyser
- An oxygen/nitrous oxide ratio monitor and controller
- A pin-index safety system for cylinders
- An alarm for failure of oxygen supply
- Ventilator disconnection alarm
- At least one reserve oxygen cylinder.

Table 5.8 Colour codes for gas conducting system

Gas	Cylinder	Pipeline
Oxygen	Black/white shoulder white	
N_2O	Blue	blue
N_2O/O_2	Blue/white shoulder	blue/white
Air	Grey/white and black shoulder	white/black
Vacuum		Yellow

Delivery pressures
Oxygen, N_2O: 400kPa
Air: 700kPa

Chest approach to erect chest X-ray

Systematic data: NAME; AGE; SEX

Denmarker

Projection: AP (portable films are taken in the resuscitation room)/PA

Technical quality
- Rotation: medial ends of clavicles equidistant from the thoracic spinous processes (T4 level)
- Penetration/exposure: lower thoracic intervertebral disc spaces visible through the heart
- Degree of inspiration: hemidiaphragms at level of 5th to 7th rib anteriorly and 9th to 10th rib posteriorly. Expiratory films cause crowding of bronchovascular markings and an appearance of hilar enlargement.

Tubes and lines
- ECG leads
- Tracheal tube
- Nasogastric tube
- Intercostal tube
- Central line
- Pacemaker.

Soft tissues of chest wall
- Contour abnormality
- Opacity: soft tissue mass, foreign body, calcification
- Radiolucency: subcutaneous emphysema; mastectomy.

Bony cage (RCSS-ribs, clavicle, scapula, sternum)
- Opacity
- Radiolucency: erosions
- Notching
- Fractures
- Missing bones: ribs; clavicles.

Mediastinum
- Opacity
- Radiolucency
- Distortion or displacement
- The right paratracheal stripe is 2–3mm in diameter.

Heart
- Cardio-thoracic ratio less than 50%, or 60% in supine film
- Normal position: two-thirds to left of midline; one-third to right of midline
- Shape
- Calcification
- Prosthetic valves.

Pleura

- Air/fluid
- Fissures: the major fissure is normally seen only on a lateral CXR.

Lungs

- Zones
- Volumes
- Hilar shadows : the left hilum is 1–2cm (up to one interspace) superior to the right hilum. The hilar shadows represent primarily the shadow of the pulmonary vessels
- Normal hilum: concave lateral border; diameter of right interlobar artery <16mm; border of pulmonary outflow tract <4cm from the midline.

Diaphragms

- Levels: the right dome is 2cm higher than the left dome at the level of 6th rib anteriorly
- Clarity of outlines: silhouette sign
- Costophrenic angles: clarity
- Subdiaphragmatic gas.

Problems of supine chest X-ray

- The patient cannot take a full inspiration
- Pulmonary vessels, especially in the upper lobes, appear dilated, leading to an erroneous impression of pulmonary venous hypertension
- Smaller lung volumes may mask lung pathology in lower lobes and alter the appearance of the visualized lungs
- The hemidiaphragms are elevated
- The mediastinum is widened
- Small pleural effusions lie in the posterior pleural space
- Small pneumothoraces move to the anterior pleural surface.

Pneumothorax on supine chest X-ray

- Hyperlucency in the lower zone
- Increased air in anterior and lateral costophrenic sulcus
    - Hyperlucency of upper abdominal quadrants and lower chest
    - Wide, deep and sometimes 'tongue-like' lateral costophrenic sulcus
    - Visualization of the anterior costophrenic sulcus
    - Sharp diaphragmatic or mediastinal contours
- Depression of the ipsilateral diaphragm
- Double diaphragm contour
- Presence of a sharply defined pericardial fat pad and a distinct cardiac apex (mediastinal structures sharply outlined by free air)
- Subpulmonic air which outlines the visceral pleura of the lung base.

Problems of portable chest X-rays

- Supine or semi-supine positioning
- Inability to hold a breath, leading to expiratory films
- Artefacts such as bandages, ECG monitoring leads, ventilator tubing
- Short tube–film distance
- Lower power output
- Longer exposure times.

Pleural fluid on supine chest X-ray

- Homogeneous opacity over lung apex (pleural cap): the apex is the most dependent portion of the thorax tangential to the frontal x-ray beam
- Increased hazy opacity of the hemithorax with preserved vascular markings
- Blunting of costophrenic angle
- Fluid lies more medially than laterally because of concavity of the posterior aspect of the pleural cavity
- Hazy diaphragm silhouette: masks posterior and medial aspects of diaphragm
- Thickening of the minor fissure
- Widened paraspinal soft tissues
- Elevated hemidiaphragm sign.

Ill patient with diffuse lung disease—chest X-ray analysis

Diffuse lung disease may involve the vessels, the alveoli or air spaces, or the supporting structures (interstitium) of the lung.

Analysis

Pattern of opacity on plain film

- Round(nodular)
- Linear
- Irregular(reticulonodular)
- Ground glass.

Location (distribution) of the disease

- Upper, middle or lower zones
- Central versus peripheral
- Diffuse.

Lung volumes

- Increased
- Decreased
- Normal.

Presence of ancillary findings

- Pneumothorax
- Pleural effusion
- Hilar adenopathy
- Bone lesions.

Alveolar disease: air space disease; airlessness; alveolar pattern; amorphous shadows; coalescing shadows; end-air space disease; ground-glass pattern; ill defined opacities; patchy density.

Interstitial disease: Kerley A, B, C lines; peribronchial or perivascular infiltration; peribronchial cuffing; honeycombing; hilar haze, perihilar infiltrates, subpleural oedema.

Causes of diffuse pulmonary opacities on chest X-ray

Alveolar

Acutely ill

- Pulmonary oedema
- Widespread pneumonic consolidation
  Pneumocystis; viral; varicella
- Goodpasture's syndrome.

Not acutely ill

- Sarcoidosis
- Lymphoma
- Alveolar proteinosis.

Interstitial

Nodular

- Miliary tuberculosis
- Sarcoidosis
- Pneumoconiosis
- Histiocytosis
- Varicella pneumonia.

Linear or reticular

- Interstitial oedema (heart failure)
- Lymphangitis carcinomatosa
- Lymphoma
- Pneumoconiosis
- Histiocytosis
- Idiopathic pulmonary fibrosis (Hamman–Rich syndrome).

Assessment of interventional procedures on chest X-ray

Tip of endotracheal tube 4–5cm above the carina with the neck in the neutral position With neck flexion and extension, the tip can move 2cm caudad and cephalad, respectively.

Tracheostomy tube tip one-third to two-thirds the distance between the tracheal stoma and carina, at about the level of the D3 body.

Central venous catheter tip beyond the last venous valve, located distal to anterior end of the first rib. Ideal position for catheter tip: just above the junction of the superior vena cava and right atrium; just below the junction of the inferior vena cava and right atrium. In adults, the catheter tip should lie no more than 2cm below a line joining the lower surfaces of the medial ends of the clavicle on a PA CXR.

Dyspnoea

First line investigations in dyspnoea

- CXR
- Spirometry: FEV, FVC, PEFR
- Pulse oximetry at rest and following exertion
- 12-lead ECG
- FBC/differential count
- U&E
- Arterial blood gases if SpO_2 <94% at rest

Dyspnoea mechanisms

Dyspnoea is the conscious appreciation of increased work done during breathing. The mechanisms involved in production of this symptom include the following.

Increased work of breathing:
- Airflow obstruction
  - Asthma
  - Chronic obstructive airways disease
  - Tracheal obstruction
- Decreased pulmonary compliance
  - Pulmonary oedema
  - Pulmonary fibrosis
  - Extrinsic allergic alveolitis
- Restricted chest expansion
  - Ankylosing spondylitis
  - Respiratory muscle paralysis
  - Kyphoscoliosis.

Increased ventilatory drive:
- Increased physiological dead space (ventilation–perfusion mismatch)
  - Consolidation
  - Collapse
  - Pulmonary thromboembolism
  - Pulmonary oedema
- Hyperventilation resulting from respiratory centre stimulation in response to chemical or neural stimuli
  - Increased arterial hydrogen ion concentration, e.g. metabolic acidosis producing air hunger (Kussmaul's breathing)
  - Increased arterial $PaCO_2$, e.g. respiratory acidosis
  - Decreased arterial PaO_2 via aortic, carotid and brainstem chemo-receptors, e.g. pneumonia, impaired oxygen delivery due to anaemia, shock and stroke
  - Increased central arousal, e.g. exertion, anxiety, thyrotoxicosis, phaeochromocytoma
  - Pulmonary J receptor discharge, e.g. pulmonary oedema.

Impaired respiratory muscle function:
- Neuromuscular disorders: poliomyelitis, Guillain–Barre syndrome, cervical cord transection, muscular dystrophies, myasthenia gravis.

Asthma

Asthma is a syndrome of variable lower airway obstruction, associated with increased reactivity and inflammation. Patients with acute severe, life-threatening and near fatal asthma require resuscitation room management. Levels of severity (British Thoracic Society)

- **Mild**: peak expiratory flow rate (PEFR) >75% of predicted or best
- **Moderate**: PEFR 50–75% of predicted or best
- **Severe**: PEFR 33–50% of predicted or best
respiration rate >25/min
heart rate >110/min
Unable to complete sentences in one breath.

Life threatening
- PEFR <33% of predicted or best
- SpO_2 <92%; PaO_2 <8kPa; normal $PaCO_2$ (4.6–6.0kPa)
- Central cyanosis
- Bradycardia
- Cardiac dysrhythmia
- Hypotension
- Confusion
- Exhaustion
- Coma
- Silent chest.

Near fatal
- Raised $PaCO_2$ and/or
- Requiring mechanical ventilation with raised inflation pressure.

Brittle
- Type I: wide PEF variability despite intense therapy: >40% diurnal variation for >50% of the time over a period >150 days
- Type 2: sudden severe attacks on a background of apparently well controlled asthma.

Immediate therapy
- High concentration (40–60%) oxygen, with the aim of maintaining an SaO_2 of ≥92%
- Inhaled beta-2 agonists: salbutamol 5mg nebulized in 5mL 0.9% saline with oxygen (or 4–6 puffs via a metered dose inhaler with a holding chamber) at a flow rate of at least 6L/min. Repeated doses should be given at 15–30min intervals if there is inadequate response to initial treatment
- Hydrocortisone 200mg IV or prednisolone 40mg orally. Oral medication is as effective as IV provided that tablets can be ingested and retained
- Ipratropium 500mcg nebulized if poor initial response to nebulized beta-2 agonist
- Magnesium sulphate 50mg/kg or 2g (8mmol) IV in 250mL normal saline over 30min as a single dose, in life-threatening or near-fatal asthma, or where there is no good initial response to inhaled bronchodilators

- Aminophylline 3–5mg/kg loading dose diluted in 20mL of 5% dextrose over 30–45min, if not already on maintenance oral therapy, followed by infusion at a rate of 0.5–1.0mg/kg/h. Continuous ECG monitoring is required for tachyarrhythmias. There is a narrow therapeutic/toxic margin
- Heliox (80:20 helium:oxygen mixture) is not currently recommended
- Portable CXRs are useful in acute severe and life-threatening attacks where pneumothorax and/or pneumomediastinum are suspected
- Seek anaesthetic support in the presence of life-threatening features
- Intubation should be undertaken by the most experienced anaesthetist available. Rapid sequence induction using ketamine 1–2mg IV and suxamethonium 1–2mg/kg is often the best option. Recent evidence suggests a possible beneficial role for non-invasive ventilation in acute asthma.

Paediatric acute asthma treatment

- Salbutamol 5mg or terbutaline 5mg nebulized in oxygen (half-dose if age <5yrs)—three back-to-back nebulizers
- Ipratropium 250mcg nebulized (500mcg if age>5yrs)
- Oral prednisolone 1–2mg/kg (maximum 40mg); hydrocortisone 4mg/kg or 50mg (2–5yrs) or 100mg (age >5yrs)
- Aminophylline 5mg/kg over 20min; infusion 1mg/kg/h
- Salbutamol infusion: initially 15mcg/kg over 10min, diluted to 10mL with normal saline, followed by an infusion of 1–5mcg/kg/min titrated to clinical response. Continuous ECG monitoring for tachycardia and tachyarrhythmias and serial electrolyte monitoring is required.

Levels of severity of asthma in children over 2 years of age

Acute severe

- Unable to complete sentences in one breath
- Too breathless to talk or feed
- Pulse >120 bpm (age >5yrs); >130 bpm (age 2–5yrs)
- Respiratory rate >30/min (age >5yrs); >50/min (age 2–5yrs).

Life threatening

- Cyanosis
- Poor respiratory effort
- Exhaustion
- Confusion
- Coma
- Hypotension
- Silent chest.

Initial ventilator settings in a paralysed or heavily sedated asthmatic patient

- FiO_2 1 initially
- Prolonged expiratory time: I:E ratio 1:3 to 1:4
- Low tidal volume: 5–7mL/kg (to avoid pulmonary barotrauma)
- Low ventilator rate: 10 cycles/min
- Set inspiratory pressure 30–35cm H_2O on pressure control ventilation or limit peak inspiratory pressure <40cm H_2O
- Minimal or no PEEP.

Problems associated with ventilation in asthma
- High airway pressures
- Dynamic hyperinflation, with positive end-expiratory alveolar pressure (auto-PEEP) which is directly proportional to tidal volume and inversely proportional to expiratory time. Auto-PEEP results from delivery of a pre-set breath before the previous expiration is completed
- Pulmonary barotrauma: pneumothorax, pneumomediastinum, interstitial emphysema, pneumoperitoneum, tension lung cyst
- Hypotension from high mean intra-thoracic pressure leading to reduced venous return.

Desaturation in the intubated asthmatic
- Asthma alone cannot explain persistent oxygen desaturation if the patient is receiving a high FiO_2. The hypoxia of asthma is due predominantly to V/Q mismatch and should respond readily to a high FiO_2.
- Right main stem intubation and pneumothorax should be considered immediately. The endotracheal tube should be placed at the 21cm mark on the incisors.

Technique for using metered dose inhalers in mechanically ventilated patients
- Ensure tidal volume >500mL (in adults) during assisted ventilation
- Aim for an inspiratory time (excluding the inspiratory pause) >0.3 of total breath duration
- Ensure that the ventilator breath is synchronized with the patient's inspiration
- Shake the metered dose inhaler vigorously
- Place the canister in the actuator of a cylindrical spacer situated in the inspiratory limb of the ventilator circuit
- Actuate the metered dose inhaler to synchronize with the precise onset of inspiration by the ventilator
- Allow a breath hold at end inspiration for 3–5s
- Allow passive exhalation
- Repeat actuation after 20–30s until the total dose is delivered.

Technique for using nebulizers in mechanically ventilated patients
- Place the drug solution in the nebulizer, employing a fill volume (2–6mL) that ensures greatest aerosol-generating efficacy
- Place the nebulizer in the inspiratory line at least 30cm from the patient Y
- Ensure air flow of 6–8L/min through the nebulizer
- Ensure adequate tidal volume (>500mL in adults). Attempt to use duty cycle >0.3 if possible
- Adjust minute volume to compensate for additional air flow through the nebulizer, if required
- Turn off flow-by or continuous-flow mode on ventilator
- Observe the nebulizer for adequate aerosol generation throughout use

Inhaler devices for asthma

- Pressurized metered dose inhalers
- Manually activated pressurized metered dose inhalers
- Breath-activated metered dose inhalers: Autohaler; Easi-breathe
- Spacer devices: holding chambers (valved): volumatic, nebuhaler, aerochamber, babyhaler; extension device: spacehaler
- Dry powder inhalers: spinhaler; rotahaler; diskhaler; accuhaler; clickhaler; turbohaler
- Nebulizers: jet; ultrasonic; open vent.

- Disconnect the nebulizer when all medication is nebulized or when no more aerosol is being produced
- Reconnect the ventilator circuit and return to original ventilator settings.

(After Phipps P, Garrard, CS, In: Ridley S, Smith G, Batchelor M, eds. *Core cases in critical care.* Medical Media Ltd: Greenwich Medical Media Ltd., 2003; Chapter 16.

Acute exacerbation of COPD

An **acute exacerbation** of COPD is a sustained worsening of the patient's condition from the stable state, and beyond the normal day-to-day variation, which is acute in onset and necessitates a change in regular medication. Exacerbations can be associated with worsening breathlessness, increased sputum volume, changing sputum colour (sputum purulence) and cough.

Causes of acute exacerbation

- Infection: bacterial; viral
- Sputum retention with lobar or segmental collapse
- Left ventricular failure
- Pulmonary embolism
- Non-compliance with medication
- Pneumothorax.

Initial management
- Controlled oxygen therapy
24 or 28% Venturi mask, or nasal cannulae: 1–2L/min; repeat arterial blood gases after 30min and titrate oxygen administration to the response; oxygen must not be withheld if there is no evidence to support chronic type 2 respiratory failure associated with depressed hypoxic drive (i.e. high pCO_2 + high HCO_3). The availability of patients' respiratory passports or Medic Alert bracelets will prove to be helpful by indicating the presence of chronic hypercapnia.
- Nebulized bronchodilators driven by air
Beta-2 agonist: salbutamol 2.5 or 5mg 2–6 hourly
Anticholinergic: ipratropium bromide 0.5mg 6 hourly
- Antibiotics: amoxicillin
- Corticosteroids: IV hydrocortisone or oral prednisolone
- Diuretics if cor pulmonale
- Consider prophylactic heparin
- Doxapram infusion if PaO_2 <6kPa and pH <7.35
2mg/mL doxapram in 500mL 5% dextrose
Load with: 15min at 4mg/min (2mL/min)
  - 15min at 3mg/min (1.5mL/min)
  - 30min at 2mg/min (1mL/min)
- Non-invasive ventilation
- If PaO_2 <6kPa , $PaCO_2$ >6.5kPa and pH <7.35 despite controlled oxygen and doxapram (type II respiratory failure).

Indications for hospital treatment for acute exacerbations of COPD

- Impaired level of consciousness
- Acute confusion
- Severe breathlessness
- Poor and deteriorating general condition
- Rapid onset of exacerbation
- Cyanosed
- $SaO_2 <90\%$
- Worsening peripheral oedema
- Already receiving long-term oxygen therapy
- Living alone/not coping at home
- Poor level of activity, bed-bound
- Significant co-morbidity, especially insulin-dependent diabetes mellitus.

Further assessment in the emergency department
- Arterial pH <7.35
- Arterial PaO_2 <7kPa
- Acute ECG changes
- Presence of changes in the CXR.

Non-invasive ventilation for COPD (see p. 188)

Type II respiratory failure with respiratory acidosis due to acute exacerbation, where:
- PaO_2 <6
- $PaCO_2$ >6.5 (progressive hypercapnia)
- pH <7.35
- Raised or normal HCO_3
- Receiving optimal medical therapy

Non-invasive ventilation should not be used where tracheal intubation and invasive ventilation is more appropriate.

Conditions
- Conscious; not confused or agitated
- Cooperative
- Able to protect airway: swallowing and cough mechanisms intact; no vomiting
- Tracheobronchial secretions not a problem; able to clear secretions
- No facial trauma/fixed upper airway obstruction/recent facial, upper airway or upper gastrointestinal surgery
- Haemodynamically stable
- Able to tolerate mask ventilation and can coordinate breathing with ventilation.

Effects
- Improved gas exchange by increasing functional residual capacity through recruitment of previously closed air-exchange (alveolar) units
- Reduced intrapulmonary shunt

- Allows normal eating, drinking and conversation
- Allows for intermittent ventilatory support
- May avert the need for invasive ventilation.

Disadvantages
- Suboptimal airway protection, with the risk of aspiration
- Can cause gastric distension
- Pressure sores over the bridge of the nose
- Lack of access to the tracheobronchial tree in the presence of excessive secretions.

Initial ventilator settings for bi-level pressure support in COPD
- Expiratory positive airway pressure   4–5cm H_2O
- Inspiratory positive airway pressure   12–15cm H_2O
- Triggers   maximum sensitivity
- Back up rate   15 breaths/min
- I/E ratio   1:3

Patients on long-term domiciliary oxygen therapy

Selected patients with chronic obstructive pulmonary disease may benefit from long-term oxygen therapy, subject to certain conditions:

Arterial blood gases on two occasions, 3 weeks apart when the patient is stable and on maximal therapy, should show:

PaO_2 ≤7.3kPa

$PaCO_2$ >6kPa

FEV 1 <1.5L

FVC <2L

Oxygen concentrators have a flow rate adjusted to give paO_2 >8kPa; this is usually achieved at a flow rate of 1.5–2L/min.

Patients on long-term oxygen therapy presenting with an acute exacerbation of COPD almost invariably require admission to hospital.

Severity of COPD based on spirometry	
Severity	FEV1.0% predicted
Mild	60–80
Moderate	40–59
Severe	<40

CPAP: type 1 respiratory failure

NIV: type 2 respiratory failure

Effects of CPAP
- Stabilizes the upper airway
- Alveolar recruitment, preventing unstable alveolar units from collapsing
- Increased functional residual capacity
- Reduced micro- and macro-atelectasis
- Reduced work of breathing in the presence of intrinsic PEEP.

Stridor

Causes of stridor

Acute upper airway obstruction due to:

- Infection: retropharyngeal abscess; epiglottitis; croup; peritonsillar abscess; Ludwig's angina; bacterial tracheitis; diphtheria
- Trauma to the upper airway
- Burns: thermal; chemical
- Foreign body aspiration
- Neoplasm
- Anaphyloxis.

Checklist for stridor

- A preceding choking or gagging episode suggests foreign body inhalation and impaction
- Oral cavity: swelling of lips, tongue, floor of mouth, soft palate (uvula, tonsils); drooling of saliva
- Neck: masses; trauma (palpable laryngeal fracture); subcutaneous air
- Drug history: ACE inhibitors; new drug ingestion
- Fever; malaise.

General considerations in stridor management

- High concentration humidified inspired oxygen
- High dose steroids: e.g. dexamethasone 10mg 6 hourly IV × 24h
- Subcutaneous/intramuscular epinephrine
- Intravenous antibiotics
- Helium–oxygen mixture
- ENT referral with a view to urgent flexible fibreoptic laryngoscopy.

Upper airway infections

Acute epiglottitis

- Affects children aged 2–7yrs, but may occur in adults
- Caused by haemophilus influenzae type b infections; the incidence has declined due to the uptake of Hib immunization
- Acute onset of high fever, sore throat, dysphagia, hoarseness or muffling of voice, barking cough, progressing to toxicity, drooling of saliva and a propensity to fatal airway obstruction.

Management

- Do not attempt visualization of the epiglottis in an awake child
- Do not attempt intravenous cannulation
- Do not force the child to lie down
- Do not perform X-rays of the neck
- Ensure ENT surgical expertise is available
- Direct laryngoscopy in the operating room after gaseous induction of general anaesthesia, progressing on to endotracheal intubation. If intubation is not possible, needle cricothyroidotomy followed by tracheostomy
- Laryngoscopy confirms the presence of a swollen cherry red epiglottis
- Antibiotics: IV beta-lactamase-resistant agent, e.g. cefuroxime 1g 8 hourly or ceftriaxone 1g IV 12 hourly.

Acute laryngotracheobronchitis (croup)

- Affects children aged 6 months to 3yrs
- Predominantly occurs in the winter, often in epidemics
- Caused by parainfluenza virus types I and II, respiratory syncytial virus, and influenza virus types A and B
- Gradual onset, often following an upper respiratory tract infection
- Barking cough, worse at night; hoarseness of voice; inspiratory stridor
- Severity can be assessed more objectively using a clinical scoring system

Clinical croup score

	0	1	2
Inspired breath sound	Normal	Harsh	Delayed
Stridor	None	Inspiratory	Inspiratory + expiratory
Cough	None	Hoarse cry	Bark
Retraction, Flaring	None	Flaring + suprasternal retraction	Flaring, suprasternal + intercostal retraction
Cyanosis	None	In room air	In 40% oxygen

Score
Mild: <2
Moderate: 2–4
Severe: ≥5.

Management
- Humidified oxygen if hypoxaemic; keep SaO_2 >92%
- Nebulized adrenaline in oxygen: 0.5mL/kg 1 in 1000 adrenaline to a maximum of 5mL in normal saline; repeated every 30min initially
- Nebulized budesonide 1–2mg 12 hourly for 48h
  Or
- Single loading dose of oral dexamethasone 0.6mg/kg (maximum of 10mg) orally, IM or IV; followed by 0.15mg/kg 6h for 48h
- Consider inhalation of helium–oxygen mixture
- Intubation and intermittent positive pressure ventilation if drowsy or exhausted, and with worsening hypoxaemia and hypercarbia.

Features of impacted laryngeal foreign body

- Hoarseness of voice
- Shortness of breath
- Aphonia
- Odynophagia
- Haemoptysis
- Croup-like cough
- Inspiratory stridor
- Ineffective cough.

Features of impacted oesophageal foreign body

- Acute onset of dysphagia
- Odynophagia
- Drooling of saliva
- Chest pain
- Shortness of breath
- Inspiratory stridor
- Subcutaneous air.

Community-acquired pneumonia

Severe pneumonia can be life threatening, and requires the rapid administration of antibiotics (diagnosis to needle time) to reduce morbidity and mortality. The presenting symptoms have traditionally allowed categorization into typical and atypical pneumonias, although the clinical relevance of this is less certain at present.

Typical
- Fever
- Chills
- Productive cough
- Pleuritic chest pain
- Malaise
- Localized crepitations
- Consolidation.

Atypical (with a predominance of extra-pulmonary manifestations)
- Subacute onset
- Chills unusual
- Fever: moderate and persistent
- Dry cough
- Pleuritic chest pain unusual
- Adolescent/young adult
- Throughout the year
- CXR: diffuse, interstitial infiltrates.

There is some overlap between these groups, and the diagnosis of typical versus atypical pneumonia is not necessarily predictive of the causative organism(s).

Further evaluation
- Contacts with similar illness
- Travel history
- Immunization history
- Past medical history
- Drug allergy
- Immune state: steroids; asplenia; chemotherapy
- Risk factors for HIV
- Exposure to wild animals/pets
- Intravenous drug abuse.

Investigations
Venous blood
- Full blood count
- Renal and liver function tests
- Blood culture
- Consider HIV testing
- Initial sample for antibody testing: *Mycoplasma, Legionella, Chlamydia*
Arterial blood gases
Sputum: Gram stain and culture
Urine: for antigens (*Pneumococcus; Legionella*)
Chest X-ray
12-Lead ECG.

Management of community-acquired pneumonia (CAP)

Mild to moderate infection
- Extended spectrum penicillin (amoxicillin) with or without a macrolide (erythromycin) orally.

Severe infection
- Parenteral therapy with second or third generation cephalosporin and a macrolide (oral or IV)
- Cefuroxime 1.5g IV 8 hourly or cefotaxime 2g IV 8 hourly + erythromycin 1g IV 6 hourly

OR
- Amoxicillin 1g IV 6 hourly + flucloxacillin 2g IV 6 hourly + erythromycin 1G IV 6 hourly.

Suspected Legionnaire's disease
- High dose parenteral erythromycin 1g. IV 6 hourly
- Consider adding oral rifampicin.

Be aware of local antibiotic protocols prior to prescribing treatment.

British Thoracic Society (BTS) guidelines for routine investigations in hospital for all patients with severe CAP

- Blood cultures
- Sputum or lower respiratory tract sample for Gram stain, routine culture and sensitivity tests
- Pleural fluid analysis, if present
- Pneumococcal antigen test on sputum, blood or urine
- Investigations for legionella pneumonia including urine for legionella antigen, sputum or lower respiratory tract samples for legionella culture and direct immunofluorescence, and initial and follow-up legionella serology
- Respiratory samples for direct immunofluorescence to respiratory viruses, *Chlamydia* species, and possibly *Pneumocystis*
- Initial and follow-up serology for atypical pathogens.

Options for respiratory management in severe CAP

- High flow oxygen therapy
- CPAP: recruits and stabilizes collapsed alveolar units
- NIV
- Intubation and mechanical ventilation: progressive hypercapnia; reduced level of consciousness; shock
- Increasing metabolic acidosis indicates the development of circulatory shock and the requirement for fluid resuscitation and inotropic support.

Determinants of severity of CAP

Clinical
Confusion (Mental Test Score ≤8)
Respiratory rate >30/min
Systolic blood pressure <90mmHg
Diastolic blood pressure <60mmHg
Age >60yrs

Laboratory
More than one lobe involved on CXR
White blood cell count <4 or >20
Serum albumin <35g/L
Urea >7mmol/L
Atrial fibrillation
Bacteraemia
SaO_2 <92%
PaO_2 <8kPa

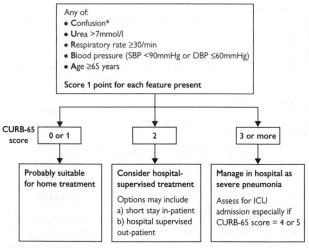

Any of:
● **C**onfusion*
● **U**rea >7mmol/l
● **R**espiratory rate ≥30/min
● **B**lood pressure (SBP <90mmHg or DBP ≤60mmHg)
● **A**ge ≥65 years

Score 1 point for each feature present

CURB-65 score

| 0 or 1 | 2 | 3 or more |

| Probably suitable for home treatment | Consider hospital-supervised treatment

Options may include a) short stay in-patient b) hospital supervised out-patient | Manage in hospital as severe pneumonia

Assess for ICU admission especially if CURB-65 score = 4 or 5 |

* Defined as a Mental Test Score of ≤8, or new disorientation in person, place or time.

Fig. 5.24 Severity assessment used to determine the management of CAP in patients admitted to hospital (CURB-65 score) updated 2004. Reproduced with permission from the British Thoracic Society.

Table 5.9 Preferred and alternative initial empirical treatment regimens and parenteral to oral switch regimens for community-acquired pneumonia updated 2004

Preferred	Alternative[a]
1. Home-treated, not severe	
Amoxicillin 500mg–1.0g tds PO	Erythromycin 500mg qds PO or clarithromycin 500mg bd PO
2a. Hospital-treated, not severe	
(Admitted for non-clinical reasons or previously untreated in the Community)	
As under Home-treated, not severe	
2b. Hospital-treated, not severe	
Either oral Amoxicillin 500mg–1.0g tds PO	*Fluoroquinolone with enhanced pneumococcal activity*
plus erythromycin 500mg qds PO or clarithromycin 500mg bd PO	e.g. levofloxacin 500mg od PO or moxifloxacin 400mg od PO (*the only such licensed agents in the UK at time of writing*)
or if IV needed Ampicillin 500mg qds IV or benzylpenicillin 1.2g qds IV	Levofloxacin 500mg od IV
plus erythromycin 500mg qds IV or clarithromycin 500mg bd IV	
3. Hospital-treated, severe	*Fluoroquinolone with enhanced pneumococcal activity*
Co-amoxiclav 1.2g tds IV	e.g. levofloxacin 500mg bd IV or PO
or cefuroxime 1.5g tds IV or cefotaxime 1g tds IV or ceftriaxone 2g od IV	*Plus*
	benzylpenicillin 1.2g qds IV
plus erythromycin 500mg qds IV or clarithromycin 500mg bd IV	
(with or without rifampicin 600mg od or bd IV)	

BTS Guidelines

Pneumocystis carinii pneumonia

Features

- An AIDS-defining illness in HIV-positive individuals
- Progressive effort intolerance over days or weeks
- Dry cough, sometimes with minimal mucoid sputum
- Fever and sweats; generalized malaise
- Minimal signs or fine, basal, end-inspiratory crackles
- Exercise-induced desaturation, demonstrated by a fall in SaO_2 on pulse oximetry.

Chest X-ray

- Diffuse reticular shadowing progressing to diffuse alveolar consolidation
- Multiple thin-walled cysts or pneumatoceles
- Intra-pulmonary nodules
- Cavitating lesions
- Lobar consolidation
- Secondary pneumothorax
- Hilar and mediastinal lymphadenopathy
- Pleural effusions are uncommon.

Management

- High inspired oxygen concentration
- Trimethoprim–sulphamethoxazole is the treatment of choice, continued for 21 days. Initially commence with trimethoprim 20mg/kg IV every 24h in two divided doses and sulphamethoxazole 100mg/kg IV every 24h in two divided doses, for 3 days
- Consider steroids for respiratory failure: methylprednisolone 40mg IV 6 hourly.

Pleural effusion

Presentation
- Progressively increasing shortness of breath
- Pleuritic chest pain
- Features of congestive heart failure.

Physical findings
- Stony dull percussion note
- Reduced tactile and vocal fremitus
- Reduced or absent air entry
- Mediastinal shift if large volume effusion >1000mL.

Causes
Transudate (protein <30g/L)
- Left ventricular failure
- Hypoalbuminaemia
- Fluid overload
- Constrictive pericarditis
- Renal failure
- Nephrotic syndrome
- Hypothyroidism
- Cirrhosis with ascites
- Superior vena cava obstruction.

Exudate (protein >30g/L)
- Post-infective (pneumonia)
- Pulmonary infarction (pulmonary embolism)
- Malignancy: metastatic (direct pleural involvement; late mediastinal involvement)
- Infections: bacterial, fungal, tuberculosis, viral, parasitic (*Entamoeba histolytica*)
- Connective tissue disorders: Systemic lupus erythematosus (SLE); rheumatoid arthritis (RA); Wegener's granulomatosis
- Drugs: nitrofurantoin; methysergide
- Primary pleural tumours: pleural mesothelioma
- Chylothorax
- Haemothorax
- Gastrointestinal disease: pancreatitis; oesophageal rupture; subphrenic abscess.

Management of pleural effusion
- Needle aspiration with a 21 gauge needle and a 20mL syringe; sitting up and leaning forwards over a bed table; tap posteriorly in the mid-scapular line one interspace below the upper limit of the dullness to percussion but above the diaphragmatic reflection of the pleura

Preliminary aspiration to confirm the presence of fluid, blood or pus while injecting local anaesthetic

- Catheter drainage with a 14 gauge intravenous cannula; remove stylet and connect the cannula to a closed pleural aspiration kit; aspirate all fluid; drainage of more than 1.5L of fluid can result in haemodynamic instability or re-expansion pulmonary oedema.

Pneumothorax

Air in the pleural space, which usually presents clinically with shortness of breath and/or pleuritic chest pain.

Classification of pneumothorax

Spontaneous

- Primary: no clinical lung disease; related to subpleural blebs and bullae
- Secondary: complication of clinically apparent lung disease, e.g. obstructive airways disease; pulmonary infections; interstitial lung disease; connective tissue disease.

Traumatic

- Penetrating chest injury
- Blunt chest injury.

Iatrogenic: central vein cannulation; pleural aspiration/biopsy; barotrauma

On an erect CXR, the pneumothorax is visualized as a visceral pleural line, with no distal lung markings. Expiratory or lateral or lateral decubitus views may aid the visualization of small pneumothoraces.

A CT scan is required to differentiate an emphysematous bulla from a pneumothorax.

Pitfalls in the recognition of pneumothorax on plain chest films

- Supine position
- Giant bullae of the lung
- Loculated pneumothorax in the presence of multiple pleural adhesions secondary to pleural disease, trauma or surgery
- Extensive surgical emphysema.

Differential diagnosis of pneumothorax on CXR

- Medial border of scapula
- Skin folds overlying the chest wall
- Companion shadows, accompanying the inferior margins of ribs
- After pleurectomy for recurrent pneumothorax.

According to the BTS guidelines, a pneumothorax is either **small**, with the distance from visceral pleural surface (lung edge) to chest wall being <2cm, or **large**, with the distance being >2cm. A 2cm width pneumothorax approximates to a 50% loss of lung volume.

Management

Primary spontaneous pneumothorax

Small: small rim of air around the lung: <2cm Observation only: small, with minimal symptoms; if admitted for observation, high flow (10L/min) oxygen.

Symptomatic: aspiration, repeated once if necessary; proceed to intercostal drainage if unsuccessful after two attempts at aspiration.

Large: aspiration; repeated once if necessary; if unsuccessful, proceed to intercostal drainage Repeat aspiration only if <2.5L of air aspirated at the first attempt.

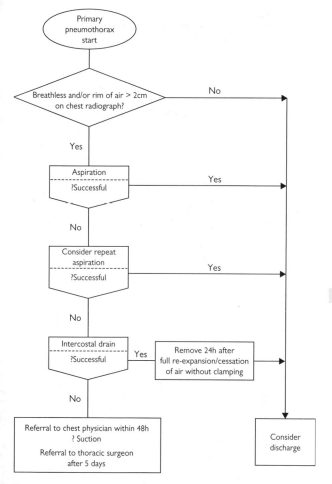

Fig. 5.25 Recommended algorithm for the treatment of primary pneumothorax.
Reproduced with permission from the British Thoracic Society.

Secondary spontaneous pneumothorax

Treat all but the smallest (apical or <1cm in depth); aspiration if not breathless initially followed by hospital admission for 24h; intercostal drain if breathless or large (>2cm).

Drainage of pneumothorax

- Check that the correct side is being treated
- The patient is in the supine position, with the head of the bed elevated 45° and the arm behind the head
- **Needle thoracentesis** through second interspace in mid-clavicular line for tension pneumothorax

Aspiration

- Via second interspace in the mid-clavicular line or via fifth interspace, using a long (30cm) catheter-over-needle device, such as an Abbocath
- (CVP line kit), or by the use of a 14 gauge venous cannula
- Initially aspirate with 20mL syringe to confirm air release
- Remove syringe and replace with three-way tap and 50mL syringe
- Aspirate air into 50mL syringe and expel. Continue until resistance is felt or >2.5L air are aspirated. The aspiration of >2.5L indicates a massive air leak for which intercostal tube placement is indicated
- Repeat CXR to confirm re-expansion.

Chest drain insertion (tube thoracostomy)

- Within the **triangle of safety** (between the infero-lateral border of the pectoralis major and the anterior border of latissimus dorsi and a line at the horizontal level of the nipples in a man and at the base of the breast in a woman) through the fifth interspace, midway between the anterior and mid-axillary lines
- Local anaesthesia, using 20mL ~1% lignocaine, of skin, subcutaneous tissues, intercostal muscles, rib periosteum and parietal pleura; advance needle along upper border of rib and aspirate air to confirm the diagnosis
- Incision <2cm in length; two mattress sutures with 1/0 or 2/0 silk at either end of the incision, leaving the ends loose
- Blunt dissection with forceps through the intercostal muscles on the superior surface of the rib down to and through the parietal pleura
- The pleural space is explored with a finger initially
- The drain is inserted with a rotatory movement until the most proximal side hole lies within the pleural cavity
- The two threads of the mattress suture will close the skin tightly around the drain; then the free ends of the sutures are left long and are looped around the drain
- The drain is secured to the chest wall with a transparent dressing
- The chest tube should fog with expiration
- Connect to a one-way valve system—either an underwater seal or a Heimlich valve; 2.5–5kPa of suction may be applied to the outlet from the underwater seal bottle if the lung does not re-expand immediately
- If dealing with pleural air only, a satisfactory alternative is to use a Seldinger technique for placement of a narrow bore tube, using a Tuohy needle, guide wire, dilator and tube sequence
- The drain bottle must always be kept below the level of the patient's thorax. The tube must never be clamped after insertion.

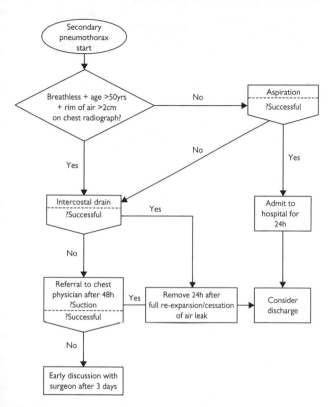

Fig. 5.26 Recommended algorithm for the treatment of secondary pneumothorax. Reproduced with permission from the British Thoracic Society.

A chest drain is made of silicone or plastic, possesses multiple drainage side holes, and has a radio-opaque line for X-ray localization. Seldinger chest drains allow for less invasive drainage of pneumothoraces.

Choice of drain size:
- <14 French: small pneumothorax
- 20–24 French: large pneumothorax
- 28 French: anticipated pleural leak.

Drainage systems
- Passive drainage with underwater seal
- Active drainage with suction-regulating device
- Portable valve system.

Indications for surgery in pneumothorax
- Persistent air leak
- Recurrent pneumothorax
- First episode in patients in whom it poses a significant occupational hazard: airline pilot; scuba diver
- First episode after prior pneumonectomy.

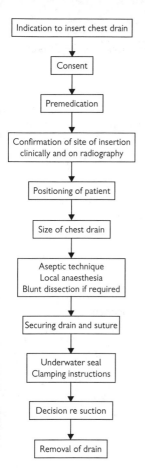

Fig. 5.27 Summary of chest drain insertion process.

Haemoptysis

Blood in the sputum is usually not a life threatening emergency, except in the context of massive haemoptysis.

Causes of haemoptysis

- Tracheobronchitis
- Bronchiectasis
- Pneumonia
- Pulmonary embolism, with or without infarction
- Tuberculosis
- Pulmonary mycetoma
- Pulmonary sequestration
- Arterio-venous malformations
- Iatrogenic.

Investigations

- Venous blood; FBC, U&E, coagulation screen
- Arterial blood gases
- 12-lead ECG
- CXR
- Sputum microscopy, culture
- Flexible fibreoptic bronchoscopy
- Selective pulmonary angiography
- High resolution CT scan.

CXR findings that might be associated with haemoptysis
- Nodule(s) or mass(es)
- Atelectasis
- Hilar/mediastinal lymphadenopathy
- Dilated peripheral airways
- Air-space consolidation
- Reticulonodular densities
- Cavity/cavities
- Hilar/mediastinal calcification.

Massive haemoptysis

Definition of massive haemoptysis
- >400mL over 3h
- >600mL over 24h

Massive haemoptysis usually arises from systemic bronchial arteries rather than the low pressure pulmonary arterial system. The amount of bleeding has no relationship to the clinical seriousness of the underlying pulmonary lesion.

Management
- High flow inspired oxygen
- Light sedation using short-acting benzodiazepines (e.g. midazolam) may be useful
- Airway control: place in lateral decubitus, with the suspected bleeding side dependent; head-down tilt; tracheal intubation, if unable to

protect airway by coughing, with a large bore (preferably 9mm tube); consider placement of a double-lumen tracheal tube
- Bronchoscopy to clear the airway, localize the site of bleeding and institute local control measures. This is best achieved by a combination of rigid and fibreoptic flexible bronchoscopy under general anaesthesia
- Control of bleeding: surgery; endobronchial and bronchoscopic techniques (balloon catheter tamponade; laser coagulation; injection of sclerosing agents; electrocautery); radiation therapy for cavitating cancer.

Indications for emergency surgery in massive haemoptysis
- >600mL blood loss in 24h
- Continued blood loss >150mL/h
- Trauma
- Tracheo-innominate artery fistula (after tracheostomy or tracheal reconstruction)
- Aorto-bronchial fistula.

Drowning

It is of academic interest only as to whether drowning was in salt water or fresh water. The only important consideration is the duration of hypoxia. The issues to be considered and dealt with include:

- Assessment and maintenance of airway patency
  - Tracheal suction
  - Tracheal intubation and assisted ventilation
- Stabilization of the cervical spine is indicated in the presence of any of the following:
  - Diving accident in shallow water
  - Water slide injury
  - Signs of injury
  - Signs of alcohol intoxication
- Management of hypothermia
- Management of fluid overload
- Management of pulmonary aspiration
- The need for prolonged cardiopulmonary resuscitation following cardiac arrest
- Infection risk from river water in particular
- There is no indication for routine steroid administration.

Drowning. *Circulation*, 2005; **112**: IV133–IV135.

Circulation management

Methods for cardiovascular system monitoring

Non-invasive

- Heart rate
- Arterial blood pressure: systolic/mean arterial pressure; postural blood pressure changes; using automated oscillometric devices (e.g. Dinamap), which can be inaccurate in low flow states, at the extremes of blood pressure and in the presence of shivering or cardiac arrhythmias. Prolonged or frequent cuff inflation can cause nerve damage
- Mean arterial pressure = diastolic BP + 1/3 (systolic BP − diastolic BP)
- ECG: lead II parallels the P wave vector, resulting in maximum P wave amplitude on the ECG
- Hourly urine output
- Skin perfusion: capillary refill time; core (tympanic) − peripheral (big toe) temperature difference
- Arterial oxygen saturation.

Invasive

- Arterial blood pressure
- Central venous pressure
- Pulmonary artery flotation catheter measurements
- Trans-oesophageal echocardiography and Doppler measurements.

Postural hypotension

- Fall in systolic blood pressure ≥20mmHg
- Fall in diastolic blood pressure ≥10mmHg
- Rise in heart rate >20 beats per min.

The technique for measurement involves measurement of blood pressure after 10min in the supine position and after 1 and 3min of standing.

Indications for cardiovascular support

Signs of impaired tissue perfusion
- Arterial hypotension:
  - Systolic blood pressure <90mmHg
  - Narrow pulse pressure
- Oliguria: <0.5mL/kg/h (older child/adult); <1mL/kg/h (young child); <2mL/kg/h(infant)
- Confusion or agitation
- Decreased conscious level
- Cold, clammy, mottled skin
- Poor filling of peripheral veins
- Increased core/peripheral temperature gradient >2°C
- Capillary refill time prolonged >3s, following 5s of local pressure
- Metabolic acidosis:
  - Base deficit more than—4mmol/L
  - Raised serum lactate >2mmol/L.

Table 6.1 Cardiovascular system monitoring methods

Parameter	Monitoring methods	Pitfalls
Heart rate	Clinical: palpation of pulse	Unreliable in AF & other irregular rhythms
	Auscultation of heart sounds	More accurate in AF
	Pulse oximeter	Finger probe unreliable with poor peripheral perfusion and patient movement
	ECG	Can double count T wave
		Lead disconnection gives asystole false alarm
Blood pressure	Non-invasive BP machine	Can also display heart rate
	Cuff methods	Incorrect cuff size
		Too narrow—falsely high
		Oversized—under-reads
	Arterial line/invasive BP	Transducer must be zeroed. Transducer height relative to patient important. Damping can occur giving low systolic reading
Circulating volume	Peripheral perfusion	Indirect indicators. Trends in CVP and response to fluid challenge more useful
	CVP measurement	

Shock

Shock is a state characterized by an imbalance between tissue oxygen delivery and tissue metabolic demands, with oxygen delivery being inadequate to meet tissue requirements.

Recognition of shock

- Breathing:
  - Increased respiratory rate
  - Increased work of breathing
- Circulation:
  - Increased heart rate
  - Reduced pulse volume
  - Reduced arterial blood pressure
  - Reduced pulse pressure (hypovolaemia) or increased pulse pressure (sepsis)
  - Mottled skin
  - Capillary refill time >2s following 5s of local pressure
- Disability:
  - Reduced conscious level
  - Coma
- Renal:
  - Oliguria/anuria.

Shock classification

Class I haemorrhage

- Blood volume loss of up to 15%
- No measurable changes in blood pressure, pulse pressure, or respiratory rate
- Minimal tachycardia with uncomplicated symptoms.

Class II haemorrhage

- 15%–30% blood volume loss
- 750–1500mL blood in a 70kg male
- Tachycardia (heart rate >100/min)
- Tachypnoea
- Decrease in pulse pressure.

Table 6.2 Relationship of palpability of pulse to systolic blood pressure

Carotid pulse	SBP ≥60mmHg
Femoral pulse	SBP ≥70mmHg
Radial pulse	SBP ≥80mmHg

These figures may not be as reliable as once thought.

Class III haemorrhage
- 30%–40% blood volume loss
- Marked tachycardia and tachypnoea
- Significant changes in mental status
- Measurable fall in systolic blood pressure.

Class IV haemorrhage
- More than 40% blood volume loss
- Life-threatening exsanguinations
- Marked tachycardia
- Significant depression in systolic blood pressure
- Very narrow pulse pressure (or an unobtainable diastolic blood pressure).

Causes of shock
Hypovolaemia
- Blood loss: absolute: external/internal bleeding
- Plasma loss: burns; capillary leak syndromes; protein-losing syndromes
- Fluid and electrolyte loss: diarrhoea and vomiting; endocrine (diabetic ketoacidosis (DKA), diabetes insipidus, adreno-cortical insufficiency).

Cardiogenic
- Contractile failure: acute myocardial infarction; cardiomyopathy
- Ventricular outflow obstruction: massive pulmonary embolism; critical aortic stenosis
- Impaired ventricular filling: cardiac tamponade
- Valve failure: acute mitral or aortic regurgitation
- Tachyarrhythmia/bradyarrhythmia

Distributive: relative blood loss
- Anaphylaxis
- Neurogenic: high spinal cord injury
- Sepsis.

Immediate goals in shock management
Haemodynamic support
- Mean arterial pressure >60mmHg
- Cardiac index >2.2L/min/m^2
- Pulmonary capillary wedge pressure = 15–18mmHg.

Initial fluid therapy

Initial bolus: 1–2L for an adult
                20mL/kg for a child
Replace each mL blood loss with 3mL crystalloid fluid: 3 for 1 rule.

Adequate urinary output
0.5mL/kg/h for adult
1mL/kg/h for child
2mL/kg/h for child under 1yr of age.

Maintain oxygen delivery
- Haemoglobin >10g/dL
- Arterial oxygen saturation >92%.

Reverse organ dysfunction
- Maintain urine output
- Reduce serum lactate
- Reverse encephalopathy.

Physiological approach to haemodynamic support in shock

Optimize preload
- Large bore intravenous access
- Crystalloid/colloid

Fluid challenge
- Improve contractility
- Inotropic support.

Optimize afterload
- Reduce an increased afterload: systemic–peripheral vasodilator; pulmonary-inhaled nitric oxide
- Increase reduced afterload: norepinephrine infusion.

Optimize rate
- Treat cardiac arrhythmia: correct metabolic disorder–acidosis; electrolyte abnormalities.

Goals to achieve adequate oxygen transport

- Cardiac index >4.5L/min/m^2
- Oxygen delivery (DO_2) >600mL/min/m^2
- Oxygen consumption (VO_2) >170mL/min/m^2
- Mixed venous oxyhaemoglobin concentration >70%
- Serum lactate <2mmol/L.

Check list for persistent hypotension

- Adequate function of monitors
- Adequate volume resuscitation
- Pneumothorax after placement of central venous access
- Occult bleeding: intra-abdominal; retroperitoneal; intra-thoracic
- Adrenal insufficiency
- Anaphylactic reaction to medication
- Cardiac tamponade (chronic renal failure).

> **A physiological approach to shock treatment**
>
> - Optimize preload
> - Reduce afterload
> - Increase myocardial contractility
> - Control cardiac dysrhythmias
> - Increase vascular resistance.

Venous access

Principles of venous access techniques

- In all but extreme emergencies, ultrasound guidance should be used for central venous access (NICE 2002)[1]
- Aseptic precautions must also be used, i.e. gown, sterile gloves, skin preparation and drapes
- The Seldinger wire method is almost universally used as it is the safest.
- Although it is now common for hospitals to stock exclusively triple and quadruple lumen catheters, the greater the number of lumens, the greater the potential for infection. The same applies to three way taps. In the presence of coagulopathy, central venous cannulation can be safe in experienced hands. However, multiple punctures can lead to haematoma, distorted anatomy and airway compromise. For this reason, it is safer to administer blood products, e.g. platelets by peripheral cannula first
- Hypovolaemic patients have collapsed veins. Large volumes of fluid resuscitation are best given through wide bore peripheral venous cannulae. It is easier to site central venous catheters after restoration of circulating volume
- Need for immediate central venous access
  - no peripheral access
  - requirement for inotropes
  - guide to intravascular volume status later
- There is no advantage to central venous catheterization for fluid administration alone
- Patients in heart failure or with severe respiratory failure do not tolerate lying flat. Close monitoring is needed during the procedure. In some cases it is preferable to use the femoral route or only obtain access after intubation and ventilation.

Types of venous cannulation devices

- Cannula over needle
- Hollow needle
- Cannula through needle: best avoided owing to the risk of catheter tip shearing and venous embolism
- Seldinger technique (catheter over guide wire), using guide wire through hollow needle followed by cannula.

---

1 NICE. Guidance on the use of ultrasound guiding devices for placing central venous catheters. Technology Appraisal Guidance No 49, September 2002.

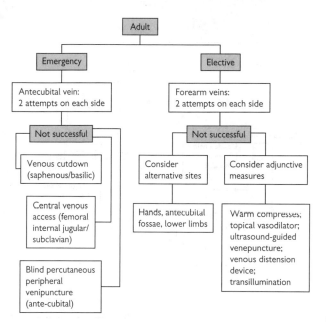

Fig. 6.1 Algorithm for peripheral venous access in adults. Reproduced with permission from the *Postgraduate Medical Journal*. In: Methods of obtaining peripheral venous access in difficult situations. *Postgraduate Medical Journal*, 1999, **75**: 459–462.

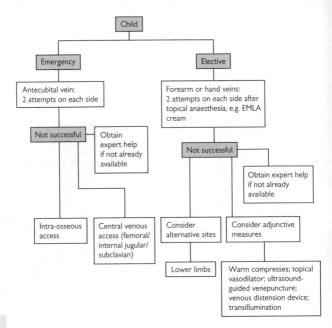

Fig. 6.2 Algorithm for peripheral venous access in children. Reproduced with permission from the *Postgraduate Medical Journal*. In: Methods of obtaining peripheral venous access in difficult situations. *Postgraduate Medical Journal*, 1999, **75**: 459–462.

Size of venous cannulae

24G orange
22G blue
20G pink
18G green
16G grey
14G cream

Over-the-needle catheters for peripheral venous access in children

Weight	Size
<10kg	24–20G
10–40kg	20–16G
>40kg	18–14G

Flow rates of water through venous cannulae

Diameter (mm)	Gauge	Length (mm)	Flow rate (mL/min)
1.0	20	32	54
1.2	18	45	80
1.7	16	45	180
2.0	14	45	270

Cannula	Flow rate (mL/min)
14G	
Short	175–200
Long	150
16G	
Short	100–150
long	20–100

Size of arterial cannulae
Adults: 20 or 22G
Term infants and children: 22G.

Size of wide bore venous cannulae
Infants: 22G
Term infants and children <2yrs: 20G
2–6yrs: 18G
Older children and adults: 16 or 14G.

Venipuncture techniques

- Over-the-needle catheter for one-step insertion
- Catheter-through-needle techniques
- Catheter-over-a-guide-wire technique (Seldinger): flexible wire catheter guide with inner core wire and outer coiled wire; flexible straight or J-shaped end; wire length at least 10cm longer than definitive catheter.

Catheter materials

- Inert: silastic: silicone elastomer or siliconized rubber
- Intermediate reactivity: Teflon, polyurethane
- Most reactive: polyvinyl chloride, polypropylene, polyethylene.

Local anaesthesia

- Prior to venous or arterial puncture, when time permits, preliminary local infiltration anaesthesia is recommended
- 1mL of 1% lignocaine is drawn up in a 2mL syringe and a 25G (orange) needle attached; alternatively a 27G needle and dental syringe may be used
- The bevel of the needle is kept parallel to the skin and the needle is advanced slowly while applying pressure to the plunger
- An intradermal bleb is created, which is usually sufficient for the subsequent puncture of a subcutaneous vein or artery.

Intraosseous access

Intraosseous access is generally considered in children aged 6yrs or under, but may have a place in the management of older children and adults.

- Support the knee and upper leg by a pillow
- Select a site in the midline of the medial flat surface of the anterior tibia 1–3cm distal to the tibial tuberosity
- Insert a 16–18G (18–20G in infants) intraosseous access needle at a 90° angle to the skin, with a firm downward pressure and twisting motion
- Advance until the cortex is penetrated, as indicated by a give, or sudden release of resistance
- The trocar is removed and a syringe is attached
- Correct placement is confirmed by aspiration of bone marrow content and by free flow of saline without subcutaneous soft tissue swelling
- The needle stands upright without support. However, protection with a dressing prevents dislodgement.

Other devices that can be used to obtain intraosseous access include simple butterfly or spinal needles, or a Jamshidi marrow aspiration needle.

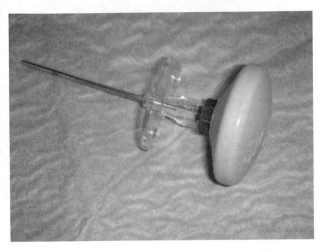

Fig. 6.3 Intraosseous needle.

Central venous access

Indications

- Rapid and reliable delivery of medications during cardiac arrest
- Haemodynamic monitoring: measurement of central venous pressure. Serial values in response to treatment are more useful than absolute values
- Delivery of potentially phlebitic intravenous fluids: vasopressors and inotropic drugs
- Administration of fluid therapy when there is a lack of or inadequate peripheral venous access
- Transvenous cardiac pacing
- Haemodialysis/plasmapheresis.

NB: tunnelled long-term lines may already be *in situ* for dialysis, chemotherapy or parenteral nutrition. Such lines should only be used if there is no available alternative access and need to be handled with meticulous asepsis. They are commonly flushed with a heparin 'lock' solution and this should be aspirated.

Pros and cons of different sites

Internal jugular

- Easy access, except where the neck is immobilized in a semi-rigid collar
- A cleaner area
- Risks of haematoma; inadvertent carotid artery puncture; and nerve injuries
- The right internal jugular vein provides a shorter and straighter path to the superior vena cava
- Lower risk of pneumothorax
- Safer in the presence of coagulopathy
- Should be avoided in the presence of either raised intracranial pressure or carotid artery disease.

Subclavian

- Easy access, with constant anatomy
- A cleaner area
- Higher risk of pneumothorax and arterial injury
- Difficult to control bleeding as the site of bleeding is not accessible for compression.

Femoral

- Easy access, especially during cardiopulmonary resuscitation
- A dirtier area, with proximity to the perineum and rectum
- Risk of inadvertent femoral artery puncture
- Radiological verification of catheter tip position is not required
- Higher thrombogenic potential.

Hazards and complications of central venous cannulation

- Failure of insertion or malposition
- Inadvertent arterial puncture
- Haematoma and haemorrhage, including haemothorax
- Pneumothorax.

Principles of central venous access techniques

- In all but extreme emergencies, ultrasound guidance should be used in preference (NICE 2002)[1]
- Aseptic precautions should be employed, i.e. gown, sterile gloves, skin preparation and drapes
- The Seldinger wire method is almost universally used as it is the safest
- Although multilumen catheters are widely used, the greater the number of lumens, the greater the potential for infection. The same applies to three-way taps which should not be routinely used.
- In the presence of coagulopathy, central venous cannulation can be safe in experienced hands. However, multiple punctures in the neck can lead to haematoma, distorted anatomy and airway compromise. For this reason, it is safer to administer blood products, e.g. platelets, by peripheral cannula first
- Hypovolaemic patients have collapsed veins. Large volumes of fluid resuscitation are best given through wide bore peripheral venous cannulae if possible. It is easier to site a central line after restoration of circulating blood volume.

Practicalities of central venous cannulation

- Correct patient positioning enhances success rates. Patients in heart failure and those with severe respiratory failure do not tolerate lying flat. In some cases it is preferable to use the femoral route or only obtain central venous access after intubation and ventilation
- 12–15cm length lines are optimal. Any longer and overinsertion is to be expected, especially when using the right internal jugular route
- Get everything ready on a sterile surface after gowning up, ensuring that flush solution and local anaesthetic are in different sized syringes to avoid confusion
- Aseptic skin preparation with 10% povidone iodine or 0.5% chlorhexidine followed by isolation of the area of interest with large sterile drapes is essential to prevent desterilization of the guidewire or catheter
- Continuous ECG monitoring is necessary during the procedure
- Secure line fixation and flushing of all lumens are essential before removing the drapes.

Internal jugular vein catheterization

- The right side is preferred as it allows more direct entry into the superior vena cava and less risk of damage to the left-sided thoracic duct. The right side is also easier to access for right handed operators
- Supine position, with pillow under shoulders to extend the neck (or no pillow at all)
- Rotation of head to opposite side
- Head-down tilt 10–15°.

---

1 NICE. Guidance on the use of ultrasound guiding devices for placing central venous catheters. Technology Appraisal Guidance No 49, September 2002.

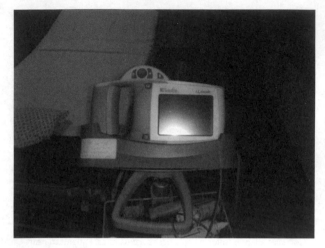

Fig. 6.4 Portable ultrasound machine.

Landmark technique
- The apex of triangle formed by lateral border of medial head and medial border of lateral head of sternomastoid muscle, and clavicle is identified as the point of entry
- Direct the needle (with attached syringe) posteriorly, at 45° angle to sagittal plane, in the direction of the ipsilateral nipple. The vein is usually punctured within 3cm below the point of entry of the needle
- The vein can alternatively be located with a small gauge (20–25G) 'seeker' needle attached to a syringe, at the apex of the triangle formed by the two heads of the sternomastoid muscle. A larger needle to introduce the guidewire is then passed adjacent to the seeker needle
- Insert the guidewire after detaching the syringe once blood is freely aspirated (in some products, the syringe barrel is hollow, permitting direct insertion of the wire). Feed with flexible J tip for ~15–20cm. A plastic straightener is used to straighten the J tip prior to introduction. The design of the J tip minimizes endothelial trauma. The straight end of the wire should not be used
- There should be no resistance to feeding the wire beyond the tip of the needle
- The wire tip will stimulate the right atrium or right ventricle causing ectopics, (sometimes VT or VF) if inserted into the heart. Watch the ECG as you advance the wire
- Remove needle over guide wire and extend skin incision with a small pointed (number 11) scalpel blade

- Advance dilator (screwing action) over the wire. The dilator should only be inserted far enough to dilate the point of entry into the vein. Do not push it all the way in. Resistance is usually from an insufficient skin incision
- Remove dilator carefully without withdrawing wire. Then insert the catheter, again using a slight twisting motion, by feeding over the wire
- Ensure that the guidewire protrudes beyond the hub of the proximal end and is held securely before advancing the tip of the catheter through the skin—otherwise the guidewire can be lost in the patient
- Remove the wire by progressively withdrawing it as the catheter is advanced
- No more than 15cm needs to be inserted
- Aspirate blood and flush the line with heparinized saline
- The catheter tip is ideally positioned in the distal superior vena cava and a CXR is required to confirm placement
- The catheter is secured to the skin by suturing through holes on the wings or around the suturing grooves on the hub
- Make sure that the catheter hub itself as well as any separate clamp are both sutured. If just the clamp is sutured, the line can slide if pulled, leading to accidental removal
- A sterile, preferably transparent, adhesive dressing is then applied to the puncture site.

Ultrasound technique
- Trendelenburg position with head turned to opposite side
- A 7.5MHz transducer covered by a sterile sheath is used to identify the common carotid artery (visualization of pulsations with real time sonography); transducer parallel to and superior to the clavicle over the groove between the two heads of sternomastoid muscle
- Internal jugular vein is identified lateral to the artery—generally larger, compressible, and changes in size with respiration and Valsalva manoeuvre
- Hold probe in non-dominant hand while imaging the vein in a transverse plane
- Centre the image over the vein
- Place needle under transducer at an angle of 70° to the skin and advance under ultrasound guidance until the tip is seen within the lumen
- Once a flash of blood is visualized, remove the probe and cannulate the vein using Seldinger technique
- Check in the longitudinal plane that the cannula lies within the vein.

Femoral vein catheterization
- The femoral arterial pulse is palpated in the groin, just distal to the inguinal ligament
- Following antiseptic skin preparation, the skin is punctured 1cm medial to the femoral artery and 2cm below the lower border of the inguinal ligament
- The needle is advanced cephalad at a 30–45° angle until free flow aspiration of blood occurs, usually at a depth of 3–4cm
- Seldinger wire technique is used for venous cannulation.

Subclavian vein catheterization

- 10–20° head-down tilt, with the head turned away to the opposite side
- Skin punctured just below the midpoint of the clavicle
- The needle is advanced towards the suprasternal notch, with continued aspiration on the attached syringe
- Once blood is aspirated, usually at a depth of 4–6cm, the syringe is detached, and the guidewire fed in 15cm
- A sequence of dilator over wire is followed by introducer sheath over wire, and then by guidewire removal.

Saphenous vein cut-down

- A 2cm incision is made 2cm anterior and superior to the medial malleolus
- A 2cm length of long saphenous vein is mobilized using blunt dissection
- The distal end of the mobilized vein is ligated
- The proximal end has a suture looped around it
- A venotomy is made with scissors
- The cannula is introduced under direct vision
- The proximal suture is tied to fix the cannula in place
- The skin is closed
- For median basilic cut-down, an incision is made three finger breadths proximal to the midpoint between the tip of the medial malleolus and the brachial pulsation.

Central venous pressure measurement

Central line information may be obtained either via a continuous waveform using a transducer attached to an oscilloscope or intermittently by a manometer system at the bedside.

- CVP is a measure of right heart filling pressure (RV preload)
- Measure at 45° head-up tilt with pressure transducer zeroed at the vertical height of the sternal angle of Louis
- In the supine position, CVP reflects transmitted intra-abdominal pressure, but postural change is a good indicator of hypovolaemia.

Saline manometer
- Check that the catheter is patent; flush if necessary
- Check zero with spirit level, using the reference point of the sternal angle
- Turn three-way tap to allow fluid to run from bag into the measuring column
- Turn tap to connect measuring column to patient and allow the level to fall; respiratory oscillations should be present
- When the level stops falling, take the measurement in cm H_2O, which can be converted to kPa or mmHg if required. Turn tap to connect patient back to the infusion and set a slow drip rate to keep the catheter patent.

Transducer measurement
- Direct readings by electronic transducers are expressed in mmHg (7.5mmHg = 10cm H_2O pressure)
- Turn tap to connect patient back to the flush set. This is commonly on a dual connector from a single pressure bag which also feeds the arterial line.

Factors affecting CVP
- Right ventricular function
- Tricuspid valve function
- Left heart function
- Pulmonary vascular resistance
- Venous return
- Pericardial pressure
- Intra-thoracic pressure.

Central venous pressure waveform
Three systolic components
- c wave: movement of the tricuspid valve annulus into the right atrium with isovolumic right ventricular contraction and tricuspid valve closure in early systole
- x descent: movement of the tricuspid valve away from the right atrium, being pulled away by the contracting ventricle, in early/mid-systole
- v wave: passive right atrial inflow in late systole prior to tricuspid valve opening.

Two diastolic components
- y descent: opening of tricuspid valve in early diastole
- a wave: right atrial contraction in end-diastole. Cannon a waves occur if the right atrium contracts against a closed tricuspid valve.

Pulmonary arterial pressure monitoring
- Generally this is undertaken in the ITU setting, but it may occasionally be used in the resuscitation room. The scope for, and clinical benefit from, this form of monitoring has been declining in recent years.

Components of multilumen venous catheter kits
These vary in sophistication of contents by manufacturer and local set-up. They may include:
- 7 French gauge(FG) triple or quadruple lumen catheter, with 20 or 30cm of usable length (ideally 15cm)
- 0.052 inch diameter guidewire with straight and J tip
- 18G thin wall needle
- 18G catheter over needle
- 7 French vessel dilator
- 22G finder needle
- Syringe and suture material.

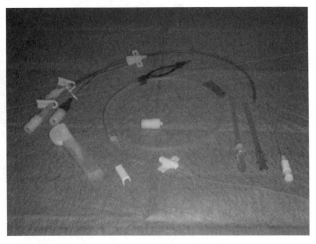

Fig. 6.5 Triple lumen catheter.

Pulmonary artery catheter

- Flexible flow-guided balloon-tipped radio-opaque flotation catheter
- 5 to 8FG sizes
- 110cm in length
- Marked at 10cm intervals with black rings, beginning at distal end
- Have up to five lumens

Proximal lumen 30cm from the tip, for CVP measurement/fluid administration—in most patients it lies within the right atrium

Distal lumen at the tip, connected to a transducer pressure monitoring system, for PAP monitoring. Inflation of the balloon occludes that pulmonary artery segment and provides an indirect measurement of the left atrial pressure (wedge pressure)

Air-balloon lumen to inflate 1mL latex rubber balloon at the tip, facilitating catheter placement. The balloon should be inflated with air prior to passage through the heart.

- Thermistor 4cm from the tip for pulmonary artery blood temperature measurement; used for thermodilution cardiac output measurements following injection of cold solution (10mL over 2–4s) through the proximal lumen
- Continuously monitor the pulmonary artery trace for spontaneous wedging
- A 7.5–9FG, 15cm, introducer sheath is inserted by Seldinger technique.

Waveform monitoring

- Each cardiac chamber has a characteristic pressure waveform
- Right ventricle: sudden increase in systolic pressure; little change in diastolic pressure compared with right atrial waveform
- Pulmonary artery: dicrotic notch in peak systolic waveform; sudden increase in diastolic pressure
- Pulmonary capillary wedge: decrease in mean pressure to <12mmHg with damping of the waveform; balloon deflation results in reappearance of the pulmonary arterial waveform and an increase in the mean pressure.

In general, the distances to reach the various areas are:
- Right atrium: 15–20cm
- Right ventricle: 30–40cm
- Pulmonary artery: 45–55cm
- Wedge: 45–60cm.

Indications

- Measurement of right atrial, right ventricular, pulmonary artery and pulmonary capillary wedge pressures
- Measurement of mixed venous (pulmonary artery) oxygen saturation
- Measurement of cardiac output by thermodilution technique
- Angiography
- Intra-cavitary electrograms
- Atrial and/or ventricular pacing.

Usage of pulmonary artery catheters is declining owing to a demonstrated lack of effectiveness.

Right heart pressures/flows

- Right atrium: 0–8mmHg
- Right ventricle
  - Systolic: 5–30mmHg
  - End-diastolic: 0–8mmHg.
- Pulmonary artery
  - Systolic: 15–30mmHg
  - Diastolic: 4–12mmHg
  - Mean: 9–16mmHg
- Pulmonary capillary wedge pressure: 2–10mmHg
- Cardiac: 2.8–4.2L/min/m² Cardiac Index.

Arterial line

Indications
1. Need for continuous beat-to-beat arterial blood pressure monitoring
   - Any unstable patient with cardiorespiratory problems
   - Inotropic support
   - All intubated, ventilated patients including severe head injury
2. Need for frequent blood sampling, especially arterial blood gas monitoring.

Sites
- Radial
- Dorsalis pedis
- Brachial
- Femoral

In patients with poor peripheral perfusion or impalpable peripheral pulses, the femoral artery is often the best choice.

Contraindications to arterial line placement
- Ischaemic extremity
- Arterial occlusive disease, embolism, microvascular perfusion problems
- Inadequate collateral flow (Allen's test)
- Presence of a vascular graft or haemodialysis access arteriovenous fistula in the upper limb
- Local sepsis: skin or soft tissue infection
- Underlying skeletal trauma.

Allen's test
The palmar arches in the hand supply the fingers via the digital arteries. These receive collateral flow from both ulnar and radial arteries. The aim is to demonstrate that all digits receive adequate perfusion even with complete radial artery occlusion.

Both ulnar and radial arteries are compressed at the wrist. The hand is exsanguinated by squeezing to form a tightly closed fist. The ulnar artery is released and the hand should rapidly 'pink up'—the ulnar artery refill time should be <5s.

There is some controversy about the reliability of the test.

Technique
- Aseptic precautions are used and local anaesthetic (1% lidocaine) injected over the site in an awake patient.
- A 20 or 22G arterial cannula (adults) or 22 or 24G cannula (children) is introduced into the radial artery of the non-dominant hand, with wrist dorsiflexed 40–60° over a towel or small pack of gauze. The cannula is inserted at an angle of 15–30°. The cannula may be threaded directly over the needle or via a guidewire
- With small vessels, it can be easier to transfix the artery intentionally, remove the needle and slowly withdraw the cannula until there is backflow of blood. At this stage, the cannula is advanced up the lumen of the artery

- The cannula and connecting tubing must be labelled as 'arterial' to avoid inadvertent intravascular injection of drugs intended for intravenous administration.

Set-up

- The cannula is connected via a three-way tap to a pressurized flushing system (normal saline is usually used; addition of heparin is generally unnecessary), incorporating a calibrated electronic pressure transducer with a disposable dome. This is in turn connected via a cable to the monitor display. The transducer dome is placed at the level of the chosen zero reference point
- The transducer is zeroed by opening the three-way tap to air whilst also open to the transducer
- The transducer converts pressure readings into electric signals. The arterial waveform and digital readings of systolic, diastolic and mean pressures are continuously displayed
- The waveform curves should be sharp with a clear upstroke (anacrotic limb) and a visible notch in the descending or dicrotic limb. A rounded peak may indicate damping due to air bubbles, blood clot or damaged cannula
- To take an arterial blood sample, clean the sampling port with an alcohol swab. Then aspirate 1–2mL blood into an ordinary syringe and discard. The sample is drawn into a pre-heparinized syringe. Air is expelled and the sample analysed rapidly. The line and the side port of the three-way tap are flushed with saline (from the pressurized bag via flow-switch) and a clean cap placed on the sampling port.

Potential complications

- Disconnection and severe blood loss or exsanguination
- Thromboembolism and ischaemia (the brachial artery is not favoured for this reason)
- Haematoma (can rarely lead to a compartment syndrome in the forearm)
- Inadvertent injection of drugs (if chemically irritant, severe ischaemia or gangrene necessitating amputation can ensue).
- Infection
- Aneurysm formation.

Table 6.3 Evaluation of hypotension

	Hypoxic	Cardiogenic	Neurogenic/vasogenic	Septic
PCWP	R	I	R	V
CO	R	Rv	N/V	I
MVO$_2$	R	R	N	I

R = reduced; I = increased; N = normal; V = variable; MV = mixed venous.

Fluid bolus in hypovolaemia

Warmed crystalloid

- Normotensive: 10mL/kg
- Hypotensive: 20mL/kg
- Known heart failure: 5mL/kg.

Normal blood volume

- Adult: 70mL/kg
- Child: 80mL/kg
- Neonate: 90mL/kg.

Daily water requirement

- 0–10kg body weight: 100mL/kg/day
- Add 50mL/kg/day for 10th–20th kg body weight
- Add 20mL/kg/day for >20th kg body weight
- Increase by 10% for each degree Centigrade above normal body temperature.

Basal requirements

First 10kg body weight: 4mL/kg
Second 10kg: 2mL/kg
Subsequent kg: 1mL/kg.

Intravenous infusions

Flow rate = volume of fluid (mL)/time for infusion (h)

Flow rate in drops/min = (volume of fluid (mL))/(total infusion time (minutes)) × calibration (drops/mL)

Drops/min = mL/min × drops/mL.

Human albumin formulations
- Dilute: 4.5 or 5% solution in saline
- Concentrated: 20 or 25% solution in saline
- Plasma protein fraction: 5% total protein (88% albumin and 12% globulins).

Table 6.4 Crystalloids

Name	Na$^+$	K$^+$	Ca^{2+}	Cl$^-$	HCO$_3^-$	Osmolality
	(all in mmol/L)					(mosmol/L)
N saline (0.9% NaCl)	154	0	0	154	0	300
Hartmann's solution	131	5	4	112	29	281
4% dextrose + 0.18% NaCl	31	0	0	31	0	284
5% dextrose	0	0	0	0	0	278

Table 6.5 Colloids (albumin, gelatins, hydroxyethyl starches, dextrans)

Name	Na$^+$	K$^+$	Ca^{2+}	Cl$^-$	HCO$_3^-$	Osmolality
	(all in mmol/L)					(mosmol/L)
Gelofusine	154	0.4	0.4	125	0	465
Haemaccel	145	5	6.2	145	0	350

Table 6.6 Colloids versus crystalloids

	Crystalloid	Colloid
Intravascular retention	Shorter	More prolonged
Peripheral oedema	Common	Possible
Pulmonary oedema	Possible	Possible
Excretion	Easy	No
Allergic reactions	No	Rare
Cost	Cheaper	More expensive

Inotropic agents

- Patients who are ill enough to require inotropic support will need continous ECG monitoring and invasive blood pressure display via an arterial line. Inotropic agents should only be commenced in conjunction with correction of hypovolaemia by fluid loading.
- All vasoactive drugs when given intravenously have the potential for sudden and profound changes in both heart rate and blood pressure. A bolus dose can precipitate cardiac arrhythmias and lead to cardiac arrest.
- Inotropes are also irritants and mostly require central venous infusion. Infusions are always given via a regulated infusion device such as a syringe driver or a volumetric infusion pump. It is essential to prime the giving set before connection to the patient at the correct infusion rate to avoid the administration of an accidental bolus dose.
- Most hospitals have standard infusion tables and concentrations based on local protocols for the available pumps.
- There is little robust evidence favouring one inotropic agent over another. Noradrenaline is often preferred in vasodilated, hypotensive patients in the context of septic shock. Patients with poor cardiac output may respond better to dobutamine or adrenaline/epinephrine. In general, the role of dopamine and dopexamine in the resuscitation room is questionable.
- The response to a given inotrope at a given concentration varies in terms of:
  - Chronotropic effect (rise in heart rate and tendency to arrhythmias)
  - Changes in regional blood flow distribution
  - Rise in blood pressure
  - Tolerance, which can develop to all catecholamines

Characteristics of an ideal positive inotropic agent

- Raises perfusion pressure by raising cardiac output rather than systemic vascular resistance; does not produce vasoconstriction
- Redistributes blood flow to vital organs
- No effect on heart rate
- Immediate onset and termination of action
- No tolerance to action
- Compatible with other vasoactive agents.

Inotropic agents

Catecholamines

- Naturally occurring sympathomimetic amines

Norepinephrine, dopamine, epinephrine

- Synthetic sympathomimetic amines

Dobutamine, dopexamine, isoprenaline, phenylephrine, methoxamine

- Phosphodiesterase inhibitors: milrinone; enoximone
- Digoxin.

Dobutamine

Synthetic catecholamine derivative of isoprenaline; a racemic mixture of the D- and L-isomers. The L-stereoisomer stimulates alpha 1 receptors The D-stereoisomer stimulates beta 1 and beta 2 receptors. It has no dopaminergic receptor activity.

The major effect is to increase myocardial contractility through beta 1 receptors. Peripheral alpha 1 and beta effects balance out, with a small net peripheral vasodilatory action. This may lead to profound hypotension in patients with intravascular volume depletion.

Dose: 5.0–20mcg/kg/min, titrated against response.

Administration

15mg/kg in 50ml 0.9% saline or 5% dextrose
(1mL/h = 5mcg/kg/min; 0.4–4.0mL/h = 2–20mcg/kg/min).

Dopexamine

A dopamine analogue with DA1, DA2 and beta 2 agonist activity. It reduces afterload via renal and mesenteric vasodilatation (beta 2 and DA1 receptor activation), positive inotropism (beta 2 activation) and natriuresis (DA1 activation).

Dose: 1.0–8.0mcg/kg/min.

Epinephrine (adrenaline)

Alpha 1 and beta agonist.
0.03–0.15mcg/kg/min.
0-15–1.0mcg/kg/min.

At lower doses it primarily stimulates beta 2 receptors, thus causing vasodilatation, followed by beta 1 stimulation with a positive inotropic and chronotropic effect. At higher doses, it predominantly stimulates alpha 1 receptors, acting as a vasopressor.

Dose: 0.3mg/kg in 50mL 0.9% saline or 5% dextrose (1mL/h = 0.1mcg/kg/min).

Norepinephrine (noradrenaline)

Alpha 1 and beta agonist.
Dose: 0.01–0.5mcg/kg/min.

Isoprenaline

Beta 1 and beta 2 agonist.
Dose: 0.02–0.20mcg/kg/min.

Dopamine

Endogenous norepinephrine precursor. Stimulates norepinephrine release from sympathetic nerves. The dose-dependent effects as described below are not specific and are subject to considerable variability of individual response. Some recent evidence suggests that renal dopamine does not work.

Dose schedules:

1–3mcg/kg/minute: dopaminergic DA1 and DA2 receptors; renal and splanchnic vasodilatation; sodium excretion; increased urine output (renal dose)
3–8mcg/kg/minute: beta 1-adrenergic receptor effects; positive inotropic effects (cardiac dose)
7–8mcg/kg/minute: alpha receptor effects; progressive pulmonary and systemic vasoconstriction.

Blood transfusion

Emergency blood transfusion options
- Fully cross matched blood: 30min
- Type-specific (ABO/Rh matched) blood partial cross-match: 10min
- Group O -ve blood: 5min. Group O -ve blood is not a panacea:
  - It is a rare blood group (~6% of the population)
  - Lack of a cross-match can lead to acute haemolysis in the presence of unrecognized red cell allo-antibodies
  - Blood is not the ideal resuscitation fluid because of its inherent viscosity.

Triggers for blood transfusion
Haemoglobin concentration—there is no absolute level that determines the need for transfusion
- Impaired cardiopulmonary reserve
- Continued blood loss
- Impaired tissue oxygenation.

Acute massive blood loss
- Loss of one blood volume within a 24h period
- Loss of >7% (adult) or 8–9% (child) of ideal body weight
- 50% blood volume loss within 3h
- Rate of blood loss: >150mL/min.

Jehovah's witnesses and blood transfusion
Basis for Jehovah's Witnesses not accepting blood:
- Since 1945, following a discussion in The Watchtower of Psalm 16 verse 4 (Their drink offering of blood I will not offer nor take up their names into my lips), Jehovah's Witnesses have refused transfused blood or blood products
- This belief is further based on: Genesis 9:3–4: But flesh with the life thereof, which is the blood thereof, shall ye not eat
- Leviticus 17: 10–16: Ye shall eat the blood of no manner of flesh: for the life of the flesh is the blood thereof: whoever eateth it shall be cut off
- Acts 15: 28–29: That ye abstain from meats offered to idols, and from blood and from things strangled

A reform movement now exists, called The Associated Jehovah's Witnesses for Reform on Blood, who are campaigning for the abolition of the blood transfusion policy.

Legal aspects of blood transfusion in Jehovah's Witnesses
- It is unlawful to administer blood to a patient who has refused it by the provision of an Advance Directive or by its exclusion in a consent form
- Properly executed Advance Directives must be respected, and special Jehovah's Witness consent forms should be widely available

- A child's right to life is paramount and must be considered before the religious beliefs of his or her parents
- If a child under 16yrs wishes to receive blood against their parents' wishes, they must be shown to be Gillick competent
- In a life-threatening emergency in a child unable to give competent consent, all life-saving treatment should be given, irrespective of the parents' wishes
- In children under 16yrs of age, if parents refuse to give permission for blood transfusion, it may be necessary to apply to the high court for a Specific Issue Order
- Except in an emergency, a doctor can decline to treat a patient if they feel pressurized to act against their own beliefs. The patient's management should be passed to a colleague.

Blood products

Red cell products
- Whole blood: 420–510mL; haematocrit (Hct) 35–45%; rarely used
- Red cell concentrate: 150–300mL; Hct 55–75%; approximate haemoglobin 20g/100mL.

Platelet concentrates

Clotting factors
- Fresh frozen plasma: 200–250mL; indicated in multiple acquired coagulation factor deficiency; liver disease; massive transfusion with coagulation factor depletion; disseminated intravascular coagulation; and for rapid reversal of warfarin effect. The use of fresh frozen plasma is, in the main, indicated when specific factor concentrates are not available. The dose is 15mL/kg body weight
- Cryoprecipitate: 20–40mL; prepared from one unit of fresh frozen plasma thawed at 4°C; indicated in some patients with haemophilia A or von Willebrand disease; fibrinogen repletion in acquired coagulopathies, including disseminated intravascular coagulation; and factor XIII deficiency.

Recombinant activated factor VII enhances haemostasis at the site of tissue bleeding without systemic activation of coagulation as it requires tissue factor to become active. It has shown an excellent safety profile in both therapeutic doses and with overdose. It may become increasingly of use as a universal haemostatic agent in major trauma with severe blood loss.

Requesting blood for transfusion

- Obtain informed consent where possible and time allows, indicating the procedure involved, the potential benefits and risks, alternatives and the potential risk of no transfusion
- Respect the autonomy of decisions by patients who take a measured decision to disallow blood transfusion, e.g. Jehovah's Witnesses
- For urgent requests, contact the blood bank by telephone
- Requests should be legibly written, and should contain:
  - The full name of the patient, correctly spelt, when available
  - A unique patient identifier (hospital number)
  - Type and number of units of blood product required
  - Time and place at which needed
  - The sample tube label should be handwritten, and should contain:
  - The full name of the patient, when available
  - Date of birth, when available
  - Date
  - Signature of the person taking the sample
- Handwritten requests are preferable to the use of pre-printed labels.

Giving blood

- Remember that ABO-incompatible transfusion can be rapidly fatal, and that the most common cause for mismatched transfusion is a clerical error
- Correct patient identification and sample labelling is essential.
- Identify the patient receiving the blood verbally, by the identity wristband, and from the medical notes, and cross-check the details with those on the completed blood request form
- Two health care professionals should confirm the identity of the patient and the destination for the cross-matched blood before commencing infusion if the patient is unresponsive or not definitively identified. Manual checklists are cumbersome and require attention to detail. In the future, the use of bar code technology with non-linear portable data format (PDF) and utilizing hand-held computers will allow safer blood transfusions.
- Use a blood-giving set. All blood products should go through a transfusion giving set with a 170–200μm filter.

Risks of massive transfusion
Hypothermia (bank blood is stored at 4°C)
Dilutional thrombocytopenia
Coagulation factor depletion
Hyperkalaemia: potassium load from stored blood
Hypocalcaemia: citrate anticoagulant binds calcium ions.

Disseminated intravascular coagulation screen
Platelet count: reduced
Prothrombin time: normal or increased
Activated partial thromboplastin time: normal or increased
Fibrinogen: reduced
Fibrin degradation products: increased
D-dimer: positive
Antithrombin III level: reduced.

Recognition of ABO-incompatible transfusion

This leads to sudden intravascular haemolysis, which can progress to cardiovascular collapse, acute renal failure and death. Early features include:
- Fever
- Chills
- Pain in the chest and low back
- Hypotension
- A sensation of impending doom.

Coagulation profile

Normal values
- Prothrombin time: 12–15s
- International normalized ratio (INR): 0.8–1.3
- Activated partial thromboplastin time: 25–40s
- Platelet count: $150–450 \times 10^9/L$
- Bleeding time: 2–9min
- Thrombin time: 10–15s
- Fibrinogen assay: 1.5–4.0g/L
- Fibrin degradation products: <1mg/L
- D-dimer <500ng/mL.

Target INR
2.0–3.0: deep vein thrombosis (DVT); pulmonary embolism (PE); transient ischaemic attack (TIA); chronic atrial fibrillation (AF)
3.0–4.5: Recurrent DVT/PE; arterial grafts; prosthetic cardiac valves.

Management of bleeding and excessive anticoagulation
- INR 3.0–6.0; target 2.5: reduce or stop warfarin
- INR 4.0–6.0; target 3.5: restart warfarin when INR <5.0
- INR 6.0–8.0; no bleeding: stop warfarin; restart when INR <5.0
- INR >8.0; no bleeding: stop warfarin; restart when INR <5.0; if other risk factors for bleeding, give vitamin K 0.5–2.5mg orally
- Major bleeding; emergency surgery, INR >2.5: stop warfarin; give prothrombin complex concentrate 50U/kg or fresh frozen plasma 15mL/kg; give vitamin K 5mg orally or IV. Prothrombin complex concentrate (factors X, IX, II and often VII) achieves complete reversal of warfarin effect within minutes; fresh frozen plasma is very slow and ineffective. Vitamin K restores coagulation factor levels in 6–12h.

Fresh frozen plasma (FFP)
Definite indications
- Single factor replacement if no specific concentrate available
- Immediate warfarin effect reversal when prothrombin factor concentrates not available
- Acute disseminated intravascular coagulation with haemorrhage
- Thrombotic thrombocytopenic purpura (with plasma exchange)
- C1 esterase deficiency if no concentrate available

Conditional use (only in the presence of bleeding and abnormal coagulation):
- Massive transfusion—when prothrombin time (PT) or partial thromboplastin time (PTT) prolonged >1.5 times normal and fibrinogen <0.8g/L
- Liver disease with abnormal coagulation and bleeding or before surgery.
- Cardiopulmonary bypass with bleeding and proven coagulation abnormalities not due to heparin
- Special paediatric indications.

No justification for use:
- Hypovolaemia
- Plasma exchange
- 'Formula' replacement
- Nutritional support
- Treatment of immunodeficiency.

Specifications for FFP

- Single donation/plasmapheresis
- Freeze plasma to −30°C within 6h of collection
- Each unit is ~280mL
- Thaw at 37°C; infuse within 2h
- Dose: 12–15mL/kg
- Use ABO compatible; AB if group unknown
- RhD compatible for women of child-bearing age
- Consider FFP with >one blood volume lost
- Single unit FFP is not virally inactivated: consider methylene blue treated (single unit) or SD-treated (pooled)
- Aim for INR and activated partial prothrombin time (aPTT) ratio <1.5.

Specifications for cryoprecipitate

- Plasma frozen quickly and then thawed slowly at 1–6°C
- Re-suspended in small volume of residual plasma (9–16mL)
- Factors VIII, fibrinogen, vWF, XIII, fibronectin in higher concentration than plasma
- 1 unit: 200–250mg fibrinogen
- Usual dose: 10–20 packs
- Aim to keep fibrinogen >1.0g/L.

> **Cryoprecipitate**
> *One unit (10–15mL)*
> 250mg fibrinogen
> 100u factor VIII
> 80u von Willebrand factor
> 40–60u factor XIII
> Shelf life 6 months.

Platelet concentrates

- 1 pool: >240 platelets x 10^9/L.
- Maintain platelets >50 or >100 if head injury
- Transfuse if anticipated platelet function abnormal: two blood volumes replaced by red cells; request platelets at levels above desired target to ensure availability.

Platelet count

>100 000/µL: normal haemostasis
<50 000/µL: prolonged bleeding after a procedure; mucosal bleeding
<20 000/µL: petechial rash; spontaneous bleeding
<10 000/µL: risk of spontaneous intracerebral haemorrhage.

Sickle cell crisis

Crises complicate homozygous sickle cell disease and can be precipitated by a number of insults including dehydration, hypoxia and sepsis.

Types of sickle cell crisis
- Painful (vaso-occlusive) crisis
- Acute chest syndrome
- Cerebral infarction
- Splenic/hepatic sequestration
- Aplastic crisis
- Haemolytic crisis
- Priapism
- Biliary colic/cholecystitis.

Investigations that may be necessary
- FBC
- Reticulocyte count
- U & E
- Liver function tests
- MSU
- Blood culture
- Arterial oxygen saturation on air
- Group and save.

Indications for CXR and arterial blood gases

- Rib, sternal and thoracic vertebral pain
- Signs of consolidation
- Respiratory rate >25/min
- Oxygen saturation <80% on air or <95% on maximal supplementary oxygen.

Principles underlying pain relief in sickle crises

- Selection of method depends on whether the pain is acute, chronic or a mixture of the two types, and on whether the patient is opioid-naïve or opioid tolerant
- The guiding principle is to use a stepwise approach
- Avoid pethidine as accumulation of the metabolite norpethidine may cause convulsions
- Diamorphine/morphine 5mg subcutaneously (SC) + cyclizine 50mg SC initially is a useful starting point. Many patients will have their own individualized analgesic protocol which should be adhered to
- Reassess pain 20min later
- Repeat dose if pain unrelieved or halve dose if pain partially relieved
- Reassess pain 20min later and repeat analgesia
- Once pain control achieved, transfer to patient-controlled analgesia system using SC diamorphine given as a variable bolus dose with a fixed lockout time.

Pain relief options
- Morphine 0.1mg/kg IV loading dose; 1mg/kg/h infusion
- Diclofenac: 1mg/kg 8 hourly orally
- Codeine phosphate: 1–2 mg/kg 6 hourly orally
- Paracetamol: 12–15mg/kg 8 hourly orally

Clinical features of acute chest syndrome
- Rib, sternal and/or thoracic vertebral pain
- Bilateral basal chest signs with new infiltrates on CXR
- Tachypnoea
- Deteriorating oxygenation
- Falling haemoglobin concentration
- Fever
- Leukocytosis.

Patho-physiology
- Bone infarction leads to atelectasis and regional hypoxia (rib, vertebral, sternal)
- Infection
- Fat embolism from necrotic bone marrow
- Pulmonary infarction due to sequestration of sickled red cells: microvascular *in situ* thrombosis
- Thromboembolic disease
- Vascular injury and inflammation.

Repeated attacks may lead to
- Chronic impairment of lung function
- Pulmonary hypertension
- Right ventricular failure.

Management
- Analgesia
- Individualized oral and IV fluids
- Parenteral broad-spectrum antibiotic therapy, including a macrolide antibiotic
- Oxygen therapy if SaO_2 <92% or arterial oxygen tension <85mmHg on room air
- Inhaled bronchodilator therapy often improves lung function
- Severe acute chest syndrome (falling arterial oxygen saturation; clinical deterioration; extensive radiological changes) is an indication for urgent exchange transfusion to reduce the level of HbS to under 20%, and thereby arrest sickling, and increase total haemoglobin (up to 14g/dL) to maintain tissue oxygenation
- Transfer to an ICU with facilities for mechanical ventilation and extra-corporeal membrane oxygenation will be required if deterioration continues.

Causes of acute anaemia
- Aplastic crisis (parvovirus)
- Sequestration crisis: splenic in infants
- Hyperhaemolysis
- Malaria
- Bleeding.

Indications for urgent exchange transfusion therapy in sickle cell disease
- Acute chest syndrome with hypoxaemia
- Stroke
- Spinal cord infarction
- Persistent priapism
- Uncontrollable non-resolving crisis with intractable pain
- Major trauma.

Objectives of transfusion
- Reduce HbS to <30%
- Improve oxygen-carrying capacity
- Remove sickle cells and reduce viscosity
- Stop autologous red blood cell production.

Electrocardiography

ECG leads

- Limb leads
  - Electrodes on right arm (red), left arm (yellow)
  - and left leg (green)
  - I
  - II
  - III
  - aVR
  - aVL
  - aVF
- Chest leads

Adhesive pre-gelled chest electrodes attached to colour-coded leads by 'clothes peg' clips

- V1: fourth intercostal space; right sternal border
- V2: fourth intercostal space; left sternal border
- V3: Midway between V2 and V4
- V4: fifth intercostal space, left mid-clavicular line
- V5: Level with V4, left anterior axillary line
- V6: Level with V4, left mid-axillary line
- V7: Level with V6 in the left posterior axillary line
- V8: Level with V7 at the left mid-scapular line
- V9: Level with V7 at the left spinal border
- Right chest leads
  - V1R: Normal V2
  - V2R: Normal V1
  - V3R: Mirror image V3
  - V4R: Mirror image V4
  - V5R: Mirror image V5
  - V6R: Mirror image V6.

Normal 12-lead ECG

- One small square: 0.04s; 1mV
- One large square: 0.20s
- Normal P wave: <0.12s wide; <2.5mm tall
- Normal PR interval: 0.12–0.20s
- Q wave abnormal in I, II, aVF and aVL if >0.04s wide or >1/4 the height of the subsequent R wave
- Normal QRS complex: 0.05–0.12s
- ST segment: isoelectric ± 1mm (0.1mV)
- Normal resting heart rate: 60–1000/min.

Normal sinus rhythm implies
- A P wave rate 60–100 beats per min with <10% variation
- P waves normal for the subject and of uniform morphology
- Each P wave followed by a narrow QRS complex
- P wave amplitude greatest in lead II
- Normal P wave orientation in the frontal plane, with the mean P wave vector pointing downward and to the left
- Constant PR interval
- Normal QRS axis
- Variation between successive beats <0.12s.

Normal P waves (sequential depolarization of right and left atria)
The first half of the P wave is produced by right atrial depolarization and the second half by left atrial depolarization.
- Normally upright in I, II, aVF, V4–V6
- May be inverted in aVR, aVL, V1 (normally inverted in aVR)
- Upright (positive), inverted (negative) or biphasic in III, aVL, V1–V3. A biphasic P wave represents right atrial activation anteriorly and left atrial activation posteriorly
- Not notched/peaked
- Frontal plane axis of 0 to +90°
- Height <2.5mm in lead II (>2.5mm reflects right atrial enlargement). The greatest amplitude is usually in II
- Width <0.12 (120ms) s in lead II (>120ms reflects left atrial enlargement; may be notched or biphasic)
- With combined atrial enlargement, the P wave is both tall and wide.

P wave abnormalities include inversion, increased amplitude, increased width, notching, biphasicity, peaking or absence. After cardiac transplantation the ECG will frequently show two distinct P waves. The P wave of the SA node of the donor heart has a constant 1:1 relationship with the QRS complex, whereas the native P wave (resulting from preservation of the recipient SA node at the superior cavoatrial junction) maintains an independent rhythm. The two SA nodes are electrically isolated by the atrial suture line.

No identifiable atrial activity (absent P waves)
- A mid-junctional pacemaker with the atria depolarized at the same time as the ventricles
- Sinoventricular conduction with the impulse reaching the atrioventricular (AV) node by way of internodal pathways without atrial depolarization
- Sinus arrest with atrial standstill (and junctional escape)
- Atrial complexes too small to see or oriented perpendicular to the lead: P waves are often very small in the elderly.

Inverted P waves
- Dextrocardia
- Junctional rhythm
- Atrial and junctional ectopics
- Incorrect placement of arm leads
- Physiological.

ECG manifestations of sick sinus syndrome

- Marked persistent sinus bradycardia <40bpm
- Sinus arrest and/or SA exit block
- Drug-resistant (e.g. atropine, isoprenaline) sinus bradyarrhythmias
- Long pause following an atrial premature contraction
- Prolonged sinus node recovery time determined by atrial pacing
- Chronic atrial fibrillation or repetitive occurrence of atrial fibrillation (less commonly, atrial flutter)
- AV junctional escape rhythm (with or without slow and unstable activity)
- Carotid sinus syncope
- Failure of restoration of sinus rhythm following cardioversion
- Brady-tachyarrhythmia syndrome
- Common co-existing AV block and/or intraventricular block.

Normal PR interval (beginning of P wave to beginning of QRS complex; PQ interval may be a more appropriate description) (onset of atrial depolarization to onset of ventricular depolarization)

The PR interval represents the physiological delay in AV conduction, allowing atrial filling of the ventricles prior to ventricular systole.
- 0.12–0.20s (120–200ms)
- Three to five small squares.

Prolonged PR interval
- Atrio-ventricular block
- Hyperthyroidism.

Short PR interval
- Junctional and low atrial rhythms
- Wolff–Parkinson–White (WPW) syndrome
- Glycogen storage disease
- Normal **QRS complex** (depolarization of ventricle; usually obscures atrial repolarization)

- <0.12s duration; normally 0.06–0.11s (60–110ms)
- Less than three small squares
- Always inverted in aVR: small or absent R
- No pathological Q waves
- No evidence of left or right ventricular hypertrophy.

Minimal frontal plane QRS amplitude
- V1, V6: 5mm
- V2, V5: 7mm
- V3, V4: 9mm

J wave, or Osborn wave
A low deflection during the terminal deflection of the QRS and in the same direction as the QRS. It is seen in hypothermia. The height of the wave is proportional to the degree of hypothermia.

Low voltage QRS complexes: <10mm in all 12-leads
- Obesity
- Old age
- Thick chest wall
- Chronic obstructive lung disease: emphysema
- Hypothyroidism
- Pericardial effusion
- Chronic constrictive pericarditis.

Q waves
A Q wave is an initiating negative deflection of the QRS complex.
It is normally present in leads I, II, aVF and left ventricular leads (V3–V6) from septal activation
- ≤0.04s wide or <25% total QRS complex duration
- ≤25% of R wave amplitude
- Depth <2mm in I and II, and <1mm in other leads.

Pathological Q waves
- Broad (0.04s or longer in duration)
- Deep (>4mm in depth)
- Usually associated with substantial loss of height of the R wave resulting in a Q wave/R wave ratio which is 25% or greater
- Frequently seen in multiple leads
- Present in leads which do not normally show wide and deep Q waves, e.g. aVR.

Causes of pathological Q waves
- Myocardial infarction
- Pulmonary embolism
- Right or left ventricular hypertrophy
- Left bundle branch block
- Cardiomyopathies
- Ventricular septal defect (in V5 and V6).

J point

- The zero reference potential for analysing current of injury
- Located at the end of the QRS complex, i.e. at the beginning of the ST segment
- In the normal ECG, the junction of the QRS complex with the ST segment (J point) is ~90°.

T waves

- Normally upright in I, II and left ventricular leads (V3–V6)
- Normally inverted in aVR. May be inverted in III, AVF, V1 and V2 in normal individuals
- Variable in all other leads: low, high, negative, positive or biphasic. Increased amplitude in aVL and aVF (if QRS >5mm)
- Height in limb leads <5mm and in precordial leads <10mm
- The height of a T wave should be at least 10% of a QRS, provided the QRS is predominantly positive with almost no S wave.

Juvenile T pattern

- Negative T waves in right precordial leads, only V1 and V2, or
- Negative T waves from V1 to V4
- Usually seen in young adults, aged 20–40 years; T wave inversion is normal in the right precordial leads in children
- The combination of negative T waves and the ST–T elevation of early repolarization resembles acute myocardial infarction.

Causes of giant T wave inversion

- Acute myocardial infarction–transmural; subendocardial
- Right ventricular hypertrophy
- Left ventricular apical hypertrophy
- Ventricular pacing
- Cerebral haemorrhage
- Hypertensive encephalopathy.

QT interval

The QT interval is measured from the beginning of the QRS complex to the end of the T wave. The interval comprises two components: the QRS duration (conduction velocity of the wave of depolarization in the bundle of His and ventricles) and the JT interval (a measure of the duration of ventricular repolarization). It is an indirect measure of the duration of ventricular action potential and ventricular repolarization.

$$QT \text{ interval} = 0.30–0.46s \ (300–460ms)$$

Most ECG machines perform an automated measurement of the QT interval

A rate-corrected QT >0.44s (in the absence of bundle branch block) is considered prolonged. In normal persons, however, the upper 95% confidence limit for QTc is 0.46s in women and 0.45s in men.

QTc values of 0.42–0.46s are diagnostically equivocal, because both LQTS gene carriers and non-carriers may exhibit QTc intervals in that normal/borderline range.

Corrected QT interval (QTc) (onset of ventricular depolarization to end of ventricular repolarisation) is obtained by Bazett's formula:

QT interval (measured in lead II) divided by the square root of the preceding R–R interval (cycle length). Inclusion of the U wave should be avoided in the measurement of the interval. Normal: 0.42s.

Heart rate	QT interval (from start of QRS to end of T wave)
60bpm	0.43s
75bpm	0.39s
100bpm	0.34s

U wave
- Normal delayed repolarization of ventricular Purkinje cells
- Represents after-depolarizations in the elderly
- Amplitude <1/3 of T wave amplitude in the same lead
- The normal polarity is in the same direction as the T wave in the limb leads

The nearly **isoelectric baseline** comprises three segments:
- ST segment: plateau of the ventricular action potential
- TP segment
- PQ segment.

ST segment monitoring

This involves automated trend analysis of the ST segment, comparing changes in the ST segment (measured 60–80ms after the J point) to the isoelectric point 40ms after the QRS complex.

ST segment elevation

The American Heart Association recommends that the PR segment (connecting the end of the P wave with the beginning of the QRS complex) should be used as the baseline and reference point for judging ST–segment elevation.

The TP segment may have to be used as the reference point for judging ST segment deviations when:
- PR interval is very short
- PR segment deviation from the baseline is present (e.g. pericarditis, AF)
- Artefact distorts the PR segment.

TP segment wander invalidates the use of the PR baseline as a reference point.

ST segment is usually isoelectric with the PR and TP segments, i.e. baseline.

Measure ST elevation at 0.04s (1mm) after the J point. Compare it with the baseline (a line drawn from the start of the P to the end of T).

The specificity of ST–T and U wave abnormalities is provided more by the clinical circumstances in which the ECG changes are found rather than by the particular changes themselves.

Primary ST–T wave abnormalities

Primary abnormalities are independent of changes in ventricular activation and may be the result of global or segmental pathological processes that affect ventricular repolarization.
- Drug effects: digoxin, quinidine, tricyclic antidepressants
- Electrolyte abnormalities of potassium, magnesium and calcium
- Intrinsic myocardial disease: myocarditis, ischaemia, infarction, infiltration, myopathy
- Neurogenic effects: subarachnoid haemorrhage, stroke, trauma, tumour.

Secondary ST–T wave changes

Secondary abnormalities are normal ST–T wave changes solely due to alterations in the sequence of ventricular activation.
- ST–T changes seen in bundle branch block: generally the ST–T polarity is opposite to the major or terminal deflection of the QRS
- ST–T changes seen in fascicular block
- ST–T changes seen in non-specific intra-ventricular conduction block
- ST–T changes seen in WPW pre-excitation
- ST–T changes in VPCs, ventricular arrhythmias and ventricular paced beats.

Causes of ST segment elevation

- Normal: male pattern: the majority of men have ST elevation of 1mm or more in the precordial leads. The ST segment is concave. Most marked in V2.
- Early repolarization
- ST elevation of normal variant
- Left ventricular hypertrophy
- Left bundle branch block

- Acute pericarditis
- Hyperkalaemia
- Brugada syndrome
- Pulmonary embolism
- Prinzmental's angina
- Acute trans-mural myocardial infarction
- Left ventricular aneurysm.

Special characteristics in ST elevation

Acute myocardial infarction
- Slow ECG evolution with localization
- Concavity downwards (convexity upwards, or straightened)
- Reciprocal ST–T changes
- Development of Q waves with QTc prolongation
- ST elevation is maximal 1h after onset. In the absence of re-vascularization, there is a gradual return to the baseline over ~10–20h.

Acute pericarditis
- Rapid ECG evolution
- Generalized, non-anatomical ST–T changes in all leads except aVR and V1
- Concavity upwards
- Often with normal QTc
- PR segment depression, a manifestation of atrial injury
- No reciprocal ST segment depression
- T waves usually low amplitude
- Heart rate usually increased.

Left ventricular aneurysm
- Chronic (>2wks after acute myocardial infarction) with no evolution
- Localized ST elevation with variable ST–T changes
- Often prolonged QTc.

Vasospasm (Prinzmetal's angina)
- Rapid ECG evolution
- Localized ST elevation
- Normal QTc.

Early repolarization
- Variable ECG evolution
- Generalized ST–T changes; widespread ST elevation, most prominent in mid-precordial leads (precordial leads > limb leads)
- J point elevation above the isoelectric line: where QRS complex ends and ST segment begins. The ST segment elevation begins at the J point. The ST segment looks like it has been lifted upwards evenly from the isoelectric baseline at the J point, preserving the normal concavity of the initial, up-sloping portion of the ST segment/T wave complex. The degree of J point elevation is usually <3.5mm
- Upward concavity of initial up-sloping part of ST segment

- Notching or irregular contour of J point (junction of R wave and S wave)
- T waves often tall and concordant with the QRS complex
- QTc normal
- Relatively fixed constant pattern
- J height/T apex in V6 (PR segment as baseline) usually <25%
- Mainly in males under age of 40
- The degree of ST elevation is greatest in the mid to left precordial leads (leads V2–V5), and found less often in the limb leads.[1]

Repolarization effects unrelated to ischaemia:
- Digitalis effect
- Bundle branch blocks
- Left ventricular hypertrophy.

Differential diagnosis of ST depression

- Normal variants or artefacts
- Pseudo-ST depression (wandering baseline due to poor skin–electrode contact)
- Physiological J point depression with sinus tachycardia
- Hyperventilation-induced ST depression
- Sub–endocardial ischaemia
- Sub–epicardial ischaemia from distant zone (reciprocal changes)
- Posterior trans–mural myocardial infarction (right precordial leads)
- Rate-related depression (tachycardia)
- RVH (right precordial leads) or LVH (left precordial leads, I, aVL) repolarization abnormality
- Digoxin effect
- Hypokalaemia
- Mitral valve prolapse
- CNS disease
- Secondary ST segment changes with intra–ventricular conduction abnormalities, e.g. right bundle branch block (RBBB), left bundle branch block (LBBB), WPW.

1 Shipley RA, Hallaran WR. The four-lead electrocardiogram in two hundred normal men and women American Heart Journal, 1936; **11**: 325–345.

Evaluation of cardiac arrhythmia

- Is a pulse palpable?
- Is the patient haemodynamically stable?
- What is the rate?
- Is the rhythm regular or irregular?
- Are the QRS complexes narrow or broad? (see below)
- Are there P waves
- Are the P waves synchronized with the QRS complexes?

Adverse signs associated with an arrhythmia

- Low cardiac output, evidenced by pallor, sweating, poor peripheral perfusion, depressed level of consciousness and hypotension (systolic blood pressure <90mmHg)
- Acute left ventricular failure
- Chest pain
- Excess tachycardia (>150/min) or bradycardia (<40/min; or <60/min if poor cardiac reserve).

Treatment aims for arrhythmia

- Restoration of sinus rhythm
- Control of ventricular rate
- Treatment of complications

ECG analysis of tachycardias

Narrow complex tachycardia

- Regular, P waves present
  - Sinus tachycardia: normal P waves
  - Paroxysmal atrial tachycardia: abnormal P waves
- Regular, no P waves
  - Atrial flutter: saw-tooth baseline
  - AV junctional tachycardia
- Irregular, P waves present
  - Multifocal atrial tachycardia: three or more P wave morphologies
- Irregular, no P waves
  - Atrial fibrillation
  - Atrial flutter with variable AV block.

Broad complex tachycardia

- Regular, no P waves/AV dissociation
  - VT
  - PSVT with aberrant conduction (bundle branch block)
  - Antidromic WPW syndrome (atrial tachycardia with pre-excitation)
- Irregular, no P waves
  - AF with bundle branch block
  - AF with WPW syndrome
  - Torsade de pointes (polymorphic VT)
  - VF.

Narrow complex tachycardia

Diagnostic approach to narrow complex regular tachycardia (see p. 80)

- Identify P wave morphology and timing
  - Sinus tachycardia: normal P wave morphology
  - Atrial tachycardia: abnormal P wave morphology
  - Junctional tachycardia

  AV nodal re-entrant: P wave hidden within QRS complex: occasionally identified as negative deflections within the QRS complex in inferior leads, or as an upright deflection immediately following the RS in V1

  Orthodromic AV re-entrant: retrograde P waves identifiable between each QRS complex, sometimes as notches at the peak or at the end of the preceding T wave
- Determine AV relationship during tachycardia
  - AV block excludes AV re-entrant tachycardia and strongly suggests the presence of atrial tachycardia
- Induction of AV block by vagal manoeuvres or adenosine:
  - Terminates junctional tachycardia
  - Reveals atrial tachycardia and atrial flutter by the transient AV block seen 10–20s after injection of adenosine.

Vagal manoeuvres for SVT

- Valsalva manoeuvre lying supine
- Unilateral carotid sinus massage
- Diving reflex: facial immersion in a basin of water at 5°C or ice pack application to the face for 10–20s.

Patterns of clinical presentation with junctional tachycardia

- WPW syndrome
- Narrow complex regular tachycardia
- Atrial fibrillation in patients with accessory pathways
- Tachycardia–mediated cardiomyopathy: persistent or incessant junctional tachycardia with progressive impairment of ventricular function.

Broad complex tachycardia (see p. 80)

Differential diagnosis of broad QRS complex tachycardia

Features suggesting VT

- Indeterminate QRS axis. Change in axis >40° to the left or right
- Evidence of AV dissociation
- Independent P waves: direct evidence of independent atrial activity. P waves may only be evident in some leads.
- Capture beats: intermittent SA node complexes transmitted to ventricle, with narrow QRS morphology. Occur earlier than expected.
- Fusion beats: combination QRS from SA node and VT focus meeting and fusing. QRS morphology is intermediate between a normal beat and a tachycardia beat
- Beat to beat variability of QRS morphology
  - Very wide QRS complexes (>140ms)
  - Same morphology in tachycardia as in ventricular ectopics
  - History of ischaemic heart disease
  - Absence of any rS, RS or Rs complexes in the chest leads
  - Concordance in chest leads: all QRS vectors either positive or negative.

Features favouring VT

- Known ischaemic heart disease
- AV dissociation: independent atrial (P wave) activity. P waves marching through tachycardia
- Fusion beats: ventricle simultaneously activated from the atria via the bundle of His and from the ventricular premature complex (VPC) (fusion of a normal and a VT beat): early beat with abnormal QRS. Appearance intermediate between a normal beat and a tachycardia beat
- Capture beats (normal independent P captures normal QRS): early beat with normal, i.e. narrow, QRS
- QRS width >140ms (3.5 small squares) with RBBB and >160ms with LBBB
- Concordance of QRS vectors in precordial leads (constant QRS axis) (all predominantly +ve or all predominantly −ve)
- QRS complex similar to VPC during sinus rhythm in the same or previous tracings
- Absence of RS in all chest leads (V1–V6)
- Bizarre frontal plane axis (aVR +ve)
- Left axis variation greater than 30° (superior axis)
- Rate commonly 150–200 beats per min.

The basic principles of treating broad complex tachycardia:
- If in doubt, treat as VT
- If superimposed on ischaemic heart disease, treat as VT until otherwise proven .

Checklist for acute tachyarrhythmia management

- Haemodynamic status: if unstable, synchronized cardioversion is indicated
- Cardiac status: angina; heart failure
- Volume status: volume depletion/overload
- Medications
- Serum electrolytes: K, Mg, Ca; keep serum K at ~4.5mmol/L or higher; keep Mg between 1 and 2mol/L
- Oxygen saturation: correct hypoxia
- Acid–base status: correct hypercarbia and acidosis
- Thyroid function.

Atrial fibrillation

Patterns of clinical presentation
- Single episode: precipitating cause (cardiac surgery, chest infection, pulmonary embolus, electrolyte disturbance)
- Paroxysmal atrial fibrillation: self-terminating and recurrent episodes
- Persistent atrial fibrillation: non-self-terminating episodes
- Permanent atrial fibrillation.

Initial assessment
- History, examination, 12-lead ECG plus CXR.
- Renal function/electrolytes, glucose, thyroid function
- Duration of AF: 0–48h or >48h since onset, but if uncertain assume >48h since onset
- Classification of AF: paroxysmal or persistent?
- Severity of symptoms/haemodynamic disturbance
- Presence of underlying cardiac disease
- Acute precipitants: respiratory tract infection, general anaesthesia, myocardial infarction/ischaemia.

Management
Electrical cardioversion is the treatment of choice in patients with known or suspected structural heart diseases, especially those with haemodynamic disturbance. 200J, followed by 360J, followed by 360J with anteroposterior paddle positions recommended. The shock should be synchronized with the R wave to avoid an R on T phenomenon, with the risk of VF.

Pharmacological cardioversion may be attempted in patients with well-tolerated AF and no evidence of heart failure. It is, however, not 100% effective. It may be negatively inotropic and may precipitate or worsen haemodynamic disturbance.

There is a risk of proarrhythmia (including organizing AF into atrial flutter with paradoxical acceleration of the ventricular rate). Class IC agents (e.g. flecainide and propafenone) are the most effective agents for achieving rapid restoration of sinus rhythm. In AF of <72h duration, IV flecainide 2mg/kg (maximum 150mg) will produce acute conversion rates of 70–80% within 0–3h of administration. IV amiodarone is associated with a lower conversion rate than class IC agents, delayed onset of action (12–24h), and ideally should be administered via central venous access.

Pharmacological cardioversion
Flecainide 2mg/kg IV over 10min(maximum 150mg) or 200–300mg PO stat (good LV function)
Amiodarone 300mg IV over 60min, then 1200mg/24h or 400mg PO tds for 7–10 days
Propafenone 2mg/kg IV over 5–10min or 450–600mg PO stat
Sotalol 20–100mg slow IV injection

DC cardioversion is more likely to be successful in atrial fibrillation if:
- Left atrial size <60mm
- Duration of atrial fibrillation <1yr
- Normal mitral valve
- Absence of major pulmonary dysfunction
- Absence of major left ventricular dysfunction.

Contraindications to cardioversion:
- Digitalis toxicity
- Untreated hyperthyroidism
- Sick sinus syndrome
- Hypokalaemia
- Prior history of recurrent atrial fibrillation after successful cardioversion.
- Presence of intra cardiac mural thrombosis

Rate control

Digoxin 0.5–1mg IV in 50ml saline over 1h
Or 0.5mg PO 12 hourly (2–3 doses)
Then 0.0625–0.25mg daily

Metoprolol 5–15mg slowly IV
Or 25–100mg tds PO

Verapamil 5mg IV over 2min repeated every 5min up to 20mg
Or 40–120mg tds PO.

Factors deciding the choice between rate or rhythm control in fast AF
- Rate control
  - Asymptomatic
  - Age >65yrs
  - Side effects from or contraindications to anti-arrhythmic therapy
  - Contraindications to or predicted failure of cardioversion
  - Duration of AF >1yr
  - Large left atrium >6cm in size
  - Relapse following or failed multiple attemps at cardioversion
- Rhythm control
  - Symptomatic
  - Age <65yrs
  - Lone AF
  - AF secondary to known precipitant: alcohol; chest infection; thyrotoxicosis
  - Presence of heart failure.

Atrial flutter

Management of atrial flutter

Three options are available to restore sinus rhythm:

- Anti-arrhythmic drug therapy: IV ibutilide (1mg, slowly over 5–10min); IV procainamide
- DC cardioversion
- Initiate rapid atrial pacing to interrupt atrial flutter.

Anti-arrhythmic drugs

Classification of anti-arrhythmic drugs

class I: sodium channel blockade

Stabilize cell membranes. Reduce the influx of sodium during depolarization (phase zero of action potential). Decrease the slope of phase zero of the action potential. Reduce conduction velocity and increase QRS duration.

IA: directly prolong repolarization; pronounced prolongation of repolarization (reflected on the ECG as a prolonged QT interval) can result in re-entrant-type ventricular arrhythmias. Linked to the development of VT of the torsade de pointes variety. Variable alpha-adrenergic blocking effects.
- Procainamide
- Quinidine
- Disopyramide
- Cibenzoline
- Pirmenol.

IB: shorten repolarization: shorten refractory period of cardiac muscle.
- Lignocaine
- Mexiletine
- Tocainide
- Phenytoin
- Ethmozine.

IC: little independent effect on repolarization. Effectively suppress VPCs. Very narrow therapeutic windows.
- Encainide
- Flecainide
- Lorcainide
- Propafenone.

Class II: beta-adrenergic blockers

Depress the SA and AV nodes. Negative dromotropic and chronotropic effects.
- Atenolol
- Metoprolol
- Propranolol.

Class III: potassium channel blockade

Reduce the duration of the action potential in all cardiac tissues. Prolong repolarization (i.e. the refractory period) in all cardiac tissue.
- Amiodarone
- Bretylium
- Sotalol.

Class IV: calcium channel blockers

Affect primarily the SA and AV nodes. Dramatically decrease conduction through the AV node. Vasodilatory and negative inotropic effects.
- Diltiazem
- Verapamil.

Specific anti-arrhythmic agents

Adenosine

Endogenous purine nucleoside with a short half-life (<5s). Adenosine receptor agonist, acting on A1 receptors in cardiac myocytes, producing a negative inotropic and chronotropic (slowed SA and AV conduction).

Rapid IV bolus of 3mg or 6mg over 1–3s followed by a 20mL normal saline flush; further doses of 6 and 12mg over 1–2min if no response observed.

Indications

- Haemodynamically stable narrow complex tachycardia
- Haemodynamically stable broad complex tachycardia of supra-ventricular origin
- Paroxysmal SVT involving a re-entry pathway involving the AV node.

Problems

- Transient side effects: flushing, dyspnoea, chest pain, headache, hypotension
- Bronchospasm
- Accelerated conduction in accessory pathways
- Prolonged effect in denervated (transplanted) heart
- Adenosine should be used with caution in asthmatics, and with atrial flutter or fibrillation in the presence of an accessory pathway.

Contraindications

- Second and third degree AV block
- Sick sinus syndrome.

Amiodarone

Broad spectrum anti-arrhythmic with class III, I, II and IV actions 300mg (5mg/kg) IV over 60min, followed by 900mg (15mg/kg) IV over 23h.

Maintenance: 600mg daily for 1 week; then 400mg daily for 1 week; followed by 200mg daily.

Indications

- Haemodynamically stable broad complex tachycardia
- Haemodynamically stable narrow complex tachycardia
- Cardiac arrest with persistent VT or VF
- Ventricular rate control/cardioversion of atrial flutter/fibrillation.

Contraindications

- Sinus bradycardia; SA exit block
- Thyroid dysfunction
- Iodine hypersensitivity
- Pregnancy.

Digoxin

Cardiac glycoside which inhibits Na^+/K^+ ATPase (the sodium pump).

Effects
- Delayed AV conduction
- Positive inotropic effect
- Increased vagal activity.

Indication: rate control of AF/flutter

Digitalization
Rapid digitalization
- 1mg in 100mL 0.9% saline infused IV over 2h
- Maintenance dose by mouth the following day.

Oral digitalization
- 500mcg (250mcg in the elderly) followed by 250mg 8 hourly for three doses
- Then 125–500mcg daily or 62.5–125mcg daily in the elderly or with renal impairment.

Plasma digoxin levels
Therapeutic: 0.8–2.0ng/ml (1.0–2.6nmol/L)
Digibind: >5.5nmol/L.

Flecainide

Class Ic agent which slows conduction in the His–Purkinje system and suppresses accessory conduction pathways. The main indication is for the termination of acute AF in patients without ischaemic or structural heart disease, i.e. with good left ventricular function.
   Dose: 2 mg/kg over 10 min, to a maximum dose of 150mg.
   Flecainide should be avoided in patients with ischaemic heart disease, heart failure or structural cardiac abnormalities.

Lidocaine

Class Ib agent. Sodium channel blocker.
- Bolus: 1.0–1.5mg/kg
- Infusion: 4mg/min for 30min, 2mg/min for 2h, reducing to 1mg/min.

Ibutilide

Class III agent which increases action potential duration and refractory period.

   Dose: weight ≥60kg, 1mg IV over 10min, repeated after 10min if required; weight <60kg, 0.01mg/kg IV.

Atrioventricular block

All P waves are conducted in first degree AV block, some but not all P waves are conducted in second degree AV block, and no P waves are conducted in third degree AV block.

First degree: prolonged conduction

- Sinus rhythm
- PR interval prolonged >0.20s (20ms) and constant
- Normal morphology of P wave, which precedes every QRS complex
- Associated bundle branch block suggests conduction delay below the AV node .

Second degree: intermittent AV conduction

Non-conducted P waves may be regular or irregular, intermittent or frequent, and preceded by either fixed or lengthening PR intervals.

Mobitz type I (Wenckebach)

- Progressive lengthening of PR interval, then dropped or non-conducted beat
- Progressive decrease in the increment of PR interval prolongation with each sinus beat: the PR interval gets longer by shorter increments until a non-conducted P wave occurs
- Progressive shortening of RR interval before AV block
- RR interval of dropped beat is less than twice the shortest cycle
- Grouped beating
- Normal morphology and axis of P waves and QRS complexes
- The AV block usually occurs in the AV node.

The prognosis is good because of the presence of subsidiary pacemakers (in the AV junction below the level of block).

Mobitz type II

- Constant PR interval before and after AV block
- Occasional non-conducted P waves with omission of QRS complex
- The AV block occurs below the AV node (in the bundle of His), and typically is accompanied by other evidence of infra-nodal conduction delay—BBB
- Significant risk for progression to complete heart block with a slow ventricular rate.

Third degree: no conduction

- No meaningful relationship between P waves and QRS complexes
- The PR interval is random
- Atrial pacemaker can be either sinus or ectopic
- Ventricular escape rhythm can have varying pacemaker sites, resulting in different rates
- The ventricular escape rhythm is slower than the atrial rhythm
- A narrow QRS with a junctional escape rhythm of 40–60 beats per min implies a nodal block, that is responsive to autonomic tone
- A wide QRS with a ventricular escape rhythm of <40 beats per min implies an infra-nodal rhythm (with a block in the His-Purkinje system) associated with a ventricular pacemaker. (See p. 79).

Indication for pacing

Indications for temporary cardiac pacing

Conduction disturbances

- Symptomatic persistent complete heart block with inferior myocardial infarction
- Complete heart block, Mobitz type II AV block, new bifascicular block or alternating LBBB and RBBB complicating acute anterior myocardial infarction
- Symptomatic idiopathic complete heart block, or high degree AV block (possible).

Rate disturbances

- Haemodynamically significant or symptomatic sinus bradycardia
- Polymorphic ventricular tachycardia with long QT interval (torsade de pointes)
- Recurrent ventricular tachycardia unresponsive to medical therapy.

External pacing

- Two large-surface low-impedance adhesive electrodes
- Positive electrode below right clavicle
- Negative electrode on left mid-axillary line lateral to the nipple
- Insert pacing lead into defibrillator port and attach electrodes to the lead
- Switch on the unit
- Adjust ECG gain to ensure sensing of any intrinsic QRS complexes
- Select DEMAND MODE, or fixed rate mode if a failing permanent pacemaker is present. In the demand mode, the sensing circuit discharges only if no cardiac depolarization is detected for a pre-set interval. This prevents an R on T phenomenon in the presence of an intrinsic normal cardiac beat. In many machines, demand mode is automatically selected
- Set pacing rate to 60–90/min
- Set pacing current at lowest setting (zero)
- Slowly increase pacing current, until electrical capture is seen on monitor. Capture is indicated by a pacing spike followed by a wide QRS complex.
- Capture typically occurs in the range of 50–100mA; the minimum current to achieve capture is the pacing threshold
- Analgesia with incremental doses of morphine or sedation with a benzodiazepine makes discomfort due to muscle contraction bearable.

Temporary transvenous pacing

In the resuscitation room, this procedure can be done by intracardiac ECG monitoring or with the aid of a portable image intensifier. The aim is to advance the electrode tip into the trabeculae carneae at the apex of the right ventricle

- Advance guidewire through needle into superior vena cava
- Remove needle
- Advance dilator with peel-away sheath
- Remove guidewire and dilator, leaving outer peel-away sheath in place
- Advance balloon-tipped pacing lead through sheath to 20cm mark
- Remove peel-away sheath
- Inflate balloon
- Attach pacemaker lead to generator
- Use DEMAND MODE
- Measure pacing threshold (minimum voltage that will capture the ventricle). This should be <1v
- Set at pacing voltage of 3v at a rate of 70/min or 10–20/min greater than the intrinsic ventricular rate
- Slowly advance watching ECG trace
- Contact with right atrium causes pacing spikes with atrial capture
- Contact with right ventricle produces broad QRS complexes preceded by a pacing spike
- When this happens, deflate the balloon and insert a further 5cm of catheter
- Placement in the trabeculae carneae of the right ventricular tip is a requisite for endocardial stimulation
- Optimal catheter tip position should allow capture at <2V. The tip should be repositioned until this electrical threshold is achieved.
- Obtain a CXR to confirm catheter position and to exclude pneumothorax.

Pacemaker impulse

- Sharp, narrow, vertically oriented spike <2ms in duration
- If it appears before a P wave, it is pacing the atrium
- If it appears before the QRS complex, it is pacing the ventricle
- The QRS complex that follows a pacing spike resembles an LBBB pattern, due to right ventricular stimulation
- There may also be changes in T wave morphology, e.g. T wave inversion and QT prolongation.

All patients with a permanent implanted pacemaker are given a **European Pacemaker Identification Card** which contains information about:

- Make of pacemaker
- Pacemaker leads: unipolar or bipolar
- Date and place of implant
- Implanting cardiologist
- Pacing mode
- Pacing rate
- Reason for pacemaker implant and symptomatology
- Follow-up data.

Permanent pacemaker nomenclature
- Position 1: chamber paced
- Position 2: chamber sensed
- Position 3: response to sensing: triggered, inhibited or dual
- Position 4: programmability or rate modulation
- Position 5: anti-tachycardia pacing.

Permanent pacemaker problems

Failure to pace

No pacing spikes, when there should be.

Causes: lead fracture or disconnection
Battery depletion; component failure: generator malfunction; oversensing; external interference (electromagnetic interference).

Failure to sense

Spikes without sensing. Constant pacemaker spikes despite ongoing intrinsic cardiac electrical activity (native P wave or QRS).

Pacemaker spikes at inappropriate times, e.g. shortly after a normal QRS complex.
* Causes: lead fracture or dislodgement
* Fibrosis around lead tip
* Battery depletion
* Pacer in asynchronous mode
* External interference
* Low amplitude intracardiac signal: low intrinsic QRS current

Failure to capture

Spikes without capture:
Pacemaker spikes but no subsequent cardiac activity (no P wave or QRS complex following it).
* Causes: lead or insulation fracture, dislodgement or disconnection
* Fibrosis around lead tip
* Myocardial perforation
* Pulse generator battery depletion
* Metabolic abnormalities, e.g. hyperkalaemia
* Medications.

Inappropriate pacemaker rate (runaway pacemaker)

Causes: pacemaker re-entrant tachycardia (acute termination with a magnet over the generator)
* Retrograde transmission of a ventricular impulse that is rapidly transmitted to the atrium.
* This is sensed by the pacemaker as a P wave. The ventricular pacemaker awaits the programmed AV interval and then fires, causing ventricular depolarization. Fast retrograde conduction again occurs, creating a self-sustaining circus movement
* Resetting from external interference
* Battery depletion.

Troubleshooting steps for pacemaker problems

Clinical assessment
* Indication for pacing
* Focused history and physical examination.

12-lead ECG
- Rate
- Pacing and sensing
- QRS axis
- Magnet response.

CXR
- Device type and location
- Proper contact between lead pins and setscrews
- Lead integrity
- Lead position.

Pacemaker interrogation
- Sensing threshold(s)
- Pacing threshold(s)
- Lead impedance
- Battery status
- Programming
- Contact the manufacturer for assistance.

Initial ECG interpretation in the presence of implanted pacemaker
- Find any portion of the ECG during which the heart is not paced, i.e. identify the intrinsic cardiac rhythm
- That portion of the ECG should be interpreted as any ECG would be: PR, QRS and QT intervals; rate; axis; voltage
- If no intrinsic rhythm is apparent, the patient may be pacemaker-dependent or the pacemaker may be programmed to stimulate faster (i.e. at a shorter cycle length) than the intrinsic rhythm
- Determine the spontaneous atrial and ventricular rhythms and look for a relationship between the two
- Assess pacemaker activity: is there one stimulus or two stimuli? If only one stimulus is present, does it result in atrial or ventricular depolarization? Is there an apparent relationship between pacemaker activity and atrial activity or ventricular activity, or both?

Knowing the patient and the pacing system

Know the patient
- Cardiac diagnosis
- Non-cardiac diagnosis
- Exposure to electromagnetic interference, e.g. workplace, hobbies, medical procedures
- Any physical trauma since prior evaluation
- Any reprogramming at other institutions since prior evaluation.

Know the pacemaker
- Manufacturer
- Model number
- Serial number
- Previously programmed values
- Previous battery status
- Device idiosyncrasies.

Know the lead or leads
- Manufacturer
- Model number
- Serial number
- Connector type
- Polarity
- Insulation material
- Fixation mechanism
- Normal radiographic appearance.

Acute coronary syndromes

Classification

- Acute myocardial infarction
- Trans-mural myocardial infarction
  - Q wave infarction
  - ST elevation myocardial infarction (STEMI)
- Non-Q wave myocardial infarction
  - Subendocardial infarction
  - Non-ST elevation myocardial infarction (NON-STEMI)
- Unstable angina.

Risk stratification

Three groups can be recognized

1 Persistent ST elevation
2 No persistent ST elevation, usually ST depression and T wave inversion
3 No acute or atypical ECG changes: in this group, a baseline and 12h negative troponin would suggest that the presenting condition is probably not an acute coronary syndrome.

Secondary clinical risk stratification of groups 2 and 3

Low risk

- New onset angina within 2 weeks to 2 months
- Deteriorating exercise tolerance in stable angina; increasing angina frequency, severity or duration; angina provoked at a lower threshold.

Intermediate risk

Angina at rest.

High risk

- Prolonged angina at rest (>20min) with ECG changes

The risk is increased further by:

- Increasing severity of ST depression and the presence of fluctuating ST changes (dynamic ST segment changes)
- An ECG pattern which precludes assessment of ECG changes
- Evidence of infarction (enzyme rise of troponin T >0.06µg/L): elevated markers of myocardial damage
- Recent infarction (early post-infarction unstable angina)
- Recurrence of angina at rest after initially settling
- Clinical evidence of left ventricular dysfunction: S3; heart failure
- Haemodynamic instability: hypotension (systolic BP <105mmHg)
- Diabetes mellitus
- Additional co-morbidity, especially renal disease.

Management of unstable acute coronary syndrome (ACS)[1]

- The initial ECG has a low sensitivity for ACS; a normal ECG does not rule out ACS
- Oxygen 2–4L/min by nasal cannula, even with normal oxygen saturation on pulse oximetry
- Opiate analgesia: diamorphine/morphine 2.5mg IV (at 1mg/min); repeated every 5min till adequate analgesia is achieved; antiemetic as required (metoclopramide 10mg)
- Continuous ECG monitoring, with serial 12-lead ECGs every 15min during ongoing symptoms
- Sublingual glyceryl trinitrate (GTN) 500mcg in pill or spray form repeated every 5min; not more than 1.5mg in 15min. Avoid nitrates if systolic BP <90mmHg or heart rate <50bpm
- Aspirin 300mg loading dose—preferably chewable aspirin; withhold if true aspirin allergy or active peptic ulcer disease
- Add clopidogrel 300mg loading dose, followed by 75mg once daily in the presence of existing aspirin therapy
- Metoclopramide 10mg IV over 2min; avoid cyclizine
- Enoxaparin 1mg/kg (100U/kg) bd SC 12 hourly
- Naloxone may be used for opiate-induced respiratory depression
- A rapid clinical assessment should be made for signs of left and/or right heart failure, and for any cardiac murmurs.

Nitrate infusion
Glyceryl trinitrate infusion
- 50mg GTN in 50mL normal saline (1mg/mL)—supplied by the manufacturer
- Start at 0.6mL/h (10mcg/min), using an infusion pump or micro-drip set
- Increase by 10mcg/min every 15min until a therapeutic effect is obtained
- The maximum dose is 200mcg/min (12mL/h)
- Titrate to 10% reduction in mean arterial pressure (MAP) if normotensive, 30% reduction in MAP if hypertensive.

Isosorbide dinitrate infusion
- Set up a concentration of 0.5mg/mL
- Start with 4mL/h, increasing up to 40mL/h, titrated against arterial blood pressure
- *Anti-ischaemic drugs*: nitrates; beta blockers; calcium antagonists
- *Anti-thrombotic drugs*: aspirin; clopidogrel; low molecular weight heparin; platelet glycoprotein IIb/IIIa inhibitors.

Relative contraindications to beta-blockers
- Heart rate <60bpm
- Systolic blood pressure <100mmHg
- Moderate to severe left ventricular failure
- Peripheral hypoperfusion

---

1 Task force on management of acute myocardial infarction of the European Society of Cardiology. Management of acute myocardial infarction in patients presenting with ST segment elevation. *European Heart Journal*, 2003; **24**: 28–66.

PR interval prolonged >0.24s
- second and third degree AV block
- Severe COPD
- Asthma
- Severe peripheral vascular disease.

Cardiac markers

Early:
- Myoglobin
  - High negative predictive value
  - Not cardiac specific
  - Universally acceptable reference standard lacking
  - Standardization between different assays is problematic
- Creatine kinase (CK) isoenzyme MB mass assays.

Later or definitive:
- CK-MB
- Cardiac troponins I and T (cTnI and cTnT)
  - Highly sensitive and moderately specific markers for myocardial cell damage
  - Similar kinetics to CK-MB
  - Increased sensitivity for minor myocardial damage
  - Have prognostic value in patients with unstable angina and non-STEMI.

Conditions associated with raised cardiac troponins

Cardiac disease and interventions
- Cardiac contusion
- Cardiac surgery
- Cardioversion and ICD (implantable cardioverter defibrillator) shocks
- Coronary vasospasm
- Dilated cardiomyopathy
- Heart failure
- Hypertrophic cardiomyopathy
- Myocarditis
- Percutaneous coronary intervention
- Post-cardiac transplantation

Table 6.7 Plasma markers of myocardial necrosis

Marker	Rise time	Peak	Return to baseline
Myoglobin	1–4h	6–7h	24h
Troponin I	3–12h	24h	5–10 days
Troponin T	3–12h	12–48h	3–4 days
CK	4–8h	12–24h	3–4 days
CK-MB	4–8h	18–36h	2–3 days
AST	8–12h	18–36h	3–4 days
LDH	8–12h	3–6 days	8–14 days

- Radio-frequency ablation
- Supraventricular tachycardia.

Non-cardiac diseases
- Critically ill patients
- High dose chemotherapy
- Primary pulmonary hypertension
- Pulmonary embolism
- Rhabdomyolysis
- Renal failure
- Subarachnoid haemorrhage
- Scorpion envenomation
- Sepsis and septic shock
- Stroke
- Ultra-endurance exercise (triathlon).

ST elevation myocardial infarction

- In the first 3h from symptom onset, primary angioplasty and thrombolysis are of similar effectiveness
- Percutaneous coronary intervention (PCI; angioplasty) is superior to thrombolysis within 3–12h of symptom onset. Primary angioplasty restores normal coronary flow in >90% of cases. All PCI facilities should be able to perform angioplasty within 90min of patient arrival
- Where thrombolysis fails, coronary angiography and PCI (rescue angioplasty) is indicated. Even after successful thrombolysis, there is still a place for angiography and PCI, if applicable owing to recurrent ischaemia.

TIMI (thrombolysis in myocardial infarction) risk score for unstable angina/non-STEMI

	Points
Age ≥65yrs	1
Documented prior coronary artery stenosis >50%	1
≥3 conventional cardiac risk factors (age, sex, family history, hyperlipidaemia, diabetes mellitus, smoking, hypertension, obesity)	1
Use of aspirin in preceding 24h	1
≥2 anginal events in preceding 24h	1
ST segment deviation (transient elevation or persistent depression)	1
Raised cardiac biomarkers	1
Range of risk score	0–7

Ammann P, Pfisterer M, Fehr T, Rickli H. Editorial. *British Medical Journal*, 2004; **328**: 1028–1029. (after cardiac troponins).

- Door to balloon time should be <90 to 120min ideally. Many centres in the UK are now providing primary PCI—be aware of local protocols and transfer policies. The benefits from primary PCI include reduced mortality, reduced recurrent ischaemia and re-infarction, reduced stroke rate, and reduced length of hospital stay.

> Myocardial infarction in the presence of LBBB ECG criteria (sensitivity 30%; specificity 90%)
> - Concordant ST deviation (in the same direction as the major QRS vector) of 1mm in any lead
> - ST depression at least 1mm in V1, V2, V3 or in II, III or aVF
> - ST elevation at least 1mm in V5
> - Very discordant ST deviation (>5mm): ST elevation >5mm in leads with negative R wave.

Detection of right ventricular and posterior wall infarction
- 15 or 18-lead ECG
- Non-standard leads: right precordial leads: V4R, V5R, V6R; posterior leads: V7, V8, V9.

Right ventricular infarction

Complicates 1/3 of inferior myocardial infarcts. Triad of:
- Hypotension, which may progress to cardiogenic shock
- Raised jugular venous pressure
- Clear lung fields.

Special features of management:
- Reperfusion with early thrombolysis or PCI
- Volume infusion to optimize right ventricular preload
- Inotropic support of the dysfunctional right ventricle
- Avoidance of preload-reducing medication such as nitrates and ACE inhibitors
- Haemodynamic monitoring.

Indications for thrombolysis

- <12h of chest pain
- ST segment elevation 0.2mV (2mm) or greater in two or more contiguous chest leads
- ST segment elevation 0.1mV (1mm) or greater in two or more contiguous limb leads
- New onset left bundle branch block—if in doubt treat as new onset and thrombolyse on clinical grounds
- Dominant R waves and 2mm ST depression in V1–V3 (posterior infarction)—posterior or right ventricular leads are helpful to clarify the diagnosis; inspecting the abnormal ECG leads in the inverted position is often helpful in addition.

Thrombolytic agents

First generation
- Streptokinase
- Urokinase.

Second generation
- Anistreplase (APSAC)
- Alteplase (tissue-type plasminogen activator; rt-PA)
- Prourokinase (Suraplase; scu-PA).

Third generation
- Reteplase (r-PA): deletion mutant of wild-type human t-PA
- Lanoteplase (n-PA): deletion mutant of t-PA
- Staphylokinase: 136 amino acid recombinant protein
- TNK-t-PA (tenecteplase): triple-site-specific mutant of t-PA.

In the UK, most centres currently use fibrin-selective third-generation agents, such as reteplase and tenecteplase[1].

Adjuncts to thrombolytic therapy
Platelet glycoprotein IIb/IIIa receptor antagonists
- Abciximab
- Tirofiban
- Lamifiban.

Characteristics of ideal thrombolytic agents
- Rapid, complete coronary flow and microcirculatory reperfusion in 100% patients: high and maintained rates of coronary artery perfusion
- Effective in dissolving older thrombi
- Long half-life to allow single IV bolus administration
- Fibrin selective
- Low incidence of intracranial and systemic bleeding
- Resistance to plasminogen activator inhibitor
- No procoagulant effect
- Low re-occlusion rate
- No effect on blood pressure
- No antigenicity
- Safe and well tolerated
- Reasonable cost.

Contraindications to thrombolysis
Absolute
- Prior haemorrhagic stroke
- Ischaemic (thromboembolic) stroke within 6 months
- Known intracranial neoplasm
- Known cerebral aneurysm or arterio-venous malformation
- Active internal bleeding, excluding menstruation
- Known bleeding disorder
- Aortic dissection.

Relative
- Warfarin with INR >2.3
- Pregnancy
- Traumatic resuscitation
- Systolic BP >180mmHg despite treatment

1 Verstraete M. Third-generation thrombolytic drugs. *American Medical Journal*, 2000; **109**: 52–58.

- Active peptic ulcer disease
- Recent (within 3wks) major surgery, organ biopsy or puncture of a non-compressible vessel
- Recent (within 2–4wks) trauma including head injury or traumatic or prolonged (>10min) CPR
- Recent (within past 6 months) gastrointestinal or genitourinary, or other internal bleeding

Do not withhold thrombolysis if unsure, but discuss the pros and cons with coronary care unit staff.

Thrombolysis regimens

Tenecteplase

Single bolus injection (500mcg/kg) over 5s
- <60kg: 30mg
- 60–69kg: 35mg
- 70–79kg: 40mg
- 80–89kg: 45mg
- >90kg: 50mg
- Total dose not to exceed 50mg.

Accompanied by low molecular weight heparin (enoxaparin 1mg/kg IV) or standard heparin (5000U IV bolus followed by an infusion of 1000 U/h) via a separate IV cannula.

Reteplase

A double IV bolus of 10U, 30min apart.

Streptokinase

1.5 million units by IV infusion in 100mL normal saline over 1h.

Alteplase

15mg IV bolus, followed by 0.75mg/kg (maximum 50mg) infusion over 30min, and then 0.5mg/kg (maximum 35mg) over 60 min.

Accompanied by unfractionated heparin IV bolus 60U/kg followed by a maintenance dose of 12U/kg.

Failure to reperfuse after thrombolysis as measured by non-resolution of ST elevation warrants consideration of percutaneous coronary intervention (rescue angioplasty).

Abciximab

- Fab fragment of chimeric human-murine monoclonal antibody 7E3
- Binds to platelet glycoprotein IIa/IIIb receptor
- Used as a bridge in the presence of delay between admission and performance of PCI in patients with acute myocardial infarction
- 250mcg/kg over 1min; followed by infusion of 125ng/kg/min (maximum 10mcg/min).

Cardiogenic shock

Cardiogenic shock can be defined as tissue hypoxia due to reduced systemic cardiac output in the presence of adequate intravascular volume. This is usually the result of severe primary cardiac pump failure.

The essential features leading to the diagnosis are:

- Persistent hypotension: systolic BP <90mmHg
- Clinical signs of a low cardiac output: impaired peripheral perfusion; reduced level of consciousness; hourly urine output <0.5mL/kg
- Raised cardiac filling pressure: clinical or radiological evidence of pulmonary oedema.

Causes of cardiogenic shock

Myocardial

- Left ventricular systolic dysfunction: acute myocardial infarction; acute myocarditis; cardiomyopathy
- Left ventricular diastolic dysfunction: hypertrophic obstructive cardiomyopathy
- Right ventricular dysfunction: acute right ventricular infarction.

Arrhythmias

- Bradyarrhythmias
- Tachyarrhythmias.

Mechanical causes

- Acute valvular dysfunction: aortic dissection with aortic regurgitation; infective endocarditis with acute mitral/aortic regurgitation; papillary muscle dysfunction or rupture with acute mitral regurgitation
- Ventricular septal rupture.

Management

- Adequate ventilation and oxygenation
- Correction of electrolyte (hyperkalaemia; hypomagnesaemia) and acid–base disorder
- Volume infusion to optimize preload (LV filling pressure)
- Hourly urine output monitoring
- Haemodynamic monitoring: arterial pressure; pulmonary artery and pulmonary capillary wedge pressures
- Control cardiac rhythm: treatment of dysrhythmias with pacing/cardioversion
- Inotropic support: dopamine; dobutamine; norepinephrine
- Vasodilators: GTN; nitroprusside
- Echocardiography.

Special measures in specialist units

- Intra-aortic balloon pump
- PCI
- Left ventricular assist devices, as a bridge to cardiac transplantation.

Myocarditis

Presentations
- Asymptomatic
- Unexplained congestive heart failure
- Rapidly progressive myocardial dysfunction and death
- Malignant cardiac arrhythmias in setting of acute febrile illness.

Features
- Fever, fatigue, malaise, chest pain, dyspnoea, palpitations
- Inappropriate sinus tachycardia out of proportion to fever
- Hypotension
- Faint heart sounds
- S3
- Transient murmurs
- Features of pericarditis.

Causes
Infection
- Virus: Coxsackie, influenza, adenovirus, echovirus, rubella
- Bacterial: *Corynebacterium diphtheriae*, *Chlamydia*, *Rickettsia*, *Coxiella burneti*
- Protozoa: *Trypanosoma cruzi*, *Toxoplasma gondii*.

Physical
Radiotherapy: breast/lung cancer; thymoma; lymphoma.

Chemical
- Lead
- Alcohol.

Drugs
- Emetine
- Chloroquine.

Investigations
- Venous blood: FBC; ESR; CK-MB; troponin I or T
- 12-lead ECG: sinus tachycardia, non-specific ST–T changes, arrhythmia, conduction block, ST elevation (mimicking myocardial infarction)
- CXR
- Echocardiography

Management
- Admission for monitoring
- Treat cardiac arrhythmias and heart failure
- Mechanical circulatory support, and even heart transplantation, may be needed in fulminant cases.

Heart failure

Classification of heart failure

Systolic dysfunction: abnormal emptying
- Loss of contractile function
  - Reduced global myocardial function: dilated cardiomyopathy
  - Reduced myocardial units: ischaemic heart disease
- Increased afterload: aortic stenosis; systemic hypertension
- Structural abnormalities: mitral regurgitation; aortic regurgitation; ventricular septal defect.

Diastolic dysfunction: increased filling pressure (impaired filling).
Primary disorder:
- Obstruction to filling: mitral stenosis; left atrial myxoma
- Reduced distensibility: hypertrophic obstructive cardiomyopathy (HOCM); amyloid and other restrictive cardiomyopathies
- Impaired relaxation: familial HOCM; ischaemia
- External compression: constrictive pericarditis; cardiac tamponade; cor pulmonale.

Secondary disorder:
- Systolic dysfunction.

Summary of symptoms in congestive heart failure

Left heart failure
- Dyspnoea on exertion
- Orthopnoea
- Paroxysmal nocturnal dyspnoea
- Nocturnal cough
- Pulmonary oedema.

Right heart failure
- Lower limb swelling
- Abdominal fullness
- Increasing girth
- Right upper quadrant discomfort
- Weight gain.

Table 6.8 Differentiation of systolic from isolated diastolic heart failure

	Systolic	Diastolic
History	Coronary disease	Hypertension
Examination	S3; cardiomegaly	S4; raised BP
CXR		
ECG	Q waves	
	Low R wave voltages	
	ST elevation	

Summary of clinical signs of congestive heart failure

Left heart failure
- Crepitations; rhonchi
- S3 gallop
- S4 gallop
- Mitral insufficiency
- Displaced, diffuse point of maximal impulse
- Pulsus alternans.

Right heart failure
- Jugular venous distension
- Tricuspid regurgitation
- Right sided S3 gallop
- Hepatomegaly
- Ascites
- Oedema of ankle, pretibial, sacral regions.

Acute left ventricular failure

Management of acute pulmonary oedema

Initial measures
- Prop up in bed—the patient in any case will usually refuse to lie flat!
- High concentration of inspired oxygen by face mask to maintain SpO$_2$ at 98% or higher
- Rapid acting loop diuretic: frusemide 40–80mg by slow IV injection (peak diuresis occurs within 30min)
- Two puffs of sublingual GTN (800mcg)
- IV GTN infusion: venodilatation and vasodilatation; GTN 1–10mg/h titrated to achieve a drop in systolic BP of >30mmHg, or a 30% fall, whichever is the least; buccal GTN 3–5mg is an alternative. Nitrate infusion should be avoided if the systolic BP is <90mmHg

- Opioids: IV morphine, which produces arteriolar and venous dilatation (reducing preload) and reduces the work of breathing; best avoided in the presence of drowsiness and exhaustion; an anti-emetic may also need to be given
- Short-acting beta-2 adrenoceptor agonist for bronchospasm: nebulized salbutamol 5mg in oxygen.

Second-line measures
- Repeated dose of diuretics—beware of inducing hypovolaemia and consequent deleterious organ hypoperfusion and sympatho-adrenal stimulation
- Urethral catheterization and hourly urine output monitoring
- Inotropic support: dobutamine 5–10mcg/kg/min
- Consider CPAP or BiPAP, which improves oxygenation, reduces the work of breathing, and reduces left ventricular preload and end-diastolic volume. Early CPAP or BiPAP may reduce the need for tracheal intubation and assisted ventilation. (See p. 188).

Third-line measures
- Invasive monitoring: arterial line; central venous line
- Venesection; rotating tourniquets
- Tracheal intubation and intermittent positive pressure ventilation
- Mechanical circulatory assist device, e.g. intra-aortic balloon pump.

Investigations in acute pulmonary oedema
- Venous blood: FBC; U&E; glucose; lipid profile; liver function tests (LTFs)
- 12-lead ECG
- CXR
- Echocardiography: for valvular pathology.

Checklist for causes of pulmonary oedema

Pulmonary oedema alone (without hypotension) in acutely ill patients:

Non-cardiac
- Volume overload
- ARDS
- Reduced tissue oncotic pressure
- Flash pulmonary oedema in renovascular disease.

Physiological considerations in management of acute pulmonary oedema

Reduce left ventricular preload
- Loop diuretics
- Vasodilators

Reduce left ventricular afterload
- Vasodilators: nitrate; nitroprusside

Inotropic support: Caution regarding provoking tachyorrhythmias

Cardiac
- Left ventricular systolic failure.
- Left ventricular diastolic dysfunction in absence of systolic dysfunction.

Pulmonary oedema and hypotension in acutely ill patients:

Non-cardiac
Septic or neurogenic shock with ARDS.

Cardiac
- Left ventricular systolic failure
- Ventricular septal defect
- Acute mitral regurgitation
- Acute aortic regurgitation.

CXR appearances in acute pulmonary oedema
- Cardiomegaly
- Pulmonary venous hypertension (pulmonary capillary wedge pressure (PCWP) 11–19mmHg): vascular redistribution
- Engorged central veins: azygos vein; superior vena cava
  - Increased flow to upper lobes (cephalization of blood flow): increased diameter in upper lobe arteries and veins (>3mm in first intercostal space)
  - Lower lobe vessels reduced in size
- Interstitial oedema (PCWP >19mmHg)
  - Peri-hilar haziness
  - Peri-bronchial cuffing: increased thickness of bronchial walls seen end-on, usually near hilum
  - Short, thin, 1–2cm. parallel lines at right angles to pleura, laterally at lung bases (Kerley B lines)
  - Pleural effusions; fluid in the major fissures
- Alveolar oedema (PCWP >25mmHg)
  - Alveolar infiltrates: bilateral, peri-hilar, symmetrical, patchy or dense (bat wing distribution)
  - With or without honeycombing, with Swiss cheese effect
  - Rapid clearing with diuretics.

Radiological clues to non-cardiogenic pulmonary oedema
- No upper lobe blood diversion or peribronchial cuffing
- Alveolar shadowing tends to be more peripheral (often with basal sparing)
- Septal lines absent.
- Heart size normal.

Aortic dissection

Dissection is the result of an intimal tear in the aorta leading to dissection of blood in a false lumen along the media, leading to distortion and reduction of the true lumen and compromise of aortic branches.

Possible clinical features

- Severe pain: sudden onset; maximal severity at onset; ripping or tearing
- Loss of pulses
- Stroke
- Acute limb ischaemia
- End-organ ischaemia
  - Myocardial infarction
  - Renal failure
  - Celiac axis or mesenteric artery occlusion
  - Paraplegia
- Aortic insufficiency
- Left haemothorax.

Classsification

- Stanford A: involves ascending aorta
- Stanford B: does not involve ascending aorta.

Management subsets

- Hypotension (rupture): Emergency surgery
- Severe co-morbid disease: Antihypertensive therapy
- Ascending aorta involvement: Urgent surgery
- Descending aorta only
  - Uncomplicated: Antihypertensive therapy
  - Complicated: Urgent surgery

Goals of medical management for distal dissection

- Peak systolic BP <100mmHg
- Pain free: titrated opioid analgesics
- Adequate renal perfusion (urine output >30mL/h)
- No evidence of cerebral hypoperfusion
- Minimized shear stress (beta blocked to <55/min).

Antihypertensive therapy

- IV beta blockade, aiming for heart rate <60/min
- If BP remains high, add a vasodilator, e.g. sodium nitroprusside.

Indications for operation in distal dissection

- Ongoing pain/progression of dissection
- Retrograde extension into the ascending aorta
- Rupture or impending rupture
- Ischaemia due to occlusion of a major branch artery.

Surgical therapy

- Treatment of choice for acute proximal dissection
- Treatment of choice for acute distal dissection complicated by the following:
  - Progression with vital organ compromise

- Rupture or impending rupture (e.g. saccular aneurysm formation)
- Aortic regurgitation
- Retrograde extension into the ascending aorta
- Dissection in Marfan's syndrome.

Medical therapy
- Treatment of choice for uncomplicated distal dissection
- Treatment for stable, isolated arch dissection
- Treatment of choice for stable chronic dissection (uncomplicated dissection presenting 2wks or later after onset).

Imaging

Trans-oesophageal echocardiography
MRI
- Excellent contrast between flowing blood and soft tissue
- Ability to image in sagittal as well as transverse planes.

Spiral CT with IV contrast enhancement
- Visualization of intimal flap
- Differentiation of true and false lumen
- Extent of dissection
- Rupture
- Involvement of branch vessels and infarction of organs.

Angiography
- Intimal flap detected in 85–90%
- Delayed filling of false lumen
- Displacement of catheter from apparent aortic wall by false lumen
- Highly accurate for entry and exit sites.

CXR
- Superior mediastinal widening
- Pleural fluid
- Separation of intimal calcification from the margin of the aortic outline
- Widening of the paravertebral stripe
- Depression of the left main bronchus.

Role of imaging
Confirmation
- Diagnosis: dissection, intra-mural haematoma, penetrating ulcer
- Location

Extent
- Intimal tear/communication.

Identification
- True lumen
- False lumen thrombosis
- Branch vessel involvement
- Extra-aortic extension.
- Pericardial effusion

Assessment
- Aortic valve
- Left ventricular function.

Abdominal aortic aneurysm

Definition of aneurysm of the abdominal aorta
- >50% of normal size (>1.5 times the normal diameter for that person)
- >3cm in diameter.

> Wall tension is proportional to vessel diameter. The incidence of rupture increases significantly when size doubles (>5cm) or when the annual increase in size >0.5cm per year.
>
> | | |
> |---|---|
> | <5cm | 4% incidence of rupture |
> | 5–7cm | 6.5% |
> | >7cm | 20% |

Presentation of leaking aneurysm
- Triad of abdominal and/or back pain, cardiovascular collapse/shock and pulsatile abdominal mass
- Severe back pain
- Ureteric colic-like pain
- Massive gastrointestinal bleeding (aorto-enteric fistula).

Causes of pain
- Acute expansion
- Sac necrosis
- Dissection
- Rupture
- Vertebral erosion.

Imaging for aneurysm
Ultrasound
Bedside ultrasound can be performed rapidly, with imaging of the abdominal aorta in the transverse and sagittal planes from the diaphragm to the bifurcation at the level of the umbilicus.

Measure transverse diameter from outer wall to outer wall, at a level just inferior to the renal arteries

Maximum aortic diameter
- Level of diaphragm 2.5cm
- Level of renal arteries 2cm
- Bifurcation 1.5–2cm
- Iliac arteries just distal to the bifurcation 1cm.

CT scan if haemodynamically stable
Definition of anatomy
- Shape
- Size
- Relationship to renal arteries and aortic bifurcation
- Thrombus
- Anatomical variants, e.g. horseshoe kidney, post-aortic left renal vein
- Leakage.

Complicated cases
- Inflammatory aneurysm
- Retroperitoneal fibrosis.

Plain abdominal X-ray—an accidental finding
- Soft tissue mass
- Curvilinear calcification especially on the lateral view (70–80% calcified)
- Loss of retroperitoneal planes (i.e. psoas margins and renal outlines) with leakage.

Management of leaking abdominal aortic aneurysm

Rapid referral to a vascular surgeon is needed as soon as the diagnosis is confirmed and surgery deemed appropriate.

As surgery may entail transfer to a vascular centre, preparations for moving the patient must be implemented quickly. In some areas, one vascular surgeon covers several hospitals and travels to the patient.

Although it is not always feasible to move a patient with a leaking aneurysm safely, transfers do take place without detriment. The balance of risks and benefits needs to be assessed on a case by case basis as described in the recent NCEPOD report.[1]

'Encouragingly, the patients in this study who were transferred did not do worse than patients directly admitted to the operating hospital. However, they are a selected group considered fit for transfer and who survived that transfer. It is difficult to be sure for an individual patient that transfer produces better results than staying put, since considerable additional risk and morbidity can result from delay and transfer, before the benefits of treatment in a specialized unit are realized. Every case is different and factors to be considered include comorbidity, the transfer distance and time and the mode of transport'

NCEPOD (2005).

Immediate priorities
- High concentration oxygen by face mask
- Two large bore (14G) IV lines in the upper extremities
- Titrated IV opioid analgesia
- Maintain systolic BP at 90mmHg; raising the BP further can convert a confined retroperitoneal leak into free intraperitoneal haemorrhage
- Venous blood for FBC, U&E, group and cross-match of 6–10 units (ensure availability of fresh frozen plasma and platelet concentrates)
- 12-lead ECG
- Check peripheral pulses
- Bedside ultrasound where available
- Rapid transfer to operating room, where arterial and CVP lines, a urethral catheter and a nasogastric tube are inserted.

Avoid vigorous fluid resuscitation, which leads to further bleeding, dislodging of haematoma, and to a dilutional coagulopathy.

---

1 NCEPOD. Abdominal arotic Aneurysm: a service in need of surgery? 2005; www.ncepod.org.uk

Poor prognostic signs
- Female sex
- Age >75yrs
- Actual aortic rupture
- CPR, especially before surgery
- Hypotension (<90mmHg) pre- and post-operatively
- Transfusion requirements in excess of 3L
- Raised serum creatinine
- Obtunded consciousness.

Withhold surgery (a surgical decision)
- Unconscious with fixed dilated pupils
- Refused elective surgery
- Widespread malignancy
- Severe degenerative neurological disorder
- Prolonged hypotension and anuria
- Severe cardiorespiratory disorder.

Treatment options for aortic aneurysm emergencies
Over one-third of emergency aortic aneurysm patients die. For patients with extensive co-morbidities and poor functional reserve, emergency aortic surgery is usually non-survivable and the best option will be to keep the patient comfortable. Leaking aneurysms in the emergency situation are currently dealt with by open surgery. Recently EVAR (endovascular aortic repair) has been used in the elective setting in patients deemed unfit for open surgery. Although at present outcomes are no better with this technique even in the elective setting, it is possible that in the future, EVAR may offer an alternative to open aortic grafting in the emergency situation.[2] In aortic aneurysm surgery overall, emergency operative mortality was 36% versus 6.2% for elective repair (NCEPOD, 2005).

2 Endovascular aneurysm repair and outcome in patients unfit for open repair of abdominal aortic aneurysm (EVAR2) randomized controlled trial. *Lancet.* 2005; **365**: 2187–92

Pulmonary embolism

Clinical syndromes

- Pleuritic chest pain ± haemoptysis: peripheral pulmonary artery occlusion with segmental **pulmonary infarction**
- Dyspnoea and hypoxia in the absence of other causes
- Circulatory collapse: large or **massive pulmonary embolism** with acute right ventricular failure—acute dyspnoea; hypotension; hypoxaemia; raised jugular venous pressure; right ventricular diastolic gallop rhythm; loud pulmonary valve closure sound
- Chronic pulmonary hypertension: progressive right ventricular failure and pulmonary hypertension.

Suspect PE in hypotensive patients in the presence of:
- Evidence of or predisposing factors for venous thrombosis
- Clinical evidence of acute cor pulmonale (acute right ventricular failure) such as distended neck veins, S3 gallop or a parasternal lift due to right ventricular pressure overload, tachycardia, tachypnoea and especially if
- ECG evidence of acute cor pulmonale manifested by a new S1–Q3–T3 pattern, new incomplete RBBB or right ventricular ischaemia.

Types of emboli

- Venous thrombus
- Right ventricular thrombus
- Septic emboli (e.g. tricuspid endocarditis)
- Fat embolism
- Air embolism
- Amniotic fluid
- Parasites
- Neoplastic cells
- Foreign materials (e.g. venous catheters).

Determinants of the effects of embolism

- The level of occlusion
- The extent of reduction in pulmonary blood flow
- The pre-existing cardio-respiratory reserve of the patient
- The humoral effect of vasoactive factors such as serotonin and thromboxane A2 released by activated platelets at the site of pulmonary artery occlusion.

Investigations

All

- CXR
- Arterial blood gases: typically show hypoxaemia and hypocapnia. However, remember that normal gases do not exclude PE. SaO_2 and the alveolar–arterial gradient is normal in 20% of patients with proven PE. Hypoxaemia can be due to low cardiac output and ventilation–perfusion mismatch.
- 12-lead ECG.

Wells' score	
Clinical signs of DVT	+3
Alternative diagnosis less probable than PE	+3
Heart rate >100/min	+1.5
Immobilization or surgery <4/52 ago	+1.5
Previous DVT or PE	+1.5
Haemoptysis	+1
Cancer	+1
Total score	
<2	Low clinical probability of PE
2–6	Intermediate probability
>6	High probability

Selected cases
- D-dimer: latex agglutination/rapid ELISA (enzyme-linked immunosorbent assay)
- Cross-linked fibrin degradation products released by the endogenous lysis of cross-linked fibrin clot—for low and intermediate probability
- Echocardiography
- V/Q scanning
- Spiral CTPA (computed tomographic pulmonary angiography).

CXR findings
- Without infarction
  - Focal pulmonary oligaemia: Westermark's sign
  - Increased hilar vessel size with abrupt tapering (knuckle sign)
  - Volume loss
- With infarction
  - Consolidation (Hampton's hump)
  - Discoid atelectasis
  - Volume loss
  - Pleural effusion.

V/Q scan
A normal perfusion scan rules out PE and makes a ventilation scan unnecessary.
- PE causes abnormal perfusion with preserved ventilation (mismatched defects)
- Parenchymal lung disease generally causes both ventilation and perfusion abnormalities (matched defects) in the same lung region
- Reverse mismatched defects: ventilation abnormality > perfusion abnormality: acute/chronic airway obstruction; mucus plug; atelectasis; pneumonia; pleural effusion.

Negative or low-probability scan: one or more minor perfusion defects or abnormalities with V/Q matches thought to represent abnormalities related to other pulmonary conditions.

Positive or high-probability scan: ≥2 large or moderate sized segmental V/Q mismatches.

Intermediate (or indefinite scan): shows features of both high and low probability scans.

Mismatched V/Q defects

A perfusion defect in area with normal ventilation strongly suggests PE without infarction.

The presence of perfusion defects larger than corresponding ventilation defects suggests pulmonary infarction.

Matched V/Q defects

- Pneumonia
- Pulmonary oedema
- Airway disease.

ECG changes in acute pulmonary embolism:

Rate and rhythm
- Sinus tachycardia
- Atrial fibrillation
- Atrial premature complexes/ventricular premature complexes.

Acute right heart strain
- Acute right axis deviation
- Right atrial enlargement
- Incomplete or complete RBBB
- New tall R wave in lead V1
- Right ventricular strain pattern
- S1–QIII–TIII pattern (10%; usually transient).

QRST changes
- ST–T wave abnormalities
- ST segment depression, flattening or elevation
- T wave inversion.

Management[1]

High probability
- High inspired oxygen concentration
- Start low molecular weight heparin: consider unfractionated heparin 80U/kg IV bolus if rapid effect required
- Consider thrombolysis, using bolus of alteplase 50mg IV, for acute massive pulmonary embolism with imminent cardio-respiratory arrest. There may be a role for alteplase 100mg IV over 90min for haemodynamically stable submassive PE, in the presence of pulmonary hypertension or right ventricular dysfunction. In specialized centres, pulmonary embolectomy following immediate femoral–femoral by-pass may be a feasible option

1 British Thoracic Society guidelines for the management of suspected acute pulmonary embolism *Thorax*, 2003; **58**: 470–483.

- Inotropic support, if required, may be best provided using noradrenaline
- Urgent echocardiography or spiral CTPA.

Low or intermediate probability
- High inspired oxygen concentration
- D-dimer assay
- Low molecular weight heparin before imaging where indicated

Table 6.9 Geneva clinical prognostic score in pulmonary embolism[2]

Points	
Cancer	+2
Heart failure	+1
Previous venous thromboembolism	+1
Systolic BP <100mmHg	+1
PaO_2 <8kPa	+1
Concomitant DVT on ultrasound	+1
Prognosis	
At low risk of poor outcome	<3
At high risk of poor outcome	≥3

2 Wicki, J, Perrier, A, Perneger, TV, *et al*; Predicting adverse outcome in patients with acute pulmonary embolism: a risk score. *Thrombosis and Haemostasis*, 2000; **84**: 548–552.

Hypertensive emergencies

Types
CNS
- Hypertensive encephalopathy
- Intracerebral haemorrhage.

Cardiovascular system
- Acute pulmonary oedema
- Myocardial ischaemia
- Aortic dissection
- Hyper-adrenergic states: cocaine; amphetamines; phaeochromocytoma; monoamine oxidase inhibitor interactions; clonidine withdrawal
- Pre-eclampsia.

Evaluation of hypertensive emergencies
- Supine and standing BP
- Optic fundi: exudates; haemorrhage; papilloedema
- Lungs: basal crepitations; CXR
- Heart: S3 gallop; murmur of aortic regurgitation (dissection); 12-lead ECG
- Abdomen: bruit; aortic aneurysm
- Peripheral pulses
- CNS: encephalopathy; stroke.

Hypotensive therapy for hypertension
Indications
- Encephalopathy: headache, lethargy, seizures
- Intracranial haemorrhage
- Aortic dissection
- Acute left ventricular failure with pulmonary oedema
- Pre-eclampsia/eclampsia.

Aim: Reduction of diastolic pressure to 110–115mmHg over 2–6h to allow restoration of the autoregulatory capacity of the vasculature. Expert medical advice is indicated before commencing therapy. Avoid oral or sublingual antihypertensive agents owing to their unpredictable effects, which are not readily titratable or reversible. Rapid reduction of BP using a bolus of diazoxide or a high dose of oral or sublingual nifedipine is particularly dangerous. Monitoring should ideally include invasive arterial blood pressure monitoring.

Intravenous hypotensive agents: *short-acting hypotensive agents should be used, allowing titration of blood pressure response to infusion rate.*

- GTN infusion may be tried initially
- Sodium nitroprusside infusion, starting at 0.3mcg/kg/min, rising by 0.5mcg/kg/min every 5min, to a maximum of 8mcg/kg/min. 50mg sodium nitroprusside can be added to 100mL 5% dextrose, yielding 500mcg/mL. Using a paediatric giving set, six microdrops yields a rate of 50mcg/min

- Labetalol 50mg over 1min, repeated after 5min if necessary to a total dose of 200mg; infusion: 200mg (20mL) added to 180mL 5% dextrose to a total volume of 200mL, giving 1mg/mL—start at 15mg/h and increase every 30min to a maximum of 160mg/h until the desired fall in BP is achieved
- Hydrallazine 5mg slow IV, followed by 5–10mg boluses as necessary every 30min.

> **Hypotensive agents**
> - Directly acting vasodilators
> - Glyceryl trinitrate: venodilator
> - Hydrallazine: arteriodilator
> - Sodium nitroprusside: arterio- and veno-dilator
>
> **Adrenergic receptor antagonists**
> - Labetalol: alpha1 and beta
> - Esmolol: beta 1
> - Phentolamine: alpha

Cardiac tamponade

- This is essentially a state of cardiogenic shock
- It should be suspected with hypotension in the presence of penetrating trauma to the chest or upper abdomen, but can arise in the absence of trauma
- Beck's triad of hypotension, muffled heart sounds and raised jugular venous pressure is rarely seen in its entirety. The absence of the diagnostic triad does not rule out the diagnosis
- Pulsus paradoxus, with an inspiratory fall in systolic BP >10mmHg, is often mentioned, but is difficult to elicit.

Causes of cardiac tamponade

Acute tamponade

Cardiac trauma

- Iatrogenic
  - Cardiac surgery
  - Cardiac catheterization
  - Cardiac pacing
- Aortic dissection
- Spontaneous bleeding
  - Anticoagulation
  - Uraemia
  - Thrombocytopenia
- Cardiac rupture post-myocardial infarction.

Subacute tamponade

- Malignancy
- Idiopathic pericarditis
- Infections: bacterial, tuberculosis
- Radiation
- Hypothyroidism
- Post-pericardiotomy
- SLE.

Presentations

- Cardiac arrest with pulseless electrical activity
- Shock
- Confusion
- Dyspnoea.

Differential diagnosis of hypotension with raised jugular venous pressure

- Cardiac tamponade
- Constrictive pericarditis
- Restrictive pericarditis
- Severe biventricular failure
- Right ventricular infarction
- PE
- Tension pneumothorax
- Acute severe asthma
- Malignant superior vena caval obstruction.

Pericardiocentesis

- Subxiphoid approach, using local infiltration anaesthesia of an area just left of the tip of the xiphisternum
- 16 or 18G polytetrafluoroethylene intravenous cannula over needle (10–15cm length) or 18G spinal needle
- Attach the cannula to a 50mL syringe via three-way stopcock
- Insert the needle at the junction between the xiphisternum and the left costal margin, at a 45° angle to the skin, aiming for the tip of the left scapula
- An ECG monitoring lead may be attached to the needle with an alligator clip, but is often misleading—ST elevation is usually taken to indicate epicardial contact by the needle
- Aspirate while advancing
- Resistance is encountered while traversing the diaphragm and pericardium
- Aspiration of fluid indicates correct placement of the cannula
- Once the cannula is in place, it may be feasible to pass a sequence of J-tipped guidewire, dilator and a 5–7 French pigtail catheter
- A three-way tap can be used to seal the cannula or catheter after securing in place.

Echocardiography for pericardial effusion and tamponade

Pericardium

- Covers the entire external surface of the heart and therefore is visualized from all standard echocardiographic acoustic windows
- A thin, usually single echogenic structure that is more obvious posteriorly than anteriorly
- Most pericardial processes are evident in the parasternal long-axis view because these processes generally result in diffuse pericardial involvement and pericardial fluid tends to accumulate in the oblique sinus posterior to the left ventricle initially as it gravitates posteriorly
- Pericardial effusion: echolucent material in the pericardial space; initial accumulation in the oblique sinus; volume >100mL leads to circumferential fluid filling the entire pericardial space; has echogenicity closer to the blood pool
- Epicardial fat leads to an echolucent space in the area of the pericardium but tends to occur anteriorly; has echogenicity between that of the blood pool and myocardium

A haemodynamically significant pericardial effusion causes right ventricular diastolic collapse—persistent inward motion of the right ventricular free wall during early to mid-diastole.

Trauma

Trauma resuscitation

- Assemble the team prior to the arrival of the patient: team leader, airway doctor, two circulation doctors, two nurses
- All members wear gloves, plastic aprons and eye protection; lead aprons are worn by key members
- The team leader assigns specific duties to individual team members
- Start stopclock on arrival
- Coordinated transfer from stretcher to trolley
- Concise handover from the ambulance crew: only one person talks, while all others listen
- Not more than six people should touch the patient at any one time
- The team is horizontally integrated, with multiple tasks being performed simultaneously rather than sequentially.
- All communications are directed to the team leader
- The list of roles listed below is issued only for guidance and is not meant to be unduly prescriptive.

Team leader

- Ensures presence of appropriate team members with assigned roles
- Takes handover from ambulance crew
- Provides hands-off supervision and takes a global perspective
- Gets team members to repeat back key orders as appropriate
- Ensures universal precautions for team members
- Decides on investigation and treatment priorities
- Communicates with relatives
- Ensures completeness of documentation
- Coordinates referrals.

Airway doctor

- Maintains airway patency, with cervical spine control; jaw thrust is permitted; head tilt or chin lift are not allowed
- Performs bag and mask ventilation
- Performs tracheal intubation
- Inserts nasogastric tube
- Inserts central and arterial lines as required.

Procedure doctor-1

- Stands on left side of patient
- Obtains IV access/bloods on left upper limb
- Chest drain insertion on left as required
- Obtains arterial blood gases/arterial line.

Procedure doctor-2

- Stands on right side of patient
- Obtains IV access/bloods on right upper limb
- Chest drain insertion on right as required
- Passes urethral catheter.

Nurses
- Airway nurse, to help airway doctor
- Procedure nurse, to help circulation doctors
- Circulating nurse
  - Documentation/coordinator
  - Liaison with relatives.

Radiographer
Obtains three standard X-ray films on all patients with blunt trauma: chest, pelvis, lateral cervical spine
More selective approach with penetrating trauma

Primary survey

Airway with cervical spine control
- Voice
- Assessment of airway patency.

Breathing
- Respiratory rate
- Breath sounds
- Position of trachea.

Circulation
- Pulse, pulse pressure, heart rate
- ECG leads, pulse oximetry, blood pressure cuff.

Disability
- AVPU (alert; responsive to verbal stimuli; responsive to painful stimuli; unresponsive)
- Pupil responses to light
- Spinal cord function.

Cervical spine control

Exposure

Cervical spine control is achieved by:
- Semi-rigid collar to restrict atlanto-occipital flexion and extension
- Sand bags on either side of the neck to prevent lateral flexion and rotation
- Forehead and chin strapping to prevent neck flexion

Patients should be taken off hard spinal boards as soon as is feasible to prevent the development of pressure sores.

Sizing of cervical collar

Measure the minimum distance between the lower surface of the mandible and the point on the top of the shoulder in which the collar will rest. This distance represents the distance between the black sizing post and the lower edge of the rigid plastic encircling band.

Log roll

- Three assistants stand on the same side of the supine patient. Each places one hand under the patient to reach to the other side—at chest, hip and knee levels. Their other hands are placed on the patient's opposite shoulder, hip and knee.
- The fourth person maintains in-line stabilization of the head and neck and issues the command to turn.
- On the command, all turn the patient toward them as one in a log rolling action. This avoids any rotation, flexion or extension of the spine.

Clinical clearing of cervical spine

- Alert mental state
- No evidence of intoxication; no sedative drugs
- No neurological symptoms
- No focal neurological deficits
- No painful distracting injuries
- No posterior midline cervical spine tenderness
- Normal head posture
- Painless full range of neck movement on removal of the collar.

Secondary survey

- Neurological: GCS
- Thorax:
  - Flail chest
  - Seat belt pattern
  - Subcutaneous emphysema
  - Haemopneumothorax
- Abdomen:
  - Seat belt pattern
  - Tenderness
- Pelvis:
  - Tenderness
  - Mobility on compression
- Perineum:
  - External genitalia
  - Perianal region
  - Digital rectal/vaginal examination as indicated.

Trauma scoring systems

Revised trauma score

The revised trauma score (RTS) is based on the weighted sum of coded values for three physiological measures.

Table 7.1 Respiratory rate (weight 0.2908)

Breaths per min	Score
10–29	4
>29	3
6–9	2
1–5	1
0	0

Table 7.2 Systolic blood pressure (weight 0.7326)

mmHg	Score
>89	4
76–89	3
50–75	2
1–49	1
0	0

Table 7.3 Glasgow Coma Score (weight 0.9368)

Range	Score
13–15	4
9–12	3
6–8	2
4–5	1
3	0

Useful details about injury circumstances

- Time
- Site
- Mechanism
- Vehicle: type of vehicle; speed of travel; position within vehicle (driver/passenger); restraint devices—seat belt, air bag deployment; helmet; ejection; type of collision—frontal, angled or rear-end; vehicle roll-over; state of vehicle—passenger compartment intrusion, steering column deformity, bull's-eye pattern of windscreen shattering
- Fall from height
- Penetrating injury: implement; gunshot weapon: type/calibre
- Environment: temperature; water; fire
- Number of persons injured or killed.

Causes of restlessness and agitation with trauma

- Hypovolaemic shock
- Hypoxia
- Hypoglycaemia
- Brain injury
- Post-ictal phase of post-traumatic seizure or post-epileptic seizure
- Uncontrolled pain
- Drug intoxication: alcohol; cocaine
- Drug withdrawal: alcohol
- Exacerbation of pre-existing mental illness
- Full urinary bladder.

Indications for tracheal intubation

Airway protection
- Airway at risk: airway burn/inhalation injury; laryngeal trauma; severe maxillofacial injury
- GCS <8
- Risk of pulmonary aspiration.

Ventilatory compromise
- Breathing impaired: major thoracic wall trauma; pulmonary contusion
- Class III or IV shock
- Apnoea.
To permit further procedures and imaging in an agitated patient.

Potential causes of shock after trauma

Hypovolaemia
- Blood loss: haemorrhage—external; abdomen; retroperitoneum; pelvis; chest
- Plasma loss: burns.

Cardiogenic
- Myocardial contusion
- Myocardial infarction
- Cardiac arrhythmia.

Distributive
- Neurogenic shock after high spinal cord injury.

Obstructive
- Tension pneumothorax
- Cardiac tamponade
- Haemothorax
- Air/fat embolism.

Head injury

Head injury accounts for 1 million attendances annually at Emergency Departments in the UK. The majority present with mild head injuries.

The principles of head injury assessment and management involve determining and managing

- The extent of primary brain injury
- The risk of secondary brain injury
- The prevention of secondary brain injury.

Primary brain injury is a process, not an event. It sets into motion a neuro-chemical cascade of secondary events which can be interrupted by optimal early management.

The underlying theme in management of head injury is to prevent secondary brain injury from

Extracranial factors

- Hypoxia
- Hyper/hypocarbia
- Hypotension
- Hypovolaemia
- Hypo/hyperthermia.

Intracranial factors

- Expanding haematoma
- Cerebral oedema
- Seizures.

Causes of deteriorating level of consciousness after head injury

- Respiratory impairment leading to hypoxia and hypercapnia
  - Central causes: drugs; brainstem injury
  - Peripheral causes: airway obstruction; aspiration of blood/vomit; chest trauma; ARDS; PE
- Hypovolaemia: blood loss; reduced cardiac output
- Seizures
- Intracranial haematoma: extradural; subdural; intracerebral
- Fluid overload: hyponatraemia
- Drugs: sedatives; analgesics
- Obstructed cerebral venous return: head-down tilt; cervical collar.

Glasgow coma scale

Eye opening

Spontaneous	4
To voice	3
To pain	2
Nil	1

Best motor response

Obeys commands	6
Localizes to pain	5
Withdraws from pain (normal flexion)	4
Abnormal flexion to pain (decorticate)	3
Extensor response to pain (decerebrate)	2
Nil	1

Best verbal response

Oriented	5
Confused conversation	4
Inappropriate words	3
Incomprehensible sounds	2
Nil	1

Range: 3–15

A GCS of 14 or under should always be broken down into its component scores to allow a precise understanding of the patient's clinical state. The denominator used should be stated.

The paediatric GCS differs with respect to the verbal score:

5	Appropriate for age; fixes and follows; social smile
4	Cries, but consolable
3	Persistently irritable
2	Restless; lethargic
1	None.

Table 7.4 GCS (Adult)

Points	Best eye	Best verbal	Best motor
6	–	–	Obeys
5	–	Orientated	Localizes pain
4	Spontaneous	Confused	Withdraws from pain
3	To speech	Inappropriate	Flexor (decorticate)
2	To pain	Incomprehensible	Extensor
1	None	None	None

Problems with the GCS
- Eye opening may be prevented by facial swelling
- Verbal response is prevented by endotracheal intubation
- Alcohol and drugs may impair verbal and motor responses
- Chronic conditions may affect the verbal, motor or eye response.

Head injury categorization	
Mild	14 or 15
Moderate:	9–13
Severe:	≤8

Management of bleeding scalp laceration
- Shave or trim hair around the wound when possible to improve visualization
- Wound edge pressure allows temporary control of bleeding
- Local infiltration with 1% lidocaine and adrenaline 1:200 000 may further help limit wound edge oozing
- Gloved finger palpation of the wound for underlying skull fracture, bony defect or foreign material
- Removal of clots manually
- Saline irrigation of the wound
- Single layer closure with interrupted monofilament 3/0 nylon. Stapled closure can be used, but never on the face or forehead
- If the wound cannot be closed without tension, a dressing should be applied and plastic surgical opinion sought.

Canadian CT head rule
CT is only required for patients with mild head injuries with any one of the following:

High risk (for neurological intervention)
- GCS <15 at 2h after injury
- Suspected open/depressed skull fracture
- Any sign of basal skull fracture
- Vomiting for ≥2 episodes
- Age ≥65yrs.

Medium risk (for brain injury on CT)
- Amnesia before impact 30min or longer
- Dangerous mechanism (pedestrian struck by motor vehicle, occupant ejected from motor vehicle, fall from height >3 feet or five stairs).

To these indications, the NICE guidelines add:
- Coagulopathy, with a history of amnesia or loss of consciousness
- Post-traumatic seizure
- Focal neurological deficit.

The Canadian CT head rules[1] are not applicable if:
- GCS <13
- Age <16yrs
- Bleeding disorder; warfarin therapy
- Obvious open skull fracture.

Signs of basal skull fracture

Anterior cranial fossa
- Bilateral periorbital ecchymoses: panda eyes
- CSF rhinorrhoea
- Anosmia.

Middle cranial fossa
- Haemotympanum
- CSF otorrhoea
- Bloody ear discharge
- Hearing loss
- Vestibular dysfunction with horizontal nystagmus
- Lower motor neuron VIIth nerve palsy
- Post-auricular ecchymosis (Battle's sign): rupture of mastoid emissary veins.

Recognition of CSF
- A double ring or halo on filter paper, from central blood and a peripheral rim of clear CSF; this is not specific
- Detection of glucose in the absence of blood admixture
- Immunofixation test to detect beta-2 transferrin, which is only present in the CSF and in the vitreous humor.

CT scan evaluation of head injury
- Extradural haematoma: hyperdense biconvex extra-axial mass lesion; contained at cranial sutures by dural insertions.
- Subdural haematoma: crescentic mass lesion; often midline shift. Hyperdense in the acute phase (<3 days), isodense in the subacute phase (3–10 days), hypodense in the chronic phase (>10 days).
- Subarachnoid blood: hyperdense blood within the basal cisterns and within the sulci over the cerebral convexities; may reflux into the ventricles.
- Cerebral contusion and haematoma.
- Cerebral oedema: diffuse cerebral swelling; loss of grey–white matter differentiation; effacement of sulci, fissures and/or basal cisterns.

1 Stiell IG, et al. The Canadian CT Head Rule for patients with minor head injury *Lancet* 2001; **357**: 1391–1396.

CT findings

Subdural haematoma

Crescentic shape

Acute (<1 week): hyperdense

Subacute (1–3wks): isodense.

Clues to identification on CT scan include:

- Increase in the size of the grey matter mantle
- Medial displacement of the cortical veins (best demonstrated on post-contrast CT)
- Evidence of space occupation

Chronic (>3wks): hypodense

Repeated episodes of bleeding may cause layering.

Extradural haematoma

- Well-defined, biconvex, lenticular, hyperdense, space-occupying mass
- Stops at the sutures
- May extend across the superior sagittal sinus after a tear involving the sagittal sinus or across the tentorium
- Poor prognosis is indicated by:
  - Size >2cm
  - The 'swirl' sign of active bleeding
  - Midline shift of >15mm
  - Brainstem distortion.

CT signs favouring the need for neurosurgical referral

- Midline shift >5mm
- Dilatation of the third ventricle
- Relative dilatation of a lateral ventricle
- Compression of the fourth ventricle
- Obliteration of the basal cisterns
- Intracranial air
- Subarachnoid haemorrhage
- Intra-ventricular haemorrhage.

Causes of unequal pupils in the presence of head injury

A >1mm difference in size should be considered to be abnormal

- Impending brain herniation (associated with depressed GCS)—a pre-terminal event
- Traumatic mydriasis from direct orbital trauma
- Mydriatic eye drops
- Glass eye
- Physiological, often congenital, anisocoria.

Management of moderate to severe head injury
Airway + cervical spine control
- Maintain airway patency
- Keep SpO_2 >95%
- If GCS <8 or >8 in the presence of combativeness, rapid sequence induction, followed by oral endotracheal intubation while maintaining in-line cervical spine mobilization.

Breathing
Assisted ventilation in the presence of an artificial airway
Maintain $PaCO_2$ between 4.0 and 4.5kPa.

Circulation
Two large bore intravenous lines
Maintain the systolic blood pressure >120mmHg.

Disability
- Document and monitor GCS
- Treat seizures with anticonvulsants
- Treat hyper/hypoglycaemia
- Treat hyperthermia
- Mannitol for raised ICP; may cause hypotension after rapid infusion, especially in volume-depleted patients.

Exposure
- Document extra-cranial injury.

Indications for tracheal intubation following head injury
Airway protection
- GCS ≤8
- Loss of protective laryngeal reflexes
- Copious oropharyngeal bleeding
- Facial injury with airway distortion or compromise.

Hypoventilation
- Hypoxaemia: PaO_2 <9kPa on room air or <13kPa on supplemental oxygen
- Hypercapnia: $PaCO_2$ >6kPa
- Spontaneous hyperventilation with $PaCO_2$ <3.5kPa
- Irregular breathing
- Chest injury.

NB. cautions with intubation. Cervical spine stabilization essential unless already cleared if basal skull fracture is suspected or present. Beware of nasotracheal tube or naso-gastric tube placement—both are contra-indicated (use orogastric tube).

Criteria for referral to neurosurgical centre

- Intracranial haemorrhage where neurosurgery is contemplated
- Lateralizing neurological signs
- Hydrocephalus
- Depressed skull fracture
- CSF leak
- Need for intracranial pressure monitoring.

The details of the case are usually discussed by telephone referral with CT images being transmitted electronically

Cerebral perfusion pressure (CPP)

The brain requires a perfusion pressure of at least 60mmHg mean to maintain normal function.

$$CPP = MAP - ICP$$

If ICP is normal, a MAP of 70–80mmHg gives adequate CPP. However, in older adults, especially those with existing hypertension, MAP of 90mmHg may be needed. If ICP is raised, then CPP will be reduced and so MAP needs to be raised to maintain an adequate CPP of at least 70–80mmHg.

Indications for ICP monitoring

- GCS sum score <8
- Abnormal CT scan of the head.

This is generally initiated in the neuro-intensive care unit, or intra-operatively.

ICP-lowering therapy is initiated when sustained measurements >20–25mmHg are present

Management of raised ICP

- Head up tilt 20–30°
- Keep $PaCO_2$ at 4.5kPa by controlled hyperventilation
- Keep sedated
- Maintain BP above mean 90–100mmHg
- Mannitol 0.25–0.50g/kg (usually 200mL 20% mannitol over 15–30min) OR 3% saline 5mL/kg—ensure a urinary catheter is in place
- Dexamethasone 8mg stat, followed by 4–8mg 6 hourly IV (for cerebral tumours); steroids are not indicated in head injury management[1]
- Consider CSF drainage.

Emergency burr hole

This is rarely indicated in the emergency department, and should only be considered in a situation of rapid clinical deterioration associated with impending brain herniation, where there is likely to be considerable delay to definitive neurosurgical management. The dilated pupil is on the side of the mass lesion. Trans-tentorial herniation is recognized by depressed level of consciousness, ipsilateral pupillary dilatation and contralateral hemiparesis/hemiplegia. The operator must be prepared to proceed to a

---

1 CRASH Trial. *Lancet* 2004; **364**: 1321–1328.

craniotomy as the clot is often solid. Furthermore, the clot may in fact be subdural, and control of bleeding in an extradural haematoma may prove difficult.

- 2cm incision down to bone
- Periosteal elevation with an elevator
- Use Hudson brace and initially drill a hole through the inner table of the skull with a skull perforator. On penetration of the inner table, the hole is enlarged with a conical burr or a Souttar's drill
- Elevate the dura with a sharp hook and incise with a small scalpel blade
- The incision is enlarged in a cruciate fashion using scissors.

Intracranial pressure	
0–15mmHg (0–2.0kPa)	Normal
15–20mmHg (2.0–2.7kPa)	Equivocal
20mmHg	Therapeutic threshold
20–40mmHg (2.7–5.3kPa)	Moderately increased
>40mmHg (>5.3kPa)	Severely increased
mmHg×1.36 = cm H_2O	

Spinal injury

Spinal cord damage is a serious threat in any patient with spinal trauma, and the consequences are devastating. For this reason, rigorous precautions are taken (including log-rolling) to minimize movement of the spine (especially the neck which is the most mobile) until the possibility of an unstable injury is excluded. If found to be present, advice is sought from a spinal centre or trauma specialist.

There are also pitfalls for the inexperienced in interpretation of spinal imaging and, again, a senior opinion is needed. The cervical spine cannot be 'cleared' and collar removed without either a clinical or a combined clinical and radiological assessment, depending on the circumstances. Most resuscitation room patients will require the latter.

Assessment of the patient with suspected spinal injury
Predictive factors in the history
- Injury mechanism
- Concurrent head injury.

Examination
- Local pain and tenderness
- Skin trauma locally over the affected spine
- Respiratory pattern and evidence of diaphragmatic breathing
- Sensation and movement: is there a demarcating level?

Cervical spine radiology in trauma
- A minimum of three views is required: lateral cross-table, antero-posterior and open mouth
- To obtain visualization of the C7/T1 junction, lateral views may have to be repeated with downward traction on the arms, or a swimmer's view obtained
- Supplementary right and left lateral oblique views may be required to demonstrate the pedicles, laminae, neural foramina and articular pillars
- Suboptimal visualization needs to be followed on by CT scanning
- Flexion–extension views are the province of the spinal specialist.

Indicators of spinal injury in an unconscious patient
- Neurogenic hypotension: hypotension and bradycardia, often with warm extremities; associated with complete cord injury at the C4–T6 level.
- Hypotension with lesions below T6 level should be considered as being due to hypovolaemia until proven otherwise
- Diaphragmatic breathing
- Priapism
- Flaccid areflexia below a well defined level (spinal shock)
- Loss of pain response below the level of the lesion
- Flexed posture of the upper limbs (loss of extensor innervation distal to C5)
- Relaxed anal sphincter.

Helmet removal

- A two person approach is recommended
- The helmet is held by one rescuer, who maintains the neck in a neutral position
- The chin strap is undone by the second rescuer, who places one hand behind the neck and the other hand around the jaw to support and maintain alignment
- The first rescuer then spreads the helmet with lateral force and gently removes it.

Lateral cervical spine X-ray assessment

Adequate lateral views should demonstrate the cervical spine from the cranio-cervical junction to the upper border of T1 vertebra

Upper cervical spine (occipital condyles to (2))

Clivo-odontoid relationship Wackenheim's clivus baseline: a line extrapolated along the posterior margin of the clivus should fall tangentially to or intersect the posterior 1/3 of the odontoid process.

C1–odontoid measurement (posterior margin of anterior arch of C1 to anterior surface of odontoid process): pre-dental space, maintained by the transverse ligament of the atlas

- 2–3mm adults
- 4–5mm children.

Retro-pharyngeal space Posterior pharyngeal wall to anterior inferior body of C2, 2–7mm adults and children.

Lower cervical spine

Anterior inferior margin of C3 to airway 4–5mm. Pre-vertebral fat stripe.

Retro-tracheal space (posterior tracheal wall to anterior inferior body of C6)

- 5–20mm adults
- 5–16mm children.

The **vertebral body lines** are smooth, lordotic and parallel.

Anterior spinal line: joins anterior aspects of vertebral bodies

Posterior spinal line: joins the posterior aspects of vertebral bodies

Spino-laminar line joins anterior margin of the junction of the lamina with the base of the spinous process (posterior wall of the spinal canal); forms a smooth, lordotic curve all the way to the posterior margin of the foramen magnum.

Facet joints

Posterior pillar line or **inter-facet line**: a line drawn tangentially to the posterior margins of the facet joints is smooth and parallel to the vertebral body lines.

Laminar clear space between the inter-facet and spino-laminar lines should be of the same density, especially between C3 and C6; no cortical bone should be present

Spinous line joins the tips of the spinous processes.

Inter-vertebral disc spaces uniform in height.

Spinous processes and **inter-spinous distances**: these distances should be approximately parallel or decrease in height from C3 downward.

AP diameter of the cervical spinal canal: defined by the posterior cortical margin of the vertebral bodies and the corresponding spinolaminar line.

Normal variants: anterior or posterior tilting of dens; aplasia or clefts in ring of C1; vascular channels; accessory ossicles; <2mm asymmetrical alignment between lateral masses of C1 and C2 on peg view, due to rotation or tilt.

Powers ratio
Ratio of distance between the basion and the posterior arch of C1 to the distance between the opisthion and anterior arch of C1. Normally <0.9

Swischuk's line[1]
Straight line from anterior cortex of spinous process of C1 to C3 (spinolaminar line of C1 to that of C3)

If it misses anterior cortex of C2 by >2mm, suspect true subluxation.

Paediatric cervical spine—special issues
- Secondary ossification centres
- Widening of the predental space, up to 5mm
- Lateral displacement of the lateral masses of C1 on C2.
- Facet joints of the upper cervical spine are less oblique (more horizontal) than in the lower cervical spine in young children. This allows considerable forward motion in flexion, especially at the C2–C3 and C3–C4 joints, creating the phenomenon of pseudosubluxation.
  - Physiological anterior subluxation of C2 on C3 occurs in 24% of children up to the age of 8yrs and of C3 on C4 in 14%. The mobility of these cervical segments has been attributed to:
  - The normal laxity of the ligaments of the cervical spine during childhood
  - The shallow angle of inclination of the inter-facetal joints at these levels.
- The C2–C3 level, the site of transition between the cervico-cranium and the lower cervical spine, acts as the fulcrum for flexion and extension. The anterior cortex of the posterior arch of C2 passes through, touches or is up to 1mm behind the posterior cervical line.
- Spinal cord injury can be present without radiological abnormality (SCIWORA). Thus, in the presence of normal radiography and neurological symptoms or signs, cervical immobilization is maintained until further investigation such as magnetic resonance imaging (MRI) scanning excludes significant spinal cord injury.

1 Swischuk LE. Anterior displacement of C2 in children: physiologic or pathologic?—a helpful differentiating line *Pediatric Radiology*, 1977; **122**: 759–763.

Open mouth view
- Atlanto-axial joints: joints open, symmetrically angled, with parallel contiguous surfaces
- Medial atlanto-dental spaces: the odontoid process is symmetrically located between lateral masses of atlas such that the medial atlanto-dental spaces are the same
- Lateral atlanto-axial margins: the lateral margins of contiguous facets of the atlas and axis should lie on the same vertical plane symmetrically
- This lateral alignment may be 'off' bilaterally
- Spinous process of axis: the typically bifid C2 spinous process should be midline in position
- In the presence of atlanto-occipital dislocation, distraction is indicated by a distance from the basion to the tip of the dens that is >12mm.

Radiological signs of cervical instability
- Angulation between vertebrae >10°
- Vertebral over-ride >3.5mm with fracture (vertebral body translation)
- Complete facetal over-ride
- Facetal joint widening or rotation
- Inter-spinous 'fanning': spinous process widening
- Malalignment of spinous processes on AP X-ray
- Lateral tilting of vertebral body on AP X-ray
- Vertebral body compression >25% of height
- Pedicle widening.

Three-Column theory of spinal stability
- Anterior 1/2 of the vertebral body and the anterior longitudinal ligament
- Posterior 1/2 of the vertebral body, the facets, facet capsules and posterior longitudinal ligament
- Spinous process, lamina and interspinous ligament.

Unstable injury
- Two-column failure
- Middle-column failure.

Five signs of instability in spinal fractures as defined by middle column disruption

Vertebral displacement >2mm
Widened interlaminar space
Widened facet joints
Disruption of posterior margin of vertebral body
Widened interpedicular distance.

Vertebral column

Posterior column
- Posterior neural arch
- Spinous processes
- Facetal articular processes
- Posterior ligamentous complex.

Middle column
- Posterior 1/3 of vertebral body and annulus fibrosus
- Posterior longitudinal ligament.

Anterior column
- Anterior 2/3 of vertebral body and annulus fibrosus
- Anterior longitudinal ligament.

Subtle injuries

From rostral to caudal, there are only seven cervico-cranial injuries that may be radiologically subtle and yet capable of causing an abnormal cervico-cranial pre-vertebral soft tissue shadow:
- Occipitoatlantal subluxation
- Occipital condylar fracture
- Lateral mass of C1 fracture
- Jefferson bursting fracture
- High dens fracture
- Low dens fracture
- Traumatic spondylolisthesis, type 1.

Spinal cord injury

When to suspect spinal trauma
- Severe facial injury
- Severe head injury/unconscious
- High energy road traffic accident
- Fall from height
- Alcohol consumption and injury, especially head injury
- Multiple injuries
- Evidence of neurological damage
- Seat belt marking across abdomen

Missed spinal cord injury is associated with
- Concomitant head injury
- Altered level of consciousness caused by alcohol or recreational drug abuse
- Incomplete neurological deficit
- Pre-existing neurological disorders.

Neurological evaluation in spinal cord injury
Motor
- C5 wrist flexion
- C6 wrist extension
- C7 elbow extension
- C8 middle finger flexion
- T1 little finger abduction
- L2 hip flexion
- L3, 4 knee extension
- L4 ankle dorsiflexion
- L5 big toe dorsiflexion
- S1 ankle plantarflexion
- S2, 3 anal sphincter.

Sensory
- C4 clavicular cape
- C5 lateral arm
- C6 thumb and index finger
- C7 middle and ring fingers
- C8 little finger
- T1 upper medial arm
- L1 pubic region and lower abdomen
- L2 anterior thigh
- L3 knee
- L4 medial lower leg
- L5 lateral lower leg and big toe
- S1 little toe and heel
- S2 posterior thigh
- S3 buttocks
- S4 perineum.

Indications for CT scan in spinal injury
- Further evaluation of fracture demonstrated on plain film
- Inadequate visualization of a spinal segment in the presence of high suspicion of fracture
- Altered mental state not allowing adequate neurological evaluation.

Aims of treatment in spinal injury
- Preservation of life: attention to ABC
- Preservation of intact neurological function
- Maintenance of spinal immobilization
- Restoration of spinal stability
- Prevention of spinal deformity
- Prevention of complications, including pressure sores from spinal board or from hard objects in the patient's pockets.

Causes of respiratory failure in spinal cord injury
- Intercostal muscle and phrenic nerve paralysis
- Atelectasis secondary to reduced vital capacity
- Ventilation/perfusion mismatch from sympathectomy/adrenergic blockade
- Increased work of breathing (because of reduced compliance)
- Decreased coughing with inability to expectorate
- Muscle fatigue.

Clinical patterns of spinal injury
Cauda equina lesions
- Asymmetrical lower limb deficits
- Radicular pain or paraesthesiae
- Usually retention of perianal sensation, bowel and bladder control.

Conus medullaris lesions
- Bilateral symmetrical lower limb deficits
- Disturbed bowel and bladder function
- Little or no radicular pain.

Mixed cauda–conus lesions
- Spinal cord injuries
- Spinal cord concussion
- Spinal shock
- Complete cord transection
- Incomplete cord transection.

Brown–Sequard syndrome
- Interruption of motor function, position, and vibration sense on same side as injury
- Interruption of pain and temperature on contralateral side.

Central cord syndrome
- Weakness more marked in arms
- Weakness more marked in distal portions of the limbs
- Urinary retention.

Anterior cord syndrome
- Immediate complete paralysis
- Impaired pinprick and light touch
- Retained position and vibration sense (dorsal column preservation).

Posterior cord syndrome
- Pain and paresthesiae
- Mild paresis.

Reversible transient syndromes of traumatic spinal cord injury
- Burning hands syndrome
- Contusio cervicalis
- Cord concussion.

The initial care and transfer of patients with spinal cord injuries

Skull traction
- Closed reduction of cervical spinal fractures, especially with facet dislocation, may commence in the resuscitation room with the application of skull callipers
- Intravenous midazolam may be required for sedation and neck muscle relaxation
- Local anaesthetic is infiltrated down to the periosteum
- Cranial pins are placed 1cm behind the external auditory canal and 2–3cm above the pinna.
- A cord is attached to the pins and passed over a pulley on the head of the bed.
- Weights are attached to the cord. Generally, one commences with 5–10lb of traction, increased in increments of 5lb (2.2kg) to a total of 10–15lb.

High dose steroid therapy
Steroids may have an anti-oedema, anti-inflammatory, anti-ischaemia and membrane stabilization effect on spinal cord injury. This is, however, an area for controversy and local policies should be observed.

Requirements
- Treatment should be started within 8h of injury
- Methylprednisolone 30mg/kg bolus IV over 15min
- Followed by 45min pause
- Then maintenance infusion of methylprednisolone 5.4mg/kg/h continued for 23h.

Beneficial effects of methylprednisolone
- Cell membrane stabilization
- Superoxide radical neutralization
- Limits lipid peroxidation
- Reduced accumulation of intracellular calcium
- Reduced release of excitatory amino acids
- Reduced tissue oedema
- May improve spinal cord blood flow.

Penetrating neck injury

Specific assessment of stable patient
- Dysphonia/aphonia
- Stridor
- Dysphagia
- Cranial nerve examination
- Examination for cervical and brachial plexus injury
- Sympathetic chain (Horner's syndrome)
- Peripheral pulses
- Carotid bruits (thrills)
- Sputum containing blood
- Subcutaneous emphysema
- Loss of air through the wound on coughing.

Indications for urgent surgery
- Active bleeding from the neck
- Shock, not responding to resuscitation
- An expanding or pulsatile haematoma in the neck
- Lost peripheral pulse
- Oropharyngeal bleeding
- Air escaping through the neck wound
- Major haemoptysis (or other evidence of airway penetration)
- Haematemesis (or other evidence of oesophageal perforation).

Clinical indications for neck exploration in the stable patient
Vascular
- Expanding haematoma
- Controlled external haemorrhage
- Diminished carotid pulse.

Airway
- Stridor
- Hoarseness
- Dysphonia/voice change
- Haemoptysis
- Subcutaneous air.

Digestive tract
- Dysphagia/odynophagia
- Subcutaneous air
- Blood in oropharynx.

Neurological
- Lateralized neurological deficit consistent with injury
- Altered state of consciousness not due to head injury.

Chest trauma

Trauma to the chest occurs as either an isolated injury, increasingly as a result of penetrating knife wounds, or in conjunction with injury to other parts of the body usually as blunt trauma, for example a pedestrian hit by a car. Remember that respiratory failure can ensue as a consequence of aspiration pneumonitis in major trauma in any unconscious patient.

Approach to clinical assessment in chest trauma

This follows the standard trauma ABCDE format for resuscitation, primary and secondary surveys.
Specific assessment of the chest follows the traditional lines of:

LOOK
- Respiratory rate and depth
- Asymmetry of chest wall expansion
- Paradoxical chest wall motion
- Entry and exit wounds on front, back and sides.

FEEL
- Tracheal deviation
- Tenderness
- Chest wall movement
- Subcutaneous emphysema
- Crepitus.

PERCUSS
- Altered percussion note: dull; resonant; hyper-resonant.

LISTEN
- Symmetry of breath sounds.

Beware of the rapid killers, identifiable in the primary survey:
- Airway obstruction
- Tension pneumothorax
- Open pneumothorax
- Massive flail chest
- Massive haemothorax
- Cardiac tamponade.

Potentially life-threatening injuries identifiable in the secondary survey
- Aortic disruption
- Myocardial contusion
- Pulmonary contusion
- Diaphragmatic rupture
- Tracheo-bronchial disruption
- Oesophageal disruption.

If peripheral venous access is problematic, femoral vein cannulation with a wide bore multilumen catheter is a safe alternative. Central venous access can be obtained in the neck if necessary after haemo- or pneumothorax has been dealt with or excluded.

Discussion with tertiary cardio-thoracic centre in chest trauma

Contact early for advice with:

- Ongoing haemothorax
- Pneumothorax with persisting air leak
- Suspected major airway injury
- Major haemoptysis
- Suspected great vessel injury.

Penetrating chest wounds

- Stab wounds below the nipple line anteriorly and the inferior angle of the scapula posteriorly may injure the diaphragm and intra-abdominal structures
- Stab wounds between the mid-clavicular lines and between the clavicle (and suprasternal notch) and subxiphoid region may involve mediastinal structures including the heart
- Abdominal stab wounds can pass through the diaphragm and penetrate the thoracic cavity from below
- An entry wound in the neck can breach the pleural cavity from above.

Trauma thoracotomy in the ED

Emergency thoracotomy sometimes needs to be performed as a life-saving procedure in the resuscitation room (or even at the scene) in the context of penetrating chest trauma. Usually, the young male victim of a chest stabbing has deteriorated rapidly with progression to cardiac arrest. The benefits of rapidly relieving a treatable problem (most probably tamponade) have to be weighed against the risks of suboptimal conditions in terms of surgical sterility, lighting, equipment, competence of available surgical staff and ability to deal with more major cardiac injury in the absence of cardio-pulmonary bypass.

The survival rate for thoracotomy after cardiac arrest in this situation remains low (~10%)

Safe transfer to a cardiothoracic centre of an unstable patient in the available time frame is usually impossible; however, depending on local arrangements and distance, a surgeon from a regional centre may be able to travel to the local ED.

Clearly, in other circumstances, thoracotomy would be undertaken in the proper environment of an operating theatre by a trained cardiothoracic surgeon.

Aims

- Relief of cardiac tamponade
  - Repair of ventricular laceration with pledgeted (Teflon or pericardial pledgets) horizontal mattress sutures
  - Repair of atrial laceration with application of a partially occluding vascular clamp followed by a running suture
- Bimanual internal cardiac massage
- Cross clamping of descending thoracic aorta to enhance cerebral and coronary perfusion and to reduce subdiaphragmatic bleeding
- Rapid control of intra-thoracic blood loss: hilar clamping for uncontrollable haemorrhage.

Indications:
- Signs of life at scene of incident
- Cardio-respiratory arrest in transit or shortly after arrival in hospital.

Contraindications:
- No signs of life at the scene
- CPR with endotracheal tube *in situ* prolonged >5min.

Procedure

- Universal precautions: visor, double gloves, apron and gown
- Left antero-lateral thoracotomy through the fifth intercostal space (just below the level of the male nipple) + sternal transection with heavy scissors and control of the divided internal mammary arteries—continued into the right chest as a clam-shell incision (mid-axillary line to mid-axillary line)
- Insert one or two large self-retaining retractors/rib spreaders and open to the full extent; this gives excellent access to four cavities: pericardial; two pleural; and peritoneal, as well as to the root of the neck
- At this stage, it should be possible to see whether the heart is 'full' (tamponade) or 'empty' (exsanguination)
- Lift up with forceps and incise pericardium with a blade, and continue the incision with scissors
- Open pericardium longitudinally with a long incision 3cm anterior and parallel to the phrenic nerve
- Evacuate clot and blood
- Ascertain the cardiac rhythm: if in asystole or fibrillation, commence gentle internal cardiac massage; for a non-perfusing ventricular arrhythmia, start with a 20J shock with one internal paddle behind the heart and the other in front
- Control ventricular bleeding with digital occlusion or a Foley urinary catheter and then suture with horizontal mattress pledgeted (Teflon or pericardial pledgets) 2/0 or 3/0 prolene on a large, round-bodied needle taking 1–2cm bites. Care should be taken to avoid the coronary vessels.
- Leave the pericardium open
- Ensure that the internal mammary arteries are ligated
- Place mediastinal and thoracic drains
- Approximate sternum by wire sutures after placing a sterile spoon (concavity facing upwards) below the sternum.

Open pneumothorax management

Occlusion of the defect with a square dressing secured on three sides, which acts as a flap valve.

Causes of shock in chest trauma

- Tension pneumothorax
- Haemothorax
- Cardiac tamponade
- Myocardial contusion
- Great vessel injury
- Air embolism

- Large lung contusion
- Diaphragmatic rupture.

Indications for thoracotomy after chest trauma

- Initial drainage >1500mL or 1000mL immediately followed by 500mL in the first hour and 250mL/h thereafter
- Drainage >500mL or >3mL/kg/h in three successive hours
- Cardiac tamponade
- Massive air leak despite adequate intercostal drainage
- Trans-mediastinal wounds
- Ruptured aorta/injury to great vessels
- Massive chest wall injury with large chest wall defect (traumatic thoracotomy)
- Clotted haemothorax
- Oesophageal rupture
  - Left pneumothorax or hydrothorax in absence of rib fracture
  - Pain or shock out of proportion to apparent injury
  - Mediastinal air
  - Gastric contents in chest drainage
- Diaphragmatic rupture
- Combined thoracic and abdominal wounds.

Features of major airway injury

- Increasing subcutaneous/deep cervical emphysema
- Pneumothorax, especially with a large and persistent air leak
- Tension pneumothorax
- Pneumomediastinum
- Pneumopericardium
- Haemoptysis
- Airway obstruction, with stridor
- Aphonia
- Difficult intubation, i.e. resistance to passing endotracheal tube beyond larynx
- Subcutaneous emphysema and/or tension pneumothorax on commencing positive pressure ventilation
- Fallen lung sign on CXR: the lung falls away from the mediastinum towards the lateral chest wall
- Persistent atelectasis.

Chest wall evaluation in trauma

- Bruising
- Seat belt marks
- Steering wheel imprint
- Penetrating wounds—remember to check the back!
- Subcutaneous air, associated with fine crepitus
- Coarse crepitus from rib fractures
- Palpable sternal fractures with overlap of fragments
- Sterno-clavicular joint dislocation
- Flail segments resulting in abnormal chest wall movements.

Pneumothorax (see also pp. 224–228)

- Usually but not necessarily accompanied by rib fractures
- Clinical signs not always present or obvious.
  - Resonant percussion
  - Reduced breath sounds
  - Reduced voice sounds
  - If under tension, trachea and mediastinum are displaced away from the affected side
- Drains are usually inserted in the mid axillary line

Apical for air
Basal for blood (haemopneumothorax).

Rib fractures and associated injuries	
First three pairs	Spinal or vascular injury; tracheo-bronchial rupture
Last three pairs	Hepatic, splenic and renal injury
Multiple sites	Flail chest
Multiple healed	Adult: alcohol abuse; child: non-accidental injury

Flail chest

A flail chest represents complete disruption of function of a segment of the chest wall. The features are:

- Two or more fractures (segmental) in three or more adjacent ribs
- Paradoxical chest wall motion: inward with inspiration and outward with expiration, associated with increased work of breathing, in a spontaneously breathing patient
- Underlying pulmonary contusion and pain restricting full inspiration are the predominant causes of hypoxia.

Management of flail chest

- Provision of adequate pain relief with titrated IV opioid analgesics
- Ventilatory support, with sedation, intubation and IPPV
- Occasionally, operative stabilization of ribs using either Kirschner wires, wire cerclage or Judet staples.

Possible CXR findings in chest trauma

- Rib/sternal fractures
- Pneumothorax
- Haemothorax
- Pulmonary contusion/laceration
- Pneumomediastinum; pneumopericardium
- Diaphragm rupture
- Traumatic aortic rupture.

Pulmonary contusion

- Homogeneous or patchy air space opacities with or without an air bronchogram
- Non-segmental distribution

- Demonstrable earlier on CT scans
- Caused by a disruption of alveolar capillary integrity resulting in intra-alveolar haemorrhage and oedema. Reduced surfactant production leads to reduction in lung compliance and consequent ventilation–perfusion mismatch.

Pulmonary laceration
- A lung space filled with blood (haematoma) or air-filled (pneumatocoele; pseudocyst)
- Ill-defined opacities or ovoid lucent lesions with or without an air-fluid level.

Management considerations for pulmonary contusion
- High flow oxygen
- Pain relief: analgesia; intecostal blocks; thoracic epidural analgesia
- Ventilatory support
- Careful fluid management
- There is no clear evidence supporting the use of steroids or antibiotics.

Diaphragm rupture
- Incomplete visualization of hemidiaphragm
- Elevation of and irregular border of hemidiaphragm
- Blunting of costophrenic angle
- Multiple lower rib fractures
- Persistent lower lobe collapse
- Persistent haemothorax
- Mediastinal shift away from injury
- Nasogastric tube in chest acvity
- Gas-filled viscera in chest
- Fluid level not across the whole hemithorax
- Apex contains compressed lung, not air.

Cardiac trauma

Blunt cardiac injury is usually self-limiting. The possibilities are:
- Myocardial contusion
- Haemopericardium (including tamponade)
- Coronary artery rupture
- Investigations.

ECG may show
- Arrhythmias
- ST elevation and T wave inversion
- Low voltage if pericardial effusion or haemopericardium

Transthoracic echocardiogram

Aortography or trans-oesophageal echocardiography

Cardiac tamponade clinical features
- Tachycardia and oliguria (not specific)
- Cardiogenic shock
- Hypotension with engorged neck veins—CVP raised if line *in situ*
- Heart sounds reduced or muffled (difficult to appreciate in a noisy resuscitation room!)
- Paradoxical pulse
- Confirmation by echocardiography (ultrasound may visualize).

Place of CPAP, NIV, and ventilation in chest injury

Positive pressure applied to the airway can potentially cause a pneumothorax in the presence of rib fractures. The clinical situation must be evaluated very carefully and the patient monitored closely for deterioration, if the need for intubation and ventilation arises (e.g. concurrent head injury).

If oxygenation is deteriorating despite high flow mask oxygen in the presence of blunt chest trauma when pneumothorax is absent, then CPAP or NIV may assist lung recruitment and lead to an improvement in PaO_2 and avoid the need for intubation. The risk of pneumothorax developing needs again to be remembered and risks weighed against potential benefit.

Ventilation in the presence of an air leak

This becomes necessary if gas exchange is poor and cannot be improved by mask oxygen

- Communication from the airways out to the pleural space with an existing pneumothorax will be worsened by positive pressure
- Bubbling from the chest drain will increase
- Underlying lung may re-collapse
- A pneumothorax can begin to tension unless the chest drain is placed on wall vacuum suction at low −ve pressure.

Role of double lumen tube for lung separation and isolation in major chest injury

Double lumen endotracheal tubes are commonly used in the specialized area of anaesthesia for thoracic surgery. They are longer than a standard endotracheal tube and the curved distal end enters the left or right main bronchus (left and right sided tubes are available), so directly intubating the bronchus. A second lumen runs alongside as far as the lower trachea. The tube has bronchial and tracheal cuffs allowing either lung to be ventilated separately.

In the emergency setting in the resuscitation room, they may not be immediately available as considerable expertise is needed for their safe use. However, using a double lumen tube can be the best eventual option in specific circumstances as below.

- If there is a major problem with one lung only and the other side is relatively unaffected, then a double lumen tube can be placed by an experienced anaesthetist to allow isolation of the 'bad' lung and more effectively ventilate the 'good' lung. This may improve stability until thoracotomy can be organized. In chest trauma, the indications are:
  - Uncontrollable major air leak from unilateral pneumothorax
  - Major haemorrhage into one lung
  - Severe unilateral contusion
- During thoracotomy, it is usually necessary to use one lung ventilation with a double lumen tube, permitting access by collapsing the lung on the affected side.

Aortic injury

Clinical features
Survivors arriving in hospital are self-selected, with contained rupture and haemodynamic stability.

Mechanisms
- Road traffic accidents: high-velocity motor vehicle collisions; ejection from the vehicle; direct impact with pedestrian
- Falls from a height >10 feet
- Crush injury
- Blast injury.

Pathophysiology
Differential deceleration and thoracic compression typically leads to aortic rupture at the isthmus.

Presentations
- Shortness of breath
- Inter-scapular back pain
- Often asymptomatic.

Physical findings
- Steering wheel impact on chest wall
- New heart or inter-scapular murmur
- Hoarseness of voice
- Hypovolaemic shock (75% are haemodynamically stable on arrival in hospital)
- Unequal upper limb pulses and BP
- Paraplegia/paraparesis.

Impending rupture:
- Left haemothorax
- Left supraclavicular haematoma
- Pseudo-coarctation: differential upper limb hypertension.

Plain chest film findings
- Widened superior mediastinum(>8cm on supine AP film; greater than the width of the underlying vertebral body on erect PA film)
- Mediastinal/chest width ratio >0.25
- Lack of clarity or continuity of contour of aortic knob
- Loss of aorto-pulmonary window
- Displacement of nasogastric tube (in oesophagus) or trachea to the right
- Depression of left main stem bronchus >140°
- Apical pleural cap (left apical haematoma)
- Loss of paraspinal pleural stripe
- Widening of right paratracheal stripe
- Indirect signs of significant thoracic trauma: fractures of first and/or second rib; multiple left-sided rib fractures; displaced sternal fracture; fracture—dislocation of lower thoracic spine
- In 2–7% cases, the CXR may be normal.

Imaging options
- Spiral CT scan
- Trans-oesophageal echocardiography
- Aortography
- Magnetic resonance aortography
- CT aortography.

CT findings
- Intimal flap
- Luminal clot
- Irregular wall or contour
- Intra-mural haematoma, dissection
- Pseudo-coarctation
- Pseudo-aneurysm
- Extravasation.

Aortographic findings
- Asymmetrical contour
- One or both acute margins
- Narrowed adjacent lumen
- Intimal flap
- Extravasation
- Overlap density
- May retain contrast.

Diagnostic algorithm
- Normal chest film: no further evaluation
- Wide mediastinum or mechanism in a stable patient: CT angiography
- Wide mediastinum, unstable patient: trans-catheter aortogram.

Pitfalls in assessing mediastinal width on plain CXR (all tend to magnify mediastinal diameters)
- Supine position
- AP projection
- Poor inspiratory effort
- Unfolded aorta
- Intravascular fluid overload
- Pre-existing mediastinal pathology.

Signs of peripheral arterial injury

Peripheral arterial injury is obvious when overt and external. It may, however, be overlooked if there is no external bleeding, peripheral ischaemia being the only finding. The clinical context is also important, there being certain forms of skeletal injury more likely to be associated with vascular injury.

Types of injury

- Simple laceration
- Laceration with partial wall loss
- Transection
- Simple contusion
- Contusion with elevated intimal flap and thrombosis
- Contusion with false aneurysm
- Contusion with spasm
- Contusion with subintimal haematoma
- False aneurysm
- Arterio-venous fistula
- Extrinsic compression.

Hard signs

- Diminished or absent pulse
- Arterial bruit or thrill: a systolic bruit suggests a false aneurysm, and a continuous bruit an arterio-venous fistula
- Active and pulsatile external haemorrhage
- Haematoma (large, expanding, pulsatile)
- Distal arterial ischaemia.
- The six Ps of acute arterial ischaemia
  - Pain
  - Pallor
  - Pulselessness
  - Paraesthesiae
  - Paralysis
  - Perishingly cold.

Soft signs

- Small stable haematoma
- History of haemorrhage at scene
- Unexplained hypotension
- Peripheral nerve deficit (injury of anatomically related nerves)
- Proximity of injury to major vascular structures
- Excessive bruising
- Decreased capillary refill.

Any major arterial injury requires surgical exploration even if bleeding has stopped, owing to the risks of secondary haemorrhage and of pseudo-aneurysm formation. Immediate control of peripheral arterial injury is usually obtained by local pressure and limb elevation. The use of proximal tourniquets and attempts at blind clamping of vessels in the emergency department are mentioned only to be condemned.

High risk limb fractures

- Supracondylar fracture of the humerus in children
- Comminuted high tibial 'bumper' fracture
- Knee dislocation.

Other associations

- Subclavian artery: first or second rib fracture
- Axillary artery: fractured clavicle
- Anterior dislocation of shoulder
- Posterior dislocation of sternoclavicular joint
- Fractured surgical neck of humerus.

Imaging techniques for arterial trauma

- Colour flow Doppler
- Duplex ultrasound
- Emergency room or operating room arteriography
- Digital subtraction arteriography
- Standard arteriography.

Compartment syndrome

Early
- More pain than expected
- Pain on passive stretch of muscles within the compartment by passive flexion and/or extension of the toes

Later
- Paraesthesia

Late
- Loss of sensation
- Muscle paralysis
- Absent peripheral pulses

Evaluation in abdominal trauma

Broadly speaking, abdominal trauma is either blunt or penetrating. Blunt abdominal trauma in particular can be difficult to evaluate owing to the presence of subtle and misleading signs, and the lack of consistent findings even in the presence of visceral injury. Thus, guarding may be related to abdominal wall trauma and is often absent in the presence of intra-abdominal blood. Signs such as distension and increasing abdominal girth are of little diagnostic value. Peritonism may be absent even in the presence of large amounts of free blood in the peritoneal cavity. The management hence needs to be guided by haemodynamic stability, with a major role for diagnostic imaging, especially CT scanning, in the stable patient. Abdominal visceral and/or vascular injury must always be suspected in the presence of unexplained hypotension. Early surgical involvement is indicated under these circumstances.

Specific clinical assessment of the injured abdomen follows the standard sequence of:

LOOK
- Abdominal wall
- Abrasions; bruises including in the flanks
- Seat belt abrasions; tyre marks; steering wheel bruises
- Entry and exit wounds
- Look at the back including gluteal regions, perineum and external genitalia
- Cover eviscerated organs with saline-moistened gauze and sterile dressings.

FEEL
- Tenderness
- Girth at umbilical level (usually unhelpful)
- Guarding
- Rebound
- Femoral pulses
- Rectal examination
- Bimanual pelvic examination.

PERCUSS
- Subtle rebound tenderness.

LISTEN
- Bowel sounds may be reduced or absent with ileus (unreliable)
- Bruits.

Prerequisites for local exploration of abdominal stab wounds (a technique developed in South Africa and the USA, where there is an epidemic of penetrating trauma).
- Haemodynamically stable patient
- No evidence of peritonism
- No indication for laparotomy
- Cooperative patient
- Experienced surgeon
- Good lighting.

The aim is to look for peritoneal penetration.

Indications for laparotomy in abdominal trauma
- Persistent/recurrent hypotension in the presence of abdominal injury
- Hollow viscus perforation
- Peritonitis
- Evisceration
- Gunshot wound
- Diaphragmatic injury.

FAST scan (Focused Abdominal Senography for Trauma)
- 2.5–5.0MHz convex array transducer
- A full urinary bladder is required to provide an acoustic window for visualisation of blood in the pelvis The procedure takes ~2–5 minutes. The four areas for scan can be denoted the four Ps: peri-hepatic, peri-splenic, pericardial and pelvic. The supine position is optimal.
- Subxiphoid area + tilt cephalad and to the left: heart (pericardial area)—sagittal or longitudinal view; probe just to the right of the xiphoid—interface of right ventricle and pericardium—focus through liver which is used as the acoustic window
- Right mid-axillary line between 11th and 12th ribs + direct medially: liver; right kidney; diaphragm; subhepatic space (RUQ)—sagittal view—Morison's pouch—interface between liver and Gerota's fascia of right kidney
- Left posterior axillary line between 10th and 11th ribs: spleen; left kidney (LUQ)—sagittal view—peri-splenic view of spleen–left kidney interface. The spleen lies more superior and posterior than anticipated.
- Midline, 4cm superior to symphysis pubis and tilt down: bladder; pouch of Douglas—transverse or coronal view—rectovesical pouch in male or cul-de-sac in female: most sensitive; can detect 200mL blood
- Ideally, hard copies should be retained of each view. If one view is unequivocally positive, it is not necessary to complete the examination.

The principle behind FAST is that haemoperitoneum collects primarily in three dependent regions: peri-hepatic, peri-splenic and pelvis. Blood appears anechoic or dark. Serial ultrasound examinations or CT scanning should be used to follow patients considered to be at high risk for intra-abdominal injury.

Causes of a false-negative FAST scan
- Short time since injury
- Amount of blood <250mL
- Retroperitoneal bleeding
- Solid viscus injury with encapsulated bleeding
- Hollow viscus injury.

Role of CT scan in abdominal trauma
- Free blood in the peritoneal cavity
- Injury to solid viscera: liver, spleen, pancreas, kidneys
- Free gas in the peritoneal cavity.

Technique for diagnostic peritoneal lavage

- Empty bladder
- Local anaesthesia with lignocaine + adrenaline
- 5cm midline vertical subumbilical incision
- Division of the linea alba
- Identification and division of the parietal peritoneum
- Introduction of a peritoneal dialysis catheter without guidewire, directed towards the pelvis
- Aspiration of free fluid: >5mL frank blood is abnormal
- If no blood is aspirated, the catheter is connected to an IV giving set and 1L normal saline rapidly infused
- The infused fluid is left *in situ* for 3min
- The fluid is then drained back by gravity into the dependent IV bag
- 20mL fluid is sent to the laboratory
- An abnormal test is indicated by:
  - The presence of enteric contents
  - RBCs >100 000/mm^3
  - WBCs >500/mm^3
  - The presence of bacteria.

Criteria for radiological imaging in suspected renal trauma:

- Penetrating trauma to the flank or abdomen regardless of the extent of haematuria. Gunshot wound to lower chest, flank or upper abdomen
- Macroscopic haematuria
- Microscopic (>5 RBC/high power field) or dipstick-positive haematuria and a systolic BP <90mmHg
- Deceleration injury, irrespective of the presence or absence of haematuria
- Major intra-abdominal injury with microscopic or dipstick-positive haematuria
- Any child (age <16) with flank or abdominal injury with any degree of haematuria.

Indications for renal exploration following trauma

- Persistent hypotension and tachycardia with failure to respond to appropriate volume replacement
- Expanding peri-renal haematoma
- Pulsatile peri-renal haematoma
- Severe urinary extravasation on IVU
- Proven renal pedicle or artery injury
- Penetrating renal trauma.

Pelvic trauma

Evaluation of pelvic fractures
- Ecchymosis or abrasion over bony prominences
- Perineal or scrotal haematoma
- Blood at anus or external urethral meatus
- Retroperitoneal bleeding
- Open fracture: always inspect the perineum
- Rectal examination
  - Anal sphincter tone
  - Prostate position and tenderness
  - Bony intrusion into the rectum
  - Blood in rectum
  - Fracture line
  - Pelvic haematoma
- Vaginal examination
- Lower limbs: circulation; neurological deficit; resting alignment; leg length discrepancy
- Pelvic skeletal instability: pressure on iliac wings.

Haemorrhage control in pelvic fracture
- Immediate external anterior pelvic fixation. As an immediate measure, pelvic stabilization by wrapping a sheet around the iliac crests and tying it tightly is a useful temporizing measure. Useful alternatives are binders, bean bags and tying the legs together. Unnecessary movement of the patient should be avoided, including leg rolling. External fixation can be difficult and carries considerable morbidity
- Pelvic angiography and embolization may be useful in specialist centres.

Features of injury to the urinary bladder
- Lower abdominal discomfort
- Inability to void urine
- Gross haematuria
- Paralytic ileus
- Abdominal distension with urine ascites
- Signs of abdominal sepsis with delayed recognition.

Urethral injury
Features:
- Blood at the external urethral meatus
- High-riding prostate
- Scrotal or perineal haematoma.

Management
Do not attempt urethral catheterization if urethral injury is suspected. Urological referral and ascending urethrography are indicated.

Acute anterior urethral injury
Contusion
- Small-bore (12 F) silicone catheter on free drainage for 10–14 days.

Extravasation (incomplete or complete disruption)
- Suprapubic catheterization
- Voiding urethrography 3–4wks later to determine urethral healing.

Posterior urethral injury
- Retrograde urethrogram if haemodynamically stable
- Placement of suprapubic catheter under direct vision at laparotomy.

Burns

Evaluation

Burns can be caused by thermal, chemical, electrical, frictional blast or radiation injury. The initial management of major burns is primarily supportive.

Airway

Inhalational injury
- Oedema of the upper airway
- Protect cervical spine: remember that burns and
- multiple trauma can co-exist (e.g. falls from burning buildings; motor vehicles catching fire; explosions)
- Early tracheal intubation for potential airway compromise (airway burns/inhalational injury); GCS ≤8.

Breathing
- 100% oxygen by reservoir face mask to keep SpO_2 >95%
- Circumferential chest wall eschar requires the performance of escharotomy.

Circulation

Hypovolaemia (associated injury, e.g. due to fall from height)
- Two large bore IV lines
- Venous blood for FBC, U&E, group and save, and carboxyhaemoglobin
- Volume replacement
- Maintain urine output 1mL/kg/h (3–4mL/kg/h if extensive muscle necrosis due to electrocution)
- Even when using a formula for fluid replacement, always titrate infused fluids to clinical response.

Disability
- A depressed or decreasing level of consciousness may relate to superadded hypovolaemia from other injury; head injury; carbon monoxide poisoning; or alcohol intoxication.

Exposure
- A resuscitation room warmed to 31°C and the use of warming blankets, help prevent hypothermia
- Loosely applied Clingfilm dressings provide temporary protection to burnt surfaces.

Features of inhalational injury
- Closed space fire
- History of enclosed space (building or vehicle) entrapment
- Extrication from smoke-filled room
- History of loss of consciousness
- Altered level of consciousness
- Circum-oral burns
- Hoarseness, or loss, of voice
- Inspiratory stridor
- Symptoms and signs of respiratory distress

- Singed nasal hairs
- Productive cough
- Soot in sputum and saliva, with soot staining of nose and oropharynx
- Buccal, glottic and pharyngeal mucosal swelling
- Bronchospasm
- Elevated venous carboxyhaemoglobin level.

House fire smoke—toxic components

- Water-soluble components: chlorine gas, ammonia, sulphur dioxide
- Lipid-soluble components: phosgene, acrolein, nitrous oxide, hydrochloric acid
- Absorbed toxins: carbon monoxide, cyanide
- Smoke is a complex aerosolized mixture of solid and microdroplet particulates in a medium of gases.

Indications for tracheal intubation

- Altered level of consciousness
- Facial/oropharyngeal burns
- Inhalational injury to the upper airway.

Evaluation of body surface area involvement

Adults

- Wallace's Rule of Nines
  - Head and neck 9%
  - Upper limbs 9% each
  - Torso anterior and posterior aspects 18% each
  - Lower limbs 18% each
  - Perineum 1%
- The hand and fingers of the patient equal ~1% of the total body surface area for that individual.

Children

- Lund and Browder chart
- Erythema should not be included in the body surface area calculation.

IV fluid replacement is required for burns involving >10% of total body surface area in children, and >15% in adults.

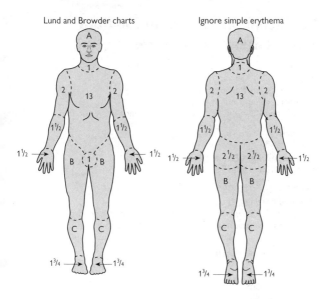

Lund and Browder charts — Ignore simple erythema

Region	Head	Neck	Ant. trunk	Post. trunk	Right arm	Left arm	Buttocks	Genitalia	Right leg	Left leg	Total burn
%											

Relative percentage of body surface area affected by growth (age in years)						
Area	**Age 0**	**1**	**5**	**10**	**15**	**Adult**
A: half of head	$9^1/_2$	$8^1/_2$	$6^1/_2$	$5^1/_2$	$4^1/_2$	$3^1/_2$
B: half of one thigh	$2^3/_4$	$3^1/_4$	4	$4^1/_2$	$4^1/_2$	$4^1/_2$
C: half of one leg	$2^1/_2$	$2^1/_2$	$2^3/_4$	3	$3^1/_4$	$3^1/_2$

Replacement formulae for fluid replacement after burns

Crystalloid

Parkland

- 4 mL/kg/% Hortmann's solution
- 1/2 total volume in first 8h after burn
- The other 1/2 in the next 16h, i.e. 1/4 in each 8h period.

Combined

Evans

- Saline 1mL/kg/% BSA for 24h +
- Colloid 1 mL/kg/% BSA for 24h.

Plasma

Muir and Barclay

- 0.5mL/kg/% BSA per period—given at 4h intervals for the first 12h, then at 6h for the next 12h (Mount Vernon formula).

Period
0	0–4h after burn
1	4–8h
2	8–12h
3	12–18h
4	18–24h
5	24–36h.

Remember to add maintenance fluid requirements.

Altered fluid resuscitation requirements

- Delay in resuscitation
- Associated visceral or skeletal trauma
- High voltage electrical injury
- Extensive muscle necrosis
- Inhalational injury
- Extremes of age.

Burn depth assessment

Partial thickness

Superficial dermal: epidermis + superficial dermis
- Red/pink, with capillary return
- Blanching on pressure
- Blister formation
- Painful to touch and pin-prick
- Heals within 14 days, with epithelial regeneration from hair follicles, sweat and sebaceous glands
- Little or no scar formation.

Deep dermal: epidermis+ dermis+ upper part of sweat glands and hair follicles
- Red, without capillary return (fixed staining); cream-coloured or white
- No blister formation
- Wet or waxy surface
- Analgesic
- Heals in 3–4wks with scar formation

Full thickness: epidermis + dermis + subcutaneous tissues
- Charred black-brown or white
- Dry, leathery layer of necrotic tissue (eschar)
- Thrombosed vessels
- No blisters
- Painless
- Granulates, with healing by wound contraction and with epithelial ingrowth from the edges
- Excise if area involved >2cm

Clues to burn depth from history

Superficial
- Flash
- Scald
- Sunburn
- Some chemicals, e.g. weak acids.

Deep
- Flame
- Electrical contact
- State of depressed consciousness: stroke; seizure; alcoholism; hypoglycaemia
- Hot fat
- Molten metal
- Clothing
- Hot water immersion
- Some chemicals: concentrated acids, alkalis.

Guides to burn depth

- Temperature of thermal agent
- Duration of contact
- Depressed level of consciousness
- Site of burn: skin thickness; tissue perfusion
- Appearance
- Pin prick test.

Referral to burns unit

- Major burns
  - >15% body surface area in adult
  - >10% body surface area in child under 10 or adult over 50
  - > 5% body surface area in infant
- Inhalational injury
- Circumferential burns
- Deep burns of scalp
- Burns of eyes
- Deep dermal or full thickness burns >1% body surface area
- Perineal or genital burns
- Non-accidental burns
- Burns of major joints.

Electrical burns
- Electro-thermal burns: flame burns
- Low voltage (<1000V) contact burns
- High voltage (>1000V) contact burns
- Flash burns
- Arc burns.

Domestic mains supply: 240V.
Common industrial supply: 415V.

Sources of electrical charge
- Household current
- Car batteries
- Arc welders
- High tension lines
- Lightning: DC discharge of static electricity between clouds and earth, lasting 1/10 000–1/1000s, and involves current of 12 000–200 000A
- Patients: electro-cautery; monitoring; diathermy.

Extent of injury depends on
- Current intensity: voltage, amperage, type (DC versus AC-tetanizing effect)
- Duration of contact with current
- Resistance at points of contact
- Efficiency of grounding
- Pathway of current through body.

Emergency Management of Severe Burns course. British Burns Association. www.britishburnsassociation.co.uk

Tissue resistance (increasing order)
- Nerve
- Blood vessel
- Muscle
- Skin
- Tendon
- Fat
- Bone.

Types of skin damage
- Contact burns: entry and exit sites
- Arc burns
- Flame burns: ignition of clothing by external high-voltage arcing.

Problems of high-voltage injuries
- Cardiac arrest is relatively common
- Cardiac arrhythmias may occur as late as 24–48h after injury
- Myoglobinuric renal failure following rhabdomyolysis
- Compartment syndromes.

Management of high-voltage injuries
- Admit to hospital
- Continuous ECG monitoring
- Hourly urine output
- Serial serum CK levels
- IV fluids
- Treat acidosis
- Treat myoglobinuria: mannitol; sodium bicarbonate.

Neurological resuscitation and management

Checklist for acute alteration in mental state

- Hypoxia
- Cardiovascular compromise
- Post-seizure
- Drug or alcohol intoxication/withdrawal/ adverse reaction
- CNS infections: meningitis; encephalitis
- Structural CNS lesion: infarct, haemorrhage, mass
- Metabolic causes: hypoglycaemia; hyperglycaemia; hyponatraemia; hypernatraemia
- Infections: chest, generalized sepsis, urinary tract
- Acute psychosis
- Head injury.

Coma

General principles

- Ensure airway patency and protect the airway
  - Intubate with GCS 8 or less if cause of coma not rapidly reversible
- Maintain ventilation and oxygenation
- Support circulation: fluid bolus of 20mL/kg if signs of shock present and assess response
- Specific measures
  - Glucose 50mL 50% dextrose IV
  - Thiamine 250mg IV (10mL high potency Pabrinex over 10min)
  - Naloxone 0.8–1.6mg IV
  - Mannitol 25–50g in 20% solution over 10–20min IV
- Clues to level of lesion in coma
  - Supratentorial: abnormal pupils; asymmetrical motor signs; focal cerebral dysfunction
  - Subtentorial: cranial nerve palsies; abnormal respiration
  - Metabolic: pupils normal or dilated ± fixed; symmetrical motor signs; myoclonus
  - Psychogenic: pupils normal or dilated; inappropriate eye closure.

Assessment and supportive management proceed simultaneously

- Airway protection
- Ventilatory support
- Circulatory support: maintenance of blood pressure
- Provision of glucose if hypoglycaemic
- Baseline vital signs
  - BP
  - Heart rate (12-lead ECG)
  - Core temperature: fever (infection; heatstroke), hypothermia
  - Respiratory rate and pattern
- Skin and mucosae: anaemia, jaundice, cyanosis
  - Bullous lesions
  - Exanthem
  - Bruising
  - Hyperpigmentation: Addison's disease
  - Puncture wounds: diabetes mellitus; recreational drug abuse
- Odour of breath: alcohol; ketones; uraemia
- Signs of head injury
- Heart auscultation: murmurs in endocarditis
- Meningism: meningitis; encephalitis; subarachnoid haemorrhage
- Optic fundi: papilloedema; subhyaloid haemorrhage; vascular or diabetic retinopathy
- Neurological assessment
  - GCS
- Brainstem function:
  - Pupillary reactions
  - Corneal responses
  - Spontaneous eye movements

- Oculocephalic responses
- Oculovestibular responses
- Respiratory pattern
- Motor function
  - Abnormal movements or postures adopted by limbs; seizures
  - Muscle tone
  - Tendon reflexes
  - Plantar responses.

Pupil responses in coma

- Pupils equal
  - Pinpoint: opiate overdose, pontine lesion; organophosphate poisoning
  - Small, reactive: metabolic encephalopathy
  - Mid-sized unreactive: midbrain lesion; reactive: metabolic encephalopathy
  - Large: drug, e.g. cocaine, ecstasy, anti-depressants, cholinesterase inhibitors
- Pupils unequal
  - Large, unreactive: third nerve palsy (uncal herniation; rupture of internal carotid artery aneurysm)
  - Small, reactive: Horner's syndrome.

Anisocoria should be considered pathological in a comatose patient.

Categories of coma

- With neck stiffness
  - With fever
  - Without fever
- With focal signs
- Without focal signs or neck stiffness.

Causes of coma

Supra-tentorial

- Subarachnoid haemorrhage
- Extradural haematoma
- Subdural haematoma
- Tumour
- Intracranial haemorrhage
- Infarct
- Abscess
- Venous sinus thrombosis
- Head injury.

Infra-tentorial

- Infarct
- Haemorrhage
- Tumour
- Inflammatory lesion.

Diffuse
- Metabolic:
  - Hypoglycaemia
  - Hyperglycaemia
  - Hyponatraemia
  - Hypernatraemia
  - Hypercalcaemia; hypocalcaemia
  - Hypoxia
  - Acidosis
  - Hepatic failure
- Toxic
- Drugs: sedative–hypnotics
- Epilepsy
- Hypothermia
- Infections
  - Meningitis
  - Encephalitis.

Investigations in coma (used selectively)
- Venous blood: FBC; U & E; glucose; culture; smear for malarial parasites; toxic screen; alcohol; carboxyhaemoglobin
- Arterial blood gases
- Neuroimaging: CT; MRI
- Lumbar puncture.

Brainstem death and organ donation

Brainstem death is the irreversible permanent destruction of the centres responsible for consciousness, breathing control, thermoregulation and essential protective reflexes. Once brainstem dead, it is impossible for life to be sustained without artificial support. Even with ventilation and inotropes, all organ systems fail after several days at the most, leading to inevitable death.

Now that intensive care ventilation is widely available, patients with no prospect of neurological recovery can be supported until brainstem death is confirmed and a decision is made to withdraw organ support. If brainstem death is confirmed, then a patient is eligible to be considered for organ donation. This process is mediated by the Transplant Co-ordinators who have continuous on-call availability for all hospitals in the UK. The NHS organ donor register records details of people wishing to donate their organs after death. Technically, this 'permission', given before death, will guide organ harvest decision (Human Tissue Act 2006).

The majority of patients presenting to the emergency department with serious neurological damage due to intracranial problems (usually spontaneous haemorrhage or massive trauma) will have evidence of residual brainstem activity and are not immediately eligible for brainstem death testing even though brainstem death may develop later.

Non-heart-beating donors

In the resuscitation room, some patients will have severe neurological damage confirmed by CT scan and at this stage will be ventilated but may have some residual brainstem activity—either spontaneous breathing or coughing. If a decision is made to discontinue ventilation and withdraw support on the grounds that the situation is non-survivable, after explanation to the family, the patient is taken off the ventilator and after death has occurred, organ harvest proceeds without the need for brainstem death testing. This technique of controlled non-heart-beating organ donation is gaining wider acceptance.

This is clearly a very sensitive area, but Transplant Coordinators in all regions are available to be contacted to initiate the approach to the family in this situation in the ED before withdrawal of treatment.

Beating heart donors

Of the small remainder of patients who clearly appear to be brainstem dead, in the resuscitation room setting, it is nearly always too early to conclude with certainty that brainstem death has occurred, and the preconditions for formal testing cannot be met so quickly.

In order to proceed to formal brainstem testing, a period of observation after definitive imaging and without sedative drugs has to elapse. This would normally take place after admission to an ICU where support is continued until organ harvest.

Sometimes, it is possible for brainstem death to be declared and organ donation agreed by the family from the resuscitation room, with the patient proceeding directly to organ harvest.

The likelihood of non-survivable brain damage needs to be communicated to the patient's family in a sensitive way. When it becomes clear that brainstem death has occurred, or is imminent, the Transplant Coordinator is contacted to make a collaborative approach to the family to request organ donation.

Pre-requisites

- Two independent consultants testing alone or together on two separate occasions
- Deep coma: no depressant/neuromuscular blocking drugs; no hypothermia; no treatable metabolic or endocrine disturbance
- Spontaneous ventilation inadequate or absent: muscle relaxants and depressant drugs excluded
- Condition due to proven irremediable structural brain damage
- Diagnostic tests
  - Absent brainstem reflexes
  - Pupils non-reactive to light
  - No corneal reflexes
  - No vestibulo-ocular reflexes: no eye movements on caloric testing
  - No conjugate eye movements in response to head turning (doll's eye reflex present)
  - No gag or tracheal suction reflexes
  - Apnoea test

No respiratory movements on disconnection from the ventilator and PCO_2 greater than threshold (6.7kPa or above).

Brain death mimics

- Hypothermia
- Acute poisoning
- Acute metabolic encephalopathy
- Related neurological disorders
- Akinetic mutism
- Persistent vegetative state
- Locked-in syndrome.

Convulsive status epilepticus

This is usually defined as a seizure lasting ≥30 min. However, for practical purposes, a seizure lasting 5 min, or two successive seizures without full recovery in between, should warrant treatment as for status.

Management
- High flow oxygen
- Intravenous line
- Capillary blood glucose
- Consider glucose 50mL 50% dextrose + thiamine 250mg IV as Pabrinex
- 2 pairs of ampoules in 50mL normal saline in the presence of suspected alcohol abuse
- Venous blood: FBC; U&E; glucose; LFT; Ca, Mg; anticonvulsant levels; clotting tests
- Arterial blood gases
- Anticonvulsants—**termination of seizure activity is the priority**

First line
- Lorazepam 4mg (0.1mg/kg) IV over 2min; repeat after 10min
- OR
- Diazepam 10–20mg (0.2–0.3mg/kg) IV at 2mg/min repeated boluses
- OR
- Diazepam 10–20mg rectal gel (0.5mg/kg) PR
- OR
- Midazolam 0.5mg/kg

Second line
- Phenytoin 15–20mg/kg IV at 25–50mg/min (do not give through the same line as other medications and do not give with glucose solutions) OR
- Fosphenytoin 15–20mg phenytoin equivalents (PE)/kg at 100–150mg PE/min OR
- Phenobarbitone 10–20mg/kg IV at 100mg/min OR
- Paraldehyde 0.4mg/kg PR (0.8mL/kg of prepared solution)

Third line
- Anaesthetic support is required for induction of general anaesthesia:
- Rapid sequence induction with thiopentone 4–8mg/kg
- Consider acyclovir, cefotaxime and erythromycin if the aetiology is uncertain, to treat for meningoencephalitis
- General anaesthesia by itself does not suppress seizure activity, and contined anticonvulsant therapy guided by EEG monitoring will be required.

Properties of lorazepam
- Slower onset of action: <5min *slower CNS penetration*
- Less lipid soluble; does not accumulate in lipid stores
- Smaller volume of distribution
- Longer duration of action: half-life 12–44h. *Longer distribution half life (3–10h)*
- *Greater affinity for benzodiazepine receptor and the GABAergic receptor.*

Properties of diazepam

Diazepam has rapid brain penetration due to high lipid solubility, a short distribution half-life (<30min) with a rapid fall in plasma levels, and a long elimination half-life (30h).

- With repeated boluses of diazepam there is a reduced volume of re-distribution, higher peak levels, prolonged action and the development of tolerance.

Table 9.1 Guidelines for treating status epilepticus in adults and children

General measures	
1st stage (0–10min)	
● Secure airway and resuscitate	*Early status*
● Administer oxygen	
● Assess cardiorespiratory function	
● Establish intravenous access	
2nd stage (0–30min)	
● Institute regular monitoring	
● Consider the possibility of non-epileptic status	
● Emergency antiepileptic drug therapy	
● Emergency investigations	
● Administer glucose (50mL of 50% solution) and/or intravenous thiamine (250mg) as high potency IV Pabrinex if any suggestion of alcohol abuse or impaired nutrition	
● Treat acidosis if severe	
3rd stage (0–60min)	
● Establish aetiology	*Established status*
● Alert anaesthetist and ITU	
● Identify and treat medical complications	
● Pressor therapy when appropriate	
4th stage (30–90min)	
● Transfer to intensive care	*Refractory status*
● Establish intensive care and EEG monitoring	
● Initiate intracranial pressure monitoring where appropriate	
● Initiate long-term, maintenance therapy	

Table 9.2 Emergency anticonvulsant therapy for convulsive status epilepticus

Premonitory stage (pre-hospital)	Diazepam 10–20mg given rectally, repeated once 15min later if status continues to threaten, or midazolam 10mg given buccally
	If seizures continue, treat as below
Early status	Lorazepam (IV) 0.1mg/kg (usually a 4mg bolus, repeated once after 10–20min; rate not critical)
	Give usual medication if already on treatment
	For sustained control or if seizures continue, treat as below.
Established status	Phenytoin infusion at a dose of 15–18mg/kg at a rate of 50mg/min or fosphenytoin infusion at a dose of 15–20mg phenytoin equivalents (PE)/kg at a rate of 50–100mg PE/min and/or phenobarbitone bolus of 10–15mg/kg at a rate of 100mg/min
Refractory status*	General anaesthesia, with one of:
	• Propofol (1–2mg/kg bolus, then 2–10mg/kg/h) titrated to effect.
	• Midazolam (0.1–0.2mg/kg bolus, then 0.05–0.5mg/kg/h) titrated to effect.
	• Thiopentone (3–5mg/kg bolus, then 3–5mg/kg/h) titrated to effect; after 2–3 days infusion rate needs reduction as fat stores are saturated.
	Anaesthetic continued for 12–24h after the last clinical or electrographic seizure, then dose tapered

* In the above scheme, the refractory stage (general anaesthesia) is reached 60–90min after the initial therapy.

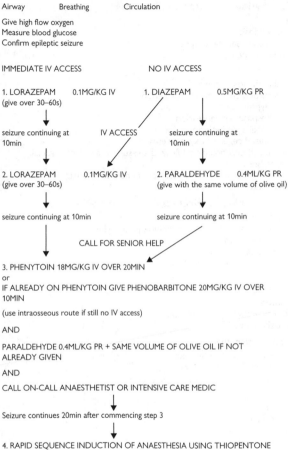

Airway   Breathing   Circulation

Give high flow oxygen
Measure blood glucose
Confirm epileptic seizure

IMMEDIATE IV ACCESS   NO IV ACCESS

1. LORAZEPAM   0.1MG/KG IV   1. DIAZEPAM   0.5MG/KG PR
(give over 30–60s)

seizure continuing at   IV ACCESS   seizure continuing at
10min   10min

2. LORAZEPAM   0.1MG/KG IV   2. PARALDEHYDE   0.4ML/KG PR
(give over 30–60s)   (give with the same volume of olive oil)

seizure continuing at 10min   seizure continuing at 10min

CALL FOR SENIOR HELP

3. PHENYTOIN 18MG/KG IV OVER 20MIN
or
IF ALREADY ON PHENYTOIN GIVE PHENOBARBITONE 20MG/KG IV OVER
10MIN

(use intraosseous route if still no IV access)

AND

PARALDEHYDE 0.4ML/KG PR + SAME VOLUME OF OLIVE OIL IF NOT
ALREADY GIVEN

AND

CALL ON-CALL ANAESTHETIST OR INTENSIVE CARE MEDIC

Seizure continues 20min after commencing step 3

4. RAPID SEQUENCE INDUCTION OF ANAESTHESIA USING THIOPENTONE
4MG/KG IV

TRANSFER TO INTENSIVE CARE UNIT

Fig. 9.1 Treatment guideline for an acute tonic–clonic convulsion including
established convulsive status epilepticus. When the protocol is initiated it is
important to consider what pre-hospital treatment has been received and to
modify the protocol accordingly. Modified form Appleton et al. 2000[1].

1 Appleton R, Choonara I, Martland T, Phillips B, Scott R, Whitehouse W. The treatment of
convulsive status epilepticus in children. The Status Epilepticus Working Party, Members of the
Status Epilepticus Working Party. *Archives of Disease in Childhood.* 2000; **83:** 415–419.

Patho-physiology of status epilepticus
Early
- Lactic acidosis
- Increased adrenergic output
- Cerebral oedema.

Late
- Cerebral hypoxia from:
  - Disturbed cerebral autoregulation
    —Hypotension
    —Respiratory depression
    —Cardiac arrhythmia
  - Increased cerebral oxygen demand
  - Reduced cerebral blood flow as a result of raised intracranial pressure
  - Excitotoxic amino acids cause direct neuronal damage, e.g. glutamate, aspartate.

Progressive physiological stages in status epilepticus
Compensation
- Increased heart rate, blood pressure, plasma glucose
- Cardiac arrhythmias
- Increased cerebral blood flow
- Rise in core body temperature
- Acidosis.

Decompensation
- Hypotension
- Loss of cerebral autoregulation
- Hypoglycaemia.

With progression, there is
- Progressive neuronal damage
- Progressive difficulty to treat.

Features of non-epileptic seizures
- Gradual onset
- Gradual offset
- Last too long
- Precipitated by suggestion
- No involvement of face
- Poorly coordinated thrashing movements
- Out of phase limb movements: movements in two arms or two legs being in opposite directions
- Side to side head movements compared with uni-directional turning in generalized tonic–clonic seizures
- Forward pelvic thrusting, as in sexual activity
- Opisthotonic posturing
- Directed motor activity: purposeful or semi-purposeful coordinated motor behaviour simulating complex partial seizures: labio-lingual movements or apparently confused behaviour such as picking objects, fumbling with clothes, undressing, etc.

- Resist eye opening
- Crying; vocalization at onset: yelling, screaming, crying, sobbing, verbal expressions of obscenities
- Lack of post-ictal period
- Lack of self injury.

Stroke

A stroke is characterized by the sudden onset of focal neurological deficit, with a characteristic temporal profile of evolution, which is of non-traumatic vascular origin. Recovery in under 24h leads to a retrospective diagnosis of TIA.

Initial evaluation

- A, B, C
- Capillary blood glucose (always beware of hypoglycaemia mimicking stroke)
- Level of consciousness: GCS
- Speech
- Swallowing
- Vision; gaze
- Facial asymmetry
- Leg and arm strength
- Sensory loss/extinction
- Limb ataxia.

The basic questions to be answered

- Is it a stroke? Rule out stroke mimics, especially hypoglycaemia
- If a stroke, is due to cerebral infarction or haemorrhage? CT or diffusion-weighted MRI
- If an infarct, is thrombolysis indicated?
- Where is the arterial or anatomical localization?

Clinical classification of stroke (Oxford Community Stroke Project)
- Anterior circulation stroke
  - Total: hemiparesis ± hemisensory loss, involving two out of face, upper limb and lower limb; homonymous hemianopia; cortical deficit, e.g. dysphasia
  - Partial: only two out of the three components of the total anterior circulation stroke syndrome
- Lacunar infarction: pure motor stroke affecting face, arm and leg; pure sensory stroke; ataxic hemiparesis–limb ataxia + ipsilateral pyramidal signs; sensorimotor stroke
- Posterior circulation stroke: ipsilateral cranial nerve palsies with contralateral motor and/or sensory deficit; bilateral motor and/or sensory deficit; cerebellar dysfunction; isolated hemianopia; cortical blindness.

Investigations after stroke

Initial

- Full blood count: polycythaemia; thrombocytopenia; thrombocytosis
- Blood glucose: hypoglycaemia; hyperglycaemia
- U & E
- INR if on warfarin
- Lipid profile

- Sickle solubility test if possible sickle cell disease
- Blood culture × 2: if febrile or endocarditis suspected
- 12-lead ECG
- Cranial CT (non-contrast).

Later
- ESR: vasculitis; endocarditis; myxoma
- CXR
- Echocardiography: suspected endocarditis, myxoma or aortic dissection
- Syphilis serology.

Remember the stroke mimics
- Mass lesions: subdural haematoma; neoplasm
- Infections: meningitis; encephalitis; brain abscess; neurosyphilis
- Metabolic disorder: hypoglycaemia; hyponatremia; hypernatremia; hyperosmolar states
- Post-ictal paralysis.

National clinical guidelines for stroke
The intercollegiate working party for stroke
Urgent brain imaging is required in the following circumstances:
- Clinical deterioration in the patient's condition
- Suspected subarachnoid haemorrhage
- Hydrocephalus secondary to intracerebral haemorrhage is suspected
- Suspected trauma
- On anticoagulant treatment, or known bleeding tendency
- Diagnosis in doubt because of other unusual features.

Initial management
- Aspirin 300mg stat
- No other drug therapy unless as part of a randomized controlled trial
- Neurosurgical opinion for cases of hydrocephalus
- Consider anticoagulation for all patients with AF; start only after excluding intracerebral haemorrhage by brain imaging and usually after 14 days
- Avoid, if possible, centrally acting drugs
- There is no licence in the UK at present for thrombolysis with alteplase, but some centres are currently providing this treatment.

All patients treated with alteplase should be registered with an international register, SITS-MOST (www.acutestroke.org). Treatment must be delivered by people who have been trained under the auspices of the British Association of Stroke Physicians (www.basp.ac.uk).

Criteria for thrombolysis for stroke
- Age >18yrs
- Onset of ischaemic stroke, <3h previously
- No haemorrhage demonstrated on CT scan
- A measurable deficit on the NIH Stroke Scale.

Surgery for haemorrhagic stroke
- Moderate to large lobar or basal ganglia haemorrhages; progressive neurological decline (with GCS between 6 and 12)
- Cerebellar haemorrhage >3cm; brainstem compression; hydrocephalus; neurological deterioration.

Stroke

Ischaemic
- Large artery atherosclerosis
- Cardio-embolism
- Small vessel occlusion

Haemorrhagic
- Parenchymal haemorrhage
- Subarachnoid haemorrhage
- Ruptured arterio-venous malformation

Subarachnoid haemorrhage

Clinical features

- Most frequent between ages of 40 and 60
- The incidence is in the range 6.0–10.6 per 100 000 persons per annum
- Sudden severe headache (explosive 'thunderclap' headache)
- Vomiting
- Neck stiffness
- Back or leg pain
- Photophobia
- Coma
- Third nerve palsy: posterior communicating artery aneurysm
- Subhyaloid haemorrhages: large, smooth-bordered
- Hypertension
- Preceding smaller bleeds: warning leaks or sentinel headaches.

Investigations

To confirm the diagnosis of SAH

CT scan positive in 95% within the first 48h after onset of headache. Non contrast-enhanced CT should be used as contrast may interfere with the detection of subarachnoid blood—contrast may show enhancement in the basal cisterns that may be mistaken for clotted blood. Subarachnoid blood may be seen in the sylvian fissures, the basal cisterns or the inter-hemispheric fissure, and over the convexities. Increased attenuation in the subarachnoid space, most commonly seen in the posterior inter-hemispheric fissure, adjacent to the falx cerebri, or layering along the tentorium cerebelli. Subarachnoid blood can be very subtle. Look in the occipital poles of the lateral ventricles for sediment and for 'fissures which have disappeared'.

- Intracerebral and/or intraventricular(with creation of fluid/fluid levels within dependent areas) blood may be demonstrated
- Giant (>25mm) thrombosed aneurysm
  - Infarction due to vasospasm
  - Secondary hydrocephalus as a result of blood in the region of the arachnoid granulations interfering with CSF reabsorption
- Lumbar puncture with xanthochromic CSF supernatant. Haemorrhagic CSF with xanthochromic supernatant: spectrophotometry for bilirubin mandatory. After SAH, haemolysis of subarachnoid erythrocytes release haemoglobin, which is converted to bilirubin. Bilirubin concen-tration reaches a maximum at 48h and may last for 2–4 weeks after extensive bleeding. Visual inspection of CSF for xanthochromia (yellow or reddish discoloration) has poor sensitivity. Spectrophotometry for haem pigments (bilirubin and oxyhaemoglobin) should be used to confirm the absence of haem pigments in CSF.

Focal signs elicited early after subarachnoid haemorrhage

Hemiparesis:
- Large subarachnoid clot in the Sylvian fissure (middle cerebral artery aneurysm)

Paraparesis:
- Aneurysm of anterior communicating artery
- Spinal arterio-venous malformation

Cerebellar ataxia and/or lateral medullary syndrome:
- Vertebral artery dissection

Third nerve palsy:
- Internal carotid artery aneurysm at posterior communicating artery origin
- Basilar artery aneurysm
- Superior cerebellar artery aneurysm
- Pituitary apoplexy

Sixth nerve palsy:
- Non-specific increase in intracranial pressure

Cranial nerve IX–XII palsies:
- Vertebral artery dissection

Table 9.3 Word Federation of Neurosurgeons (WFNS) grading for subarachnoid haemorrhage

Grade	GCS	Motor deficit
I	15	Absent
II	13 or 14	Absent
III	13 or 14	Present
IV	7–12	Absent/present
V	3–6	Absent/present

Other investigations

U & E: hyponatraemia may develop; Toxicology screen: cocaine and amphetamine use suspected; 12-lead ECG: ST changes, tall T waves, prolonged QRS complex or QT interval (catecholamine surge as a result of hypothalamic dysfunction, stimulating alpha-adrenergic receptors in the myocardium). The catecholamine surge may lead to cardiac arrhythmias and subendocardial ischaemia.

Initial coma

- Massive intra-ventricular haemorrhage and acute hydrocephalus
- Early seizures
- Raised ICP and global ischaemia.

Worsening coma

- Acute hydrocephalus
- Cardiac arrhythmias
- Severe electrolyte or acid–base abnormality
- Seizures
- Rebleed
- Delayed cerebral ischaemia
- Temporal lobe haematoma.

Physical findings in patients with SAH

Likely location of aneurysm can be predicted by focal deficit
- Neck rigidity—any
- Reduced level of consciousness—any
- Retinal and subhyaloid haemorrhage—any
- Third nerve palsy—posterior communicating artery
- Sixth nerve palsy—posterior fossa
- Bilateral weakness in legs or abulia—anterior communicating artery
- Nystagmus or ataxia—posterior fossa
- Aphasia, hemiparesis or left sided visual neglect—middle cerebral artery.

Meningitis

Meningitis can be difficult to diagnose, especially in the early stages. Presentation varies with age and immune status of the patient. Classical signs of meningism are often absent, particularly in infants and young children, as well as the elderly. A high index of suspicion is needed in the unwell toxic-looking patient.

Clinical features
Early
- Fever
- Irritability
- Headache
- Stiff neck
- Photophobia
- Nausea and vomiting
- Relative preservation of mental status
- Lack of major focal neurological signs
- No papilloedema

Late
- Seizures
- Cranial nerve palsies
- Deafness
- Impaired consciousness
- Focal neurological signs.

Signs associated with neck stiffness
Brudzinski sign
Flexion of the neck with the patient supine causes flexion of the knees and hips.

Kernig sign
With the patient supine and with the hips and knees flexed, there is pain on knee extension.

Signs of meningeal irritation in infants under 24 months: loss of appetite, high-pitched cry, irritability, vomiting, altered sleep pattern
   Signs of meningeal irritation in older children: the absence of neck stiffness does not exclude meningitis

Lumbar puncture
- Strict aseptic procedure
- An imaginary line between the posterior iliac crests identifies the L3–L4 interspace
- 1% lignocaine + 25G needle local anaesthesia
- A 20G spinal needle with stylet in place is advanced perpendicular to the axis of the spine, with the bevel horizontally oriented, with firm and steady pressure

- A sensation of give or a pop occur on entering the ligamentum flavum, between the laminae, which is entered at a depth of 5cm
- The stylet is removed to confirm CSF flow
- A manometer is attached via a stopcock and two-way tap; the pressure should be <20cm H_2O
- Keep supine for 30min after the procedure

Contraindications to lumbar puncture

- GCS ≤8
- Deteriorating GCS
- Focal neurological signs
- Shock; haemodynamic instability
- Dilated pupil: unilateral/bilateral
- Abnormal breathing pattern
- Abnormal posture.
- Papilloedema; bulging fontanelle
- Clinical evidence of systemic meningococcal disease
- Coagulopathy
- Skin infection at puncture site.

Diagnosis on CSF

- Gram's stain of centrifuged sediment
- Bacterial specific capsular antigen tests
- Latex particle agglutination kits
- Countercurrent immunoelectrophoresis tests
- ELISA
- Bacterial culture
- Bacterial nucleic acid detection
- Polymerase chain reaction (PCR).

Other investigations in meningitis

Venous blood

- Glucose, FBC, aPTT, PT, thrombin time (TT), U & E, C-reactive protein (CRP)
- Bacterial cultures
- Bacterial PCR
- Viral PCR
- Viral serology
- Bacterial serology.

Arterial blood gases

Throat and stool

- M, C & S (Microscopy, Culture and Sensitivity)
- Viral culture.

Urine

- Rapid antigen tests.

CT in bacterial meningitis
- Accumulation of exudates with widening of cisterns and sulci
- Meningeal and ependymal enhancement
- Subdural effusion
- Cortical infarction
- Enlarged ventricles.

Management of suspected bacterial meningitis
- No features of raised ICP, shock or respiratory failure:
- IV 2g ceftriaxone (third-generation cephalosporin) immediately after lumbar puncture; add ampicillin if <3 months old to cover *Listeria*. Consider dexamethasone 0.15mg/kg qds for 4 days, especially where pneumococcal meningitis is suspected if lumbar puncture will be delayed for >30min, IV antibiotics should be administered first
- Signs of raised ICP, IV 2g cefotaxime/ceftriaxone Careful volume resuscitation elevation of the head by 30°, early elective endotracheal intubation and ventilation
- A normal CT scan does not exclude raised ICP.

Heparin is indicated in the presence of infective sinus thrombosis, even in the presence of haemorrhages on CT scan.
See www.meningitis.org

Chemoprophylaxis
- Rifampicin 600mg 12 hourly for 2 days
- Ciprofloxacin 500mg single dose orally
- Ceftriazone 250mg single dose IM.

Passage of antibiotics into the CSF depends on
- Degree of meningeal inflammation
- Integrity of blood–brain barrier
- Lipid solubility: choroidal epithelium is highly impermeable to lipid-insoluble molecules
- Ionic dissociation at blood pH
- Protein binding
- Molecular size
- Drug concentration in serum.

Antibiotic passage into the CSF
- Penetration even when meninges are not inflamed
  - Chloramphenicol
  - Isoniazid
  - Pyrazinamide
  - Metronidazole
- Penetration only when meninges are inflamed, and used in high doses
  - Most beta-lactams
  - Quinolones
  - Rifampicin
- Poor penetration under all circumstances
  - Aminoglycosides
  - Macrolides.

Acute weakness

Causes of acute weakness in previously healthy patients

- Anterior horn cell
  - Poliomyelitis
  - Motor neuron disease (subacute)
- Nerve
  - Acute inflammatory demyelinating polyneuropathy (Guillain–Barre syndrome)
  - Tick paralysis
  - Diphtheria
  - Heavy metal intoxication
- Neuromuscular junction
  - Myasthenia gravis
  - Drug–induced myasthenia
  - Eaton–Lambert syndrome
  - Botulism
  - Organophosphate poisoning
- Muscle
  - Polymyositis
  - Periodic paralysis
  - Toxic myopathy
  - Neuroleptic malignant syndrome
  - Malignant hyperthermia
  - Myoglobinuria/rhabdomyolysis.

Localization of lesions producing weakness

Upper motor neuron
- Increased tone of clasp-knife type (spasticity)
- Weakness most evident in anti-gravity muscles
- Increased (brisk) reflexes
- Clonus
- Extensor plantar responses.

Lower motor neuron
- Fasciculation
- Reduced tone(flaccidity)
- Weakness
- Wasting
- Reduced or absent reflexes
- Flexor or absent plantar responses.

Primary muscle disorders
- Wasting
- No fasciculation
- Weakness
- Tone normal or reduced
- Reflexes normal or reduced.

Neuromuscular junction lesions
- Prominent, variable and fatiguable weakness
- Normal muscle bulk, tone and reflexes
- Ocular, bulbar and small muscles of the hand particularly affected
- No sensory deficit.

Non-organic weakness
- Collapsing quality with sudden giving way
- Variable non-anatomical distribution
- Muscle bulk, tone, reflexes and plantar responses normal.

Guillain–Barre syndrome

Clinical features

- Acute rapidly progressive symmetrical neuromuscular paralysis
- Weakness of at least two limbs, commonly all four, which may be distal, proximal or both
- Tendon reflexes diminished or absent
- Mild sensory symptoms: e.g. paraesthesiae in the hands and feet
- Dull aching pain in the lower back, flank and thighs
- Ventilatory failure
- Increased CSF protein with normal or slightly raised white cell count.

Management

Airway

- Supplemental oxygen.

Breathing

- Repeated measurements of forced vital capacity
- Intubation + assisted ventilation for a rapidly falling vital capacity or a vital capacity <20mL/kg.

Criteria for diagnosis

Required:

- Progressive motor weakness of at least two limbs and/or truncal or bulbar weakness
- Areflexia, usually complete, or distal areflexia with reduced biceps and knee jerks

Strongly suggestive:

- Mild sensory symptoms and signs
- Relative symmetry of weakness
- Progressive motor involvement (2–4 weeks) followed by a plateau and gradual complete recovery
- Cranial nerve involvement, especially bilateral facial paralysis
- Autonomic system involvement: autonomic dysfunction
- Absence of fever at onset
- Increased CSF protein

Inconsistent with diagnosis:

- Marked, persistent asymmetry of weakness
- Sudden onset of bowel or bladder dysfunction
- Sharp sensory level
- >50 mononuclear cells/mm^3 of CSF

Poor prognostic features on presentation

- Rapid onset
- Requirement for ventilation (bulbar compromise, reducing vital capacity, respiratory failure)
- Age >40yrs
- Extensive spontaneous fibrillation in distal muscles suggesting denervation
- Axonal variant (often with preceding *Campylobacter jejuni* infection)

Circulation
- Continuous ECG monitoring
- Low molecular weight heparin SC for DVT prophylaxis.

Disability
- Splinting of joints
- Analgesia.

Specific measures
- IV immunoglobulin 0.4g/kg daily for five consecutive days OR
- Plasma exchange: five 50mL exchanges over 8–13 days.

Myasthenia gravis

Myasthenia gravis—clinical features of crises

Crises in myasthenia gravis are characterized by sudden worsening of respiratory function, with the development of profound muscle weakness, which involves skeletal and bulbar muscles. The distinction between myasthenic and cholinergic crises is not easy, and all patients should be treated as though they were suffering from a myasthenic crisis in the absence of evidence to the contrary. A positive response, with reduction in muscle weakness, to a bolus of 2mg IV edrophonium is seen with a myasthenic crisis.

Myasthenic crisis
- Poor cough
- Unable to handle oral secretions
- Dysphagia
- Profound weakness
- Cyanosis
- Sweating
- Increased pulse rate and BP
- Respiratory distress/arrest.
- Improvement with edrophonium.

Cholinergic crisis
- Abdominal cramps
- Diarrhoea; nausea + vomiting
- Excessive secretions, including salivation
- Reduced pulse rate and blood pressure
- Miosis
- Muscle fasciculations
- Sweating
- Weakness
- Deterioration with edrophonium.

Management of myasthenic crisis
- Tracheal intubation + ventilatory support if unable to clear oropharyngeal secretions. Patients may be excessively sensitive to non-depolarizing neuromuscular blocking agents, which should ideally be used in small titrated doses
- Plasma exchange
- Immunosuppression
- DVT prophylaxis: SC heparin.

Sedatives

All benzodiazepines have anxiolytic, hypnotic, sedative, anticonvulsant, skeletal muscle relaxant and amnestic properties.

- Diazepam: onset in 2–3min; peak effect: 3–5min; metabolite desmethyldiazepam has half-life of 96h; rapid brain uptake and redistribution to inactive tissues; long elimination half-life
- Lorazepam: half-life of 14h
- Midazolam: half-life of 2–3h; onset in 2min, peak action in 5–10min, offset in 25–45min; inject 2mg (1mg in the elderly) over 30s; pause for 90s to assess for relaxation, drowsiness or slurred speech. For further sedation, inject 1mg increments every 30s until sedation is adequate. Generally a total dose of 5mg is adequate to achieve satisfactory conscious sedation.
- Ketamine 2–3mg/kg IM (three strengths 10mg/mL—IV; 50mg/mL and 100mg/mL—IM); onset 3–5min; offset 20–30min (IV) or 45–90min (IM).

Requirements for conscious sedation

- AMPLE history
- High dependency area
- Tilt trolley
- Venous access
- Supplemental oxygen
- Pulse oximetry
- ECG, BP and respiratory rate monitoring
- High volume suction
- Direct visual, auditory and tactile contact
- Airway equipment
- Resuscitative drugs
- Reversal drugs: flumazenil; naloxone.

Flumazenil

- Benzodiazepine receptor antagonist, used for reversal of benzodiazepine-induced conscious sedation. It may be employed for pure benzodiazepine overdose.
- Benzodiazepine antagonism starts within 1–2min after IV injection, reaching a peak in 6–10min, and lasting 1h.
- 200mcg IV over 15s
- 100mcg boluses at 1min intervals
- Usual maximum dose: 300–600mcg
- Seizures may result if it is used in the presence of physical dependence on benzodiazepines, or in the presence of mixed overdoses.

Conscious sedation

A state of depression of the CNS enabling treatment to be carried out, while allowing the patient to respond to verbal command throughout the period of sedation. The essential requirements are:

- Maintenance of protective airway reflexes
- Retention of the ability of the patient to maintain a patent airway independently and continuously

- Retention of the ability of the patient to respond appropriately to physical stimulation or a verbal command
- It is important to avoid oversedation, with the attendant risks of airway obstruction and respiratory depression.

Factors increasing sensitivity to drugs used for conscious sedation

- Advanced age
- Hypovolaemia
- COPD
- Liver disease
- Renal disease
- Poor ventricular function
- Drug interactions.

Discharge home after sedation

- Stable vital signs
- Alert and oriented
- Able to take fluids and medications by mouth
- Ability to mobilize consistent with pre-procedure status
- Minimal or no nausea and vomiting
- Able to receive, comprehend and retain discharge information
- Responsible person to accompany patient home.

Analgesia

Principles of selection of medication

Pain is what the patient feels, hence pain-relieving medication must be titrated to relieve the patient's self-reporting of pain as being experienced.
Mild pain: paracetamol; ibuprofen
Moderate pain: codeine
Severe pain: morphine.

Non-opioid analgesia

- Paracetamol 500–1000mg orally 4 hourly; 1–2g rectally 4 hourly; 15mg/kg orally 4 hourly
- Aspirin 600–1200mg 4 hourly
- Ibuprofen 400–800mg 4–6 hourly; 20mg/kg/24h
- Naproxen 250mg 6–8 hourly; 500–1000mg rectally 6–8 hourly
- Indomethacin 25–50mg 12 hourly; 100mg rectally once daily
- Ketorolac 30–60mg IV 6 hourly.

Opioid antagonism

Naloxone 400–800mcg slowly IV or 800–1200mcg IM or SC; onset of action: <60s; duration of action: 30–45min. Incremental bolus doses of 200–400mcg can be given every few minutes until ventilation improves. Naloxone may be repeated as required to a maximum of 10mg. When dealing with addicts, it is useful to combine 800mcg IV with 800mcg IM to allow for anticipated self-discharge after partial recovery.

Failure of full arousal after naloxone administration suggests a mixed overdose, an overdose of partial opioid agonist/antagonist (buprenorphine) or hypoxic brain damage.

Intranasal naloxone, commencing with 2mg delivered by a nasal mucosal atomizer device may be used in the pre-hospital situation.

> ### Treatment of opioid overdose with naloxone—JRCALC guidelines
>
> - Use minimum effective dose (this may involve small incremental doses)
> - If patient is dependent on opioids, give slowly and prepare for agitation
> - If there are long-acting opioids present (e.g. methadone), consider IV infusion
>
> Monitor vital signs and SpO_2 until the patient is conscious and is breathing adequately without naloxone

Safe discharge home after naloxone

- Mobile unaided
- GCS 15
- SpO_2 on room air >95%
- Respiratory rate >10 and <20/min
- Temperature >35°C and <37.5°C
- Pulse rate >50 and <100/min.
- Naloxone has a half-life of 1h
- Its effects last 2–3h, which is shorter than the duration of action of many opiates
- If relapse occurs after the first response to naloxone, a continuous IV infusion may be started using 2/3rds of the dose required to initially waken the patient given over each hour.

Opioid analgesics

- Pure agonists
  - Morphine 0.10–0.15mg/kg IV (titrated in 1–2mg increments); 0.20–0.30mg/kg IM
  - Diamorphine
  - Fentanyl
  - Alfentanil
- Partial agonists and mixed agonists/antagonists
  - Nalbuphine
- Pure antagonists
  - Naloxone
  - Tramadol.

Methods of opioid administration

- IV titration
- Patient-controlled analgesia pump
- Intra-spinal
- Continuous IV infusion
- SC/IM
- On demand (PRN) and intermittent dosing
- Balanced analgesia.

Table 9.4 Opioid analgesia

Agent	Incremental IV bolus	Patient-controlled analgesia bolus	Lockout period
Morphine	2.5mg	1mg	5min
Diamorphine	1mg	0.5mg	5min
Pethidine	5–10mg	10–20mg	5min
Fentanyl	25–50mcg	10–30mcg	5min
Alfentanil	250mcg		
Remifentanil	0.5mcg		
Tramadol	50mg		10–20min

Analgesic adjuncts

Anti-emetics

- Prochlorperazine 12.5mg IM
- Promethazine 25–50mg IV/IM
- Metoclopramide 5–10mg IV/IM.

Anxiolytics

- Diazepam 5–10mg IV/IM
- Midazolam 0.5–2mg IV/IM
- Lorazepam 0.5–2mg IV/IM
- Oxazepam 15–30mg orally.

Entonox

- An inhaled mixture of 50% nitrous oxide and 50% nitrogen, yielding an FiO_2 of 0.5
- The mixture is self–administered by the patient from a single cylinder, using a mask or mouthpiece.
- A demand valve ensures that gas mixture only flows when a negative inspiratory pressure is generated by the patient
- Administration requires a conscious and cooperative patient
- Has a rapid onset and offset of action
- Absolute contraindications include pneumothorax, barotrauma and acute gastric dilatation.

Properties of nitrous oxide

- A colourless and odourless gas
- Has good analgesic properties
- Can diffuse into closed air spaces, leading to significant clinical consequences; contraindicated in the presence of pneumothorax
- Produces minimal cardiovascular depression.

Paediatric analgesia

Mild pain

- Oral/rectal paracetamol 20mg/kg; then 15mg/kg 4–6 hourly and/or
- Oral ibuprofen 5–10mg/kg 6–8 hourly.

Moderate pain

- As for mild pain, plus
- Oral/rectal diclofenac 1mg/kg 8 hourly and/or
- Oral codeine phosphate 1mg/kg 4–6 hourly
- Ketorolac 1mg/kg; then 0.5mg/kg 6 hourly.

Severe pain

- Consider entonox as holding measure
- Intra-nasal diamorphine 0.2mL and/or
- IV morphine 0.1–0.2mg/kg.

Intra-nasal diamorphine

Dilute 10mg diamorphine powder with the specific volume of water. Instil 0.2mL of the solution into one nostril, using a 1mL syringe (gives 0.1mg/kg in 0.2mL). A current inexplicable shortage of diamorphine has affected clinical usage.

Weight (kg)	Volume of water (mL)
10	1.9
15	1.3
20	1.0
25	0.8
30	0.7
35	0.6
40	0.5
50	0.4
60	0.3

Sedation/anxiolysis
- Oral midazolam 0.5mg/kg
- Ketamine 4mg/kg IM or 1–2mg/kg IV; atropine 0.02mg/kg.

Anti-emetics
- Vestibular nuclei and labyrinth:
  - histamine 1 antagonists: cyclizine, promethazine; anti-cholinergic (muscarinic) M3 antagonists: hyoscine, atropine, glycopyrrolate
- Visceral afferents:
  - Serotonin (5–HT_3) receptor antagonists: ondansetron, granisetron, tropisetron
- Vomiting centre:
  - H1 antagonists and muscarinic acetylcholine (M3) antagonists
- Chemoreceptor trigger zone:
  - Dopamine D2-receptor antagonists: metoclopramide, domperidone.

Safe doses of local anaesthetics
Lignocaine
- 3mg/kg up to 200mg: without adrenaline
- 5mg/kg up to 500mg: with adrenaline.

Prilocaine
- 6mg/kg up to 400mg: without adrenaline
- 8mg/kg up to 600mg: with adrenaline.

Bupivacaine
- 2mg/kg up to 150mg: with/without adrenaline.

Chapter 10

Renal, endocrine and metabolic management

Oliguria

An approach to oliguria

- Recognition: urine output <0.5mL/kg/h
- Exclude obstruction: catheterize bladder; consider abdominal ultrasound to evaluate bladder size if difficult to palpate and/or percuss
- Exclude nephrotoxins: review current medications
- Ensure adequate renal perfusion: correct dehydration, hypotension, low cardiac output
- Differentiate pre-renal uraemia and renal disease
- Consider a trial of diuretic therapy
- Consider renal replacement therapy.

Suprapubic catheterization

Confirm the presence of a distended bladder; in case of doubt, ultrasound may be useful

- Two finger breadths above the symphysis pubis in the midline
- Local anaesthetic infiltration, confirming presence of urine by aspiration on the needle used for infiltration
- Direct needle towards the symphysis
- Trocar and catheter assembly is introduced into the bladder.

Acute renal failure

Investigations in acute renal failure

- Urine: microscopy; culture
- Venous blood: FBC; U & E; glucose; LFTs; coagulation screen; inflammatory markers; Ca, PO_4; blood culture if sepsis suspected; CK (rhabdomyolysis); CRP (vasculitis; sepsis); hepatitis serology; autoantibodies
- Arterial blood gases/venous bicarbonate
- 12-lead ECG
- CXR
- Renal ultrasound.

Diagnostic questions in suspected acute renal failure

- Is renal function impaired?
- Is it pre-renal azotaemia?
- Is renal blood flow impaired—arterial or venous?
- Is there outflow obstruction?
- Is there intrinsic renal disease?

Possible signs on examination

- Skin: rash of allergy; palpable purpura (vasculitis); livedo reticularis and digital infarction (athero-emboli)
- Eyes: fundi
- Lungs: crepitations; rubs
- Heart: hypertension; pericardial disease; jugular venous pressure
- Vascular system: bruits; pulses; abdominal aortic aneurysm
- Limbs: oedema; pulses; compartment syndrome
- Nervous system: focal findings; asterixis; Mini-Mental State
- Urinalysis.

Altered blood urea:serum creatinine ratio in acute renal failure

High (>20:1)
- Pre-renal azotaemia: dehydration
- Catabolic drug use: glucocorticoids
- Catabolic states: sepsis, burns, early phase of starvation
- Hyperalimentation with high amino acid load, high protein intake
- Gastrointestinal bleeding
- Intra-peritoneal leak of urine

Low (<20:1)
- Malnutrition: reduced protein intake; advanced starvation
- Liver failure
- Volume expansion
- Following dialysis
- Interference in creatinine estimation by ketone bodies and cefotaxime

	Pre-renal	Acute tubular necrosis
U/P creatinine ratio	>40	<10
U/P urea ratio	>20	<10
U/P osmolality ratio	>1.1	<1.1
Urine specific gravity	>1.015	<1.010
Fractional sodium excretion (%)	<1	>2
Urine sodium concentration	<10mmol/L	>25mmol/L

Renal support

Indications for urgent renal replacement therapy in acute renal failure
- Hyperkalaemia: K^+ >6.5mmol/L
- Oliguria unresponsive to fluid challenge
- Severe metabolic acidosis: pH <7.2 with normal $PaCO_2$
- Fluid overload with PE
- Urea >50mmol/L
- Creatinine >500µmol/L.

Renal replacement therapy
- Intermittent haemodialysis ± ultrafiltration
- Slow continuous ultrafiltration
- Arterio-venous haemofiltration
- Veno-venous haemofiltration
- Arterio-venous or veno-venous haemodiafiltration
- Peritoneal dialysis.

Indications for renal replacement therapy
- Oliguria <0.5mL/kg/h (<200mL/12h)
- Anuria (<50mL/24h)
- Hyperkalemia >6.5mmol/L resistant to drug therapy
- Severe acidosis: pH <7.0
- Azotaemia: rising plasma urea and/or creatinine; urea >30mmol/L
- Severe salt and water overload unresponsive to diuretics
- Plasma sodium >155mmol/L or <120mmol/L
- Uraemic symptoms: pericarditis; neuropathy; encephalopathy
- Drug overdose with dialysable toxins.

Established acute renal failure
- Dilute urine: specific gravity <1.010
- Urine iso-osmotic with plasma: 290mosmol/L
- High urine sodium content: >35mmol/L
- Low urine: plasma urea ratio: <3:1
- Low urine urea: <185mmol/L.

Management issues in acute renal failure
- Fluid management: strict input–output chart and daily body weight measurement
- Pre-renal/early intrinsic failure: IV isotonic fluid bolus
- Increased intravascular volume: frusemide 1–2mg/kg IV; if no response after 4–6h a repeat dose of up to 5mg/kg may be attempted
- Established: fluid intake (enteral + IV) to compensate for insensible free water loss (300–350mL/m^2/day)+ urine output every 2–4h. Replace insensible losses with 5% dextrose and other losses with replacement fluids approximating the electrolyte composition

Fluid management in acute renal failure

* Input: oral/IV
* Output:
Urine output: replace the amount lost
Insensible losses: 6–8mL/kg/24h
Pyrexia: 200mL per 1°C elevated temperature per 24h
Blood losses: replace estimated blood loss
Other losses: vomiting; nasogastric tube; diarrhoea

* Treat electrolyte disorders
  * Hyperkalaemia
  * Hyper/hyponatraemia
  * Hyperphosphataemia
  * Hypocalcaemia
* Treat acid–base abnormalities
* Treat hypertension: antihypertensive medication (labetalol, sodium nitroprusside, nicardipine) infusion
* Treat symptomatic anaemia: packed red cell transfusions
* Review medications and dosage schedules; stop nephrotoxin administration; give drugs in doses appropriate for their clearance
* Early nutritional support
* Search for and aggressively treat infections.

Investigations in acute renal failure

* History
* Chart review for recent inpatients
* Physical examination
* Investigations for post-renal aetiology:
  * Bladder catheter + urine output measurement
  * Renal ultrasound scan
* Investigations for pre-renal aetiology:
  * Haemodynamic assessment
  * Urine output
  * Blood and urine chemistry
* Investigations for intrinsic renal aetiology
  * Urinalysis
  * Rheumatological studies
  * Renal biopsy.

Causes of acute renal failure

Pre-renal acute renal failure

* Intravascular volume depletion: haemorrhage; vomiting; third space losses; burns; fever; diarrhoea
* Low cardiac output: congestive cardiac failure; myocardial ischaemia
* Reduced renal perfusion with normal/high cardiac output: sepsis
* Drugs: NSAIDs; ACE inhibitors.

Intra-renal
- Tubular:
  - Ischaemic acute tubular necrosis: shock
  - Nephrotoxic acute tubular necrosis: aminoglycosides; radiocontrast agents; myoglobinuria; haemoglobinuria; chemotherapeutic agents
- Glomerular:
  - Rapidly progressive glomerulonephritis
  - Acute proliferative glomerulonephritis
- Vascular: vasculitides; haemolytic-uraemic syndrome/thrombotic thrombocytopenic purpura; cholesterol emboli; vascular trauma
- Tubulo-interstitial disease: allergic interstitial nephritis; granulomatous interstitial nephritides; transplant rejection
- Thrombotic microangiopathy.

Post-renal
- Neoplasm: prostate; cervix; colorectal
- Dysfunctional bladder: anticholinergic drugs; catheter obstruction; benign prostatic hyperplasia
- Papillary necrosis
- Nephrolithiasis
- Abdominal compartment syndrome.

Hepatorenal syndrome
- Chronic liver disease with ascites
- Urine sodium <10mmol/L
- Urine: plasma osmolarity and creatinine ratios >1
- Normal central venous pressure; no diuresis on central volume expansion
- Poor prognosis.

Water balance

Dehydration

Degrees
Body weight loss <5%: no clinical signs
- 5–10%: loss of skin turgor; sunken eyes and fontanelles; dry mucous membranes
- >10%: shock.

Types
- Isotonic
- Hypotonic
- Hypertonic.

Elements of volume replacement
- Estimated deficit expressed as percentage of body weight
- Maintenance
- Ongoing abnormal losses during treatment
- Serum osmolality = $2 \times (Na^+ + K^+)$ + urea + glucose
- $(Na^+ + K^+)$ are multiplied by 2 to allow for an equimolar concentration of anions.

Sodium disorders

Hyponatraemia

Hyponatremia refers to a serum sodium <130mmol/L and reflects a deficit of sodium relative to water. Total body sodium may be low, normal or high. True hyponatraemia is produced by either sodium loss in excess of water or by water gain in excess of sodium.

Normal/high serum osmolality
- Restore volume and free water deficit
- Treat hyperglycaemia
- Treat for non-sodium solute, e.g. toxin ingestion.

Low serum osmolality—true hyponatraemia
- Elevated total body sodium:
  - Diuretics
- Normal total body sodium:
  - Restrict free water
  - Loop diuretic: frusemide
  - Demeclocycline
- Low total body sodium:
  - Restore circulating volume
  - Minimize sodium losses
- Treat adrenocortical insufficiency.

Key elements in the evaluation of hyponatraemia
- Volume status
- Serum osmolality
- Urine sodium
- Renal, hepatic, cardiac, thyroid and pituitary function.

Immediate therapy for serum sodium <120mmol/L, or rapid decrease in serum sodium at >0.5mmol/L/h, and CNS manifestations: hypertonic saline (3%) to increase serum sodium to 120–125mmol/L over 6h; too rapid correction can cause osmotic demyelination syndrome (central pontine myelinolysis).The usual administration rate is 25–100mL/h. The rate of correction should be 1–2mmol/L/h.

Classification

- Isotonic hyponatraemia: pseudohyponatraemia in hyperlipidaemia or hyperproteinaemia
- Hypertonic or translocational hyponatraemia: no change in total body sodium or total body water; osmotically active substances draw intracellular water into the extracellular space, diluting plasma solute
- Hypotonic or true hyponatraemia: increase in free water relative to sodium in the extracellular fluid
- Euvolaemic: normal total body sodium: Syndrome of inappropriate antidiuretic hormone secretion (SIADH); acute water intoxication (psychogenic polydipsia)
- Hypovolaemic: low total body sodium: reduced extracelluar fluid (ECF) volume: fluid loss + volume replacement with hypotonic fluids
- Hypervolaemic: high total body sodium: increase in total body sodium and total body water, with the water gain exceeding the sodium gain: fluid overload.

Management

Euvolaemic: fluid restriction to 1L per day; demeclocycline (inhibits ADH action on distal tubule).

Hypovolaemic: replacement of salt and water with isotonic saline and in rare cases with hypertonic saline.

Hypervolaemic: treat the underlying disease with fluid restriction and diuretics.

The severity of signs and symptoms depends on the rapidity of development and on the degree of decline in plasma osmolality. With reduction in plasma osmolality, an osmotic gradient develops across the blood–brain barrier, resulting in water movement into the brain. This carries the risk of cerebral oedema and herniation. Neurological manifestations do not occur until serum sodium falls below 125mmol/L .

Hypertonic (3%) saline (513mmol Na/L)

Dose = 0.6 × body weight(kg) × desired Na concentration
(130mmol/L) – actual Na concentration

Administered over 30–90min 1mL/kg/h of 3% saline will raise serum sodium by ~1mmol/L/h

Rate of sodium replacement in mmol/h = 0.6 × body weight

(total body water) × desired correction rate (0.5–1.0mmol/L/h)

The rate of correction should not be more than 2mmol/L/h and not more than 12mmol/L in the first 24h, to avoid central pontine myelinolysis (CPM, osmotic demyelination syndrome). CPM leads to pseudobulbar palsy, quadriplegia, a locked-in state and other neurological sequelae.

The volume of 3% saline (in mL) which will raise the serum sodium by 1mmol/L is twice the total body water in litres.

Free water deficit in litres = (actual serum Na – desired Na) × 0.6 × weight in kg

Total body water = 0.6 × body weight in kg in adults
Adult: 50–60% of body weight in kg
Infant <1yr: 80–85% of body weight in kg
Children >1yr: 70–75% of body weight in kg
Reduced by 5–10% in obese, females and the elderly

Fractional sodium excretion = (urine Na/urine creatinine) × (plasma creatinine/plasma Na)

A high fractional sodium excretion indicates natriuresis.

Risk factors for neurological sequelae following treatment of symptomatic hyponatraemia
- Hyponatraemia present >48h
- Overcorrection
- Rapid correction (faster than 1–2mmol/L/h)
- Underlying disease: malnutrition; alcohol abuse; malignancy; associated hypoxic event.

Hypernatraemia

Hypernatraemia is defined as a serum sodium level >150mmol/L. This is produced by a deficit of water relative to sodium. Total body sodium can be high, normal or low.

Water deficit in hypernatraemia

((serum Na − 140)/140) × total body water

where total body water is 50% of lean body mass in men and 40% of lean body mass in women. The serum sodium should not be lowered by more than 15mmol/day.

Classification

Hypovolaemic hypernatraemia: low total body sodium; losses of hypotonic fluid from the kidneys or gastrointestinal tract; correct volume deficit with isotonic saline.

Hypervolaemic hypernatraemia: high total body sodium; hypertonic fluid gain (3% saline; 8.4% sodium bicarbonate); discontinue offending agents and remove excess sodium with diuretics and 5% dextrose.

Euvolaemic hypernatraemia: normal total body sodium; diabetes insipidus; replace water deficit with 5% dextrose; hormone (vasopressin) replacement.

Potassium disorders

Hypokalaemia

Serum potassium <3.5mmol/L.

Classification

- Transcellular shift from ECF to intracellular fluid (ICF): alkalosis; hormones (insulin, catecholamines); beta-2 agonists
- Reduced intake
- Increased losses: renal; gastrointestinal
- Potassium chloride is supplied as ampoules of 20mmol in 10mL or 1g (13.5mmol) in 10mL.

Safe rules for IV potassium administration:
- Urine output >40mL//h
- <40mmol added to 1L
- Rate of administration <40mmol/h.

Oral replacement: potassium chloride (Sando-K) two tablets four times a day = 96mmol K.

Hyperkalaemia

Serum potassium >5.5mmol/L.

Classification

- Pseudo-hyperkalaemia: haemolysis; excess tissue breakdown
- Transcellular shifts: metabolic acidosis; insulin lack; rhabdomyolysis; tumour lysis syndrome
- Serum potassium rises by 0.3mmol/L for every 0.1 increase in pH above normal
- Increased intake
- Reduced excretion.

Treatment

In the absence of cardiac toxicity, treatment is focused on correction of the underlying cause. The presence of ECG changes indicates the need for immediate therapeutic measures.

Antagonize membrane effects (membrane stabilization)
- 5–10mL 10% calcium gluconate or 3–5mL 10% calcium chloride over 10–20min, with continuous ECG monitoring

Stimulate the cellular uptake of potassium
- Actrapid insulin 20U in 200mL 10% dextrose over 30–60 min.

Glucose is administered to prevent insulin-induced hypoglycaemia
- 8.4% sodium bicarbonate 50mL (50mmol) IV.

Increase potassium elimination from the body
- Cation exchange resin: calcium resonium 15g orally/30g rectally 8 hourly; each 1g of resin contains 1mmol of sodium and can exchange for 1mmol of potassium
- Nebulized beta-2 agonist: salbutamol 5mg
- Dialysis (haemodialysis or peritoneal dialysis) or haemofiltration.

Sequence of ECG changes in hyperkalaemia
- Peaked T waves
- Widening of PR interval
- Flattening of QT interval
- Loss of P waves
- Sine waves
- Asystole.

Medications inducing hyperkalaemia

- Potassium supplements
- Salt substitutes
- Potassium-sparing diuretics
- ACE inhibitors
- Suxamethonium
- Methicillin
- Arginine hydrochloride
- Mannitol
- Heparin
- Digoxin overdose
- Cyclosporin
- Aqueous penicillin G

Hypercalcaemic crisis

Hypercalcaemia can be defined as a total serum calcium level >2.55mmol/L.

Causes
- Malignancy
- Hyperparathyroidism
- Vitamin D/A intoxication
- Granulomatous diseases, e.g. sarcoidosis
- Renal failure
- Hyperthyroidism
- Adrenocortical insufficiency
- Thiazide diuretics
- Prolonged immobilization.

Clinical features
These are non-specific and include:
- Neurological: lethargy, confusion, irritability, coma
- Gastrointestinal: anorexia, nausea, vomiting, constipation
- Renal: nephrogenic diabetes insipidus, nephrocalcinosis, nephrolithiasis

Investigations
- Venous blood: FBC; U&E; calcium; parathyroid hormone (PTH); LFTs; thyroid function tests (TFTs)
- Plasma/urine protein electrophoresis: for multiple myeloma
- CXR
- 24h urine calcium
- End-organ damage: renal ultrasound; skeletal X-rays; markers of bone turnover.

Management
- IV hydration, with 4–6L of fluid, usually normal saline, to expand the plasma volume
- Forced saline diuresis, using saline and frusemide 40mg 4 hourly
- Specific treatment depends on the underlying cause of hypercalcaemia
- Drugs to inhibit osteoclastic bone resorption: bisphosphonates; calcitonin; mithramycin; glucocorticoids
- If serum calcium >4.5mmol/L, 500mL of 0.1M neutral phosphate over 6–8h
- Pamidronate 60mg in 500mL saline over 4h
- Calcitonin 3–4U/kg IV followed by 4U/kg SC 12 hourly
- Dialysis for patients in renal failure
- Steroids for malignancy: hydrocortisone 200–400mg IV daily.

Calcium data

Plasma

- Total calcium 2.12–2.60mmol/L
- Ionized calcium 1.10–1.35mmol/L
- Magnesium 0.65–1.05mmol/L
- Alkaline phosphatase 30–110U/L

Urine

- Calcium: 2.5–10mmol/24h (male); 2.5–90mmol/24h (female)
- Phosphate: 16–32mmol/24h

Hypoglycaemia

Definition

Blood glucose <3.5mmol/L; this is not an absolute value, as patients may differ in the threshold at which hypoglycaemia becomes symptomatic. It is essential to know the capillary blood glucose in any patient presenting with seizures, altered behaviour, coma or unexplained focal neurological deficit.

Symptoms and signs in acute hypoglycaemia

Autonomic (adrenergic)
- Tremor
- Sweating
- Anxiety, nervousness
- Pallor
- Nausea, vomiting
- Tachycardia
- Palpitations
- Shivering
- Hunger
- Increased pulse pressure.

Neuroglycopenic
- Impaired concentration
- Confusion
- Headache
- Irrational, uncharacteristic or inappropriate behaviour
- Difficulty in speaking and thinking
- Non-cooperation or aggression
- Drowsiness, progressing to coma
- Focal neurological signs, including transient hemiplegia; bizarre signs
- Focal or generalized convulsions
- Permanent neurological damage if prolonged, severe hypoglycaemia.

Non-specific
- Hunger
- Weakness
- Blurred vision.

Initial measures

- Oral glucose 20–30g
Sources of 10g carbohydrate: two teaspoons of sugar; three small sugar lumps; three Dextrosol tablets; 90mL Coca Cola; 15mL Ribena; 60mL Lucozade; 200mL milk
- Buccal carbohydrate as Hypostop or Lucozade
- IM glucagon 1mg.

Unable to swallow

- IV dextrose 50mL 50% in large vein (25g), followed by saline flush.
- Neonates/infants: 5mL/kg 10% dextrose
- Older children: 2mL/kg 25% dextrose.

Discharge criteria following a symptomatic hypoglycaemic episode
• Brief episode
• Full neurological recovery
• Able to eat
• No major co-morbidities that require hospital admission
• Cause of the episode found and addressed
• Treatment plan to prevent future episodes understood by the patient
• Hypoglycaemia accidental
• Relapse unlikely—no long-acting insulin or oral agent, nor prolonged excretion or metabolism
• Ability to do home glucose monitoring
• Responsible person to be with the patient
• Follow-up arranged.

Table 10.1 Insulins

Category	Action	
	Onset (min)	Duration (h)
Rapid	10–20	2–6
Rapid-intermediate	10–20	8–16+
Short	15–60	4–8
Short-intermediate	15–60	8–16+
Intermediate	60–120	8–16+
Long	120–240	16–30
Very long	60–120	24+

Examples of insulin (with generic type)
• Rapid: Aspart, lispro
• Rapid-intermediate: Novomix, Humalog
• Short (regular): Actrapid. Humulin-S, Insuman Rapid
• Short-intermediate (regular–isophane (nph) mixture): Mixtard, Humulin M2/3/5, Insuman Comb
• Intermediate (isophane (NPH)): Insulatard, Humulin I, Insuman Basal
• Long (crystalline zinc suspensions-lente): Ultratard, Humulin Zn,
• Very long: Glargine.

Inhaled insulins
• Exubera Inhale
• AERx Aradigm
• Alkermes
• Aerogen.

Diabetic ketoacidosis

Diabetic ketoacidosis is a major cause of death in type 1 diabetics and warrants intensive replacement and supportive therapy.

Clinical presentation

- Polyuria, polydipsia
- Nausea, vomiting
- Hyperventilation (Kussmaul's breathing)
- Abdominal pain
- Confusion; depressed level of consciousness; coma
- Dehydration
- Hypovolaemic shock.

Evaluation

- Capillary blood glucose initially
- Venous blood glucose, U&E, FBC; the blood glucose may only be in the high normal range in patients with liver disease, starvation (with low carbohydrate intake) or prolonged vomiting
- Venous blood gases to assess acid–base status; arterial blood gases only if ventilation or oxygenation a concern
- Hourly venous blood glucose + potassium.

Diagnosis

- Capillary/venous blood glucose ≥11.0mmol/L
- Capillary/venous blood pH <7.3
- Ketones in the urine.
- Other investigations that may be needed:
  - Septic screen: urine microscopy and culture; blood culture; CXR
  - Serum lactate
  - Serum amylase.

Management

- Large bore venous cannula
- Supplemental high flow oxygen
- ECG monitoring: T wave for potassium
- Nasogastric tube on free drainage if reduced alertness
- Urinary catheter if haemodynamically unstable
- Hourly capillary blood glucose
- Two hourly U & E and blood gases
- Hourly neurological observations
- Serial urine ketones
- DVT prophylaxis
  The key elements of management are:
- Fluids + insulin + potassium

Fluids

Fluids (requirement = deficit + maintenance)

(deficit = % dehydration × body weight (kg))

1L 0.9% saline over 30min

Then 1L 0.9% saline + KCl over 1h

Then 1L 0.9% saline + KCl over 2h

Then 1 litre 0.9% saline + KCl over 4h

Continue saline infusion until blood glucose = 10mmol/L . Then change to 5% or 10% dextrose.

Insulin

50U actrapid insulin made up to 50mL with 0.9% saline in a syringe pump (1mL = 1U)

Bolus of 6U followed by an infusion of 6U/h (0.1U/kg/h) initially.
Half-life of circulating insulin: 5 min.

Sliding scale

Blood glucose	Units per hour
≤4.0	increase IV dextrose infusion to 30%
4.1–7.0	0.5
7.1–11.0	1.0
11.1–14.0	4.0
14.1–17.0	6.0
≥17.1	8.0

Potassium
- Start KCl once serum potassium is confirmed to be normal or low
- 20mmol/h is an average dose.

Sodium bicarbonate
- Consider if profound acidosis (pH <6.9), guided by expert advice
- 200mL 2.74% $NaHCO_3$ over 30–60min (mmol = 0.15 × body weight in kg × base deficit in mmol/L)
- Avoid 8.4% $NaHCO_3$ if possible
- Only consider repetition if pH remains ≤ 6.9.

Cerebral oedema
- Falling level of consciousness and headache associated with improved metabolic control
- CT scan
- Mannitol (20%) 2.5mL/kg (0.5g/kg) over 15min; repeated as required 6 hourly
- Fluid restriction: replace deficit over 72h rather than 24h
- Tracheal intubation + controlled hyperventilation to reduce $PaCO_2$ to 3.5–4.0kPa.

Hyperglycaemic non-ketotic coma

Precipitating factors
- Drugs: beta-blockers; thiazide or loop diuretics; steroids
- Enteral or parenteral feeding
- Excessive IV glucose administration
- Post-cardiac surgery
- Being in a nursing home.

Features
- Metabolic complication of type 2 diabetes
- Marked hyperglycaemia (>25–30mmol/L)
- Marked osmotic symptoms during the preceding days: thirst, polyuria
- Dehydration
- Impaired consciousness
- Acute intercurrent illness (especially sepsis).

Biochemical features
- Severe hyperglycaemia
- Hyperosmolarity
- Severe volume depletion with pre-renal uraemia
- Electrolyte depletion
- Minimal or absent ketosis

> Plasma osmolality = $2 \times$ (sodium + potassium) + urea + glucose (in mmol/L)

Management
As for diabetic ketoacidosis, but:
- Use half normal (0.45%) saline if plasma sodium >150mmol/L
- Start insulin pump at 2u/h
- Aim for fall in osmolality of 15mOsmol/kg/h
- Low molecular weight heparin for thromboprophylaxis
- Monitor plasma potassium.

Addisonian crisis (acute adrenocortical failure)

It is easy to overlook the diagnosis of adrenocortical failure in the unwell patient, as the clinical features are non-specific. It always needs to be thought of, especially when the anticipated response to fluid replacement is incomplete.

Causes of adrenal crisis
- Stress + latent adrenocortical insufficiency: trauma; surgery; infection; prolonged fasting
- Sudden steroid withdrawal: replacement; suppression
- Bilateral adrenalectomy
- Excision of unilateral functioning adrenal tumour
- Pituitary necrosis
- Injury to both adrenals: trauma; haemorrhage; anticoagulant therapy; thrombosis; infection; metastatic carcinoma.

Consider adrenocortical insufficiency
- History of steroid therapy (within past year) or presence of Cushingoid features
- Hypotension with history of chronic weight loss and weakness
- Unexplained hypotension or volume depletion, gastrointestinal signs and symptoms, delirium and fever
- Hyperkalaemia and hyponatraemia, especially in presence of chronic renal failure
- Hypotension with hyperpigmentation
- Hyponatraemia with hypoglycaemia or eosinophilia
- Hypotension co-existing with absent axillary or pubic hair in female
- Unexplained hypotension unresponsive to aggressive fluid replacement and to vasoactive drugs.

Pathogenesis of features of adrenal crisis

- Glucocorticoid deficiency: generalized weakness, anorexia, nausea and vomiting, hypoglycaemia, refractory hypotension, postural hypotension, shock
- Mineralocorticoid deficiency: dehydration, hyperkalaemia, hyponatraemia, acidosis, pre-renal azotaemia

Management

Blood for serum cortisol and adrenocorticotrophic hormone (ACTH): a random serum cortisol <100nmol/L is diagnostic; a plasma ACTH >100nmol/L indicates primary adrenocortical failure
- Check the patient's belongings for evidence of steroid use, as in tablets, creams, inhalers, and for the possession of a steroid card or a Medic-Alert bracelet
- Glucocorticoid: hydrocortisone 200mg (2mg/kg) IV bolus, then 100mg IM 6 hourly for 48h, or until oral replacement is possible

- IV fluid resuscitation: boluses of colloid (e.g. 500mL gelofusine) or crystalloid (1L 0.9% saline)
- Mineralocorticoid: fludrocortisone 50mg
- Treat hypoglycaemia
- Treat cause of crisis.

Equivalent steroid dosages

- Prednisolone 5mg
- Prednisone 5mg
- Hydrocortisone 20mg
- Methylprednisolone 4mg
- Betamethasone 750mcg
- Cortisone acetate 25mg
- Triamcinolone 4mg.

Hypothermia

Hypothermia is defined as a core (rectal/tympanic) temperature <35°C. Risk factors include extremes of age (infancy and the elderly), intoxication (alcohol, drugs), malnutrition and chronic illness. Contributory environmental and social factors include inadequate domestic heating, inadequate clothing and self-neglect.

Initial management for all hypothermic patients
- Remove wet garments
- Protect against heat loss and wind chill (use blankets and insulating equipment)
- Maintain horizontal position
- Avoid rough movement and excess activity
- Monitor core temperature, with a low reading rectal thermometer
- Continuous ECG monitoring; a 12-lead ECG may show sinus bradycardia, J waves, AF with slow ventricular response, and other atrial arrhythmias, which usually respond to rewarming.
- IV access; any administered IV fluids should be passed through a blood warmer; central venous access may be required
- Venous blood analysis may show raised or low potassium, raised urea and creatinine, and raised CK
- Defibrillation is often best postponed until the core temperature is ≥30°C
- If in cardiac arrest, continue resuscitation at least until core temperature >32°C.

The choice of further management depends on the core temperature.

External passive rewarming: core temperature 32–35°C
- Remove wet clothing and dry; avoid iatrogenic burns to the skin
- Wrap in warmed blankets/foil
- Warm environment
- Infra-red (radiant) heat.

Active surface rewarming
- Warm air heating blanket: Bair Hugger: heated air forced by a compressor through a blanket; air exits through apertures on the patient side of the cover, allowing convective heat transfer).

Active core rewarming: core temperature <32°C
- Warmed (37°C) IV fluids
- Warmed (42°C) and humidified gases for ventilation
- Warmed (42°C) fluid instillation in body cavities: pleural or peritoneal lavage
- Colonic irrigation
- Cardio pulmonary by-pass or continuous veno-venous haemofiltration.

Indications for active rewarming
- Cardiovascular instability
- Moderate/severe hypothermia: <32°C
- Inadequate rate or failure to rewarm
- Endocrine insufficiency
- Traumatic or toxic peripheral vasodilatation.

ECG changes in hypothermia
- Sinus bradycardia
- T wave inversion
- Prolonged QT interval
- Osborn J waves: most prominent in the mid- to lateral precordial leads; elevation of initial portion of ST segment; may be associated with reciprocal J point depression in aVR and V1
- Ventricular premature beats
- VF.

Checklist of risk factors in old age:
- Cognitive impairment
- Autonomic impairment
- Hypothalamic dysfunction
- Inadequate clothing
- Inadequate heating
- Immobility
- Falls
- Alcohol
- Hypothyroidism
- Drugs with vasodilator properties
- Socio-economic deprivation.

Frostbite

Features of frostbite

Mild injury
- Bright red and warm
- Pain
- Paraesthesiae
- Rapid onset of oedema
- Large vesicles early
- Superficial eschar later.

Deep injury
- Deep purple and red
- Minimal pain
- Small haemorrhagic wounds
- Slow onset of oedema
- Deep structures demarcate and mummify.

Management of frostbite

- Elevate the limb and leave uncovered at room temperature
- Leave haemorrhagic blisters intact.

Heat stroke

Features of heat stroke

- Exposure to heat stress: exogenous or endogenous
- Signs of severe CNS dysfunction
  - Seizures
  - Delirium
  - Coma
- Core temperature >40.5°C (105°F); usually 40–47°C
- Dry, hot skin is common; sweating may persist
- Marked rise in liver transaminases.

Methods of cooling

Based on conductive cooling

External:

- Cold water immersion
- Application of cold packs or ice slush over part or whole of the body
- Use of cooling blankets.

Internal:

- Iced gastric lavage
- Iced peritoneal lavage.

Based on evaporative or convective cooling

- Fanning the undressed patient at room temperature 20–22°C
- Wetting of body surface during continuous fanning
- Use of a body-cooling unit: a special bed that sprays atomized water at 15°C and warm air at 45°C over the whole body surface to keep the temperature of wet skin between 32 and 33°C.

Rhabdomyolysis

An acute increase in serum concentrations of CK to more than five times the upper normal limit—and when myocardial infarction has been excluded as a cause (CK-MB fraction <5%).

Visible myoglobinuria occurs when urinary myoglobin exceeds 250mcg/mL (normal <5ng/mL), corresponding to the destruction of >100g of muscle. Myoglobinuria can be inferred by a positive urine dipstick test for haem, in the absence of red cells on urine microscopy.

All causes of rhabdomyolysis lead to a critical increase in sarcoplasmic calcium and intracellular damage by activation of calcium-dependent proteases and phospholipases.

Causes

Ischaemia

- Compression injury
- Compartment syndrome.
- Vascular injury; reperfusion.

Muscle activity/injury

- Seizures
- Burns
- Electric injury
- Lightning
- Prolonged immobilization
- Pressure from hard surfaces in comatose patients.

Drugs

- Alcohol
- Opiates
- Cocaine
- LSD
- Amphetamines and ecstasy: serotonergic drugs
- Lipid-lowering drugs: statins
- Neuroleptic malignant syndrome: dopaminergic blockade; withdrawal of dopaminergic agents.

Infection

- *Escherichia coli*
- *Salmonella.*

Metabolic disease

- Diabetic ketoacidosis
- Hyperosmolar non-ketotic coma
- Genetically determined metabolic myopathy: glycolytic enzyme deficiencies; fatty acid oxidation disorders; mitochondrial myopathies.

Miscellaneous

- Limb tourniquet
- Arterial embolism.

Investigations

- CK/creatine phosphokinase × 5 upper limit of normal; peaks at 1–3 days; declines from 3–5 days
- U & E: hyperkalaemia; early hypocalcaemia; late hypercalcaemia; hyperuricaemia; hyperphosphataemia
- Arterial blood gases: metabolic acidosis
- Urinalysis: proteinuria, haematuria, myoglobinuria.

Clinical features

Muscular

- Pain
- Weakness
- Tenderness
- Stiffness.

Urinary

- Dark urine.

Non-specific

- Malaise
- Fever
- Tachycardia
- Nausea and vomiting.

Treatment

- Hydration: aim for urine output >300mL//h until urine is myoglobin, free, monitoring CVP, pulmonary artery occlusion pressure (intravascular volume expansion)
- Reduce hyperthermia
- Correct electrolyte imbalance:
  - Hyperkalaemia: glucose + insulin
  - Hyperphosphataemia: oral phosphate-binding agent (calcium carbonate)
  - Hypocalcaemia: normally corrects with correction of hypophosphataemia
- Correct acidosis
- Alkalinize urine with sodium bicarbonate to prevent dissociation of myoglobin into nephrotoxic metabolites
- Consider diuretics to dilute nephrotoxic substances
- Dantrolene sodium can reduce calcium-mediated myolysis
- Continuous haemofiltration or haemodialysis for uncontrolled hyperkalaemia, uraemic encephalopathy, acidosis or fluid overload.

Toxicology

Introduction to poisoning

Most poisoning episodes are self-limiting, requiring attention to maintaining airway patency, adequacy of ventilation and adequate tissue perfusion. In many instances, precise identification and quantification of the ingestion is not required to guide the treatment, which is essentially supportive and symptomatic.

Supportive care in acute poisoning

Airway patency and protective reflexes

- Suction
- Positioning: left lateral decubitus
- Oropharyngeal airway
- Endotracheal intubation after rapid sequence induction.

Breathing

- Oxygen
- Assisted ventilation

Circulation

- IV line(s)
- Head-down tilt
- Plasma volume expanders
- Vasoactive drugs: noradrenaline; dobutamine
- Urine output monitoring.

Symptomatic treatment

- Seizures
- Anticonvulsants
- Cardiac arrhythmia
- Correction of hypoxia or acidosis
- Hyperthermia
- Hypothermia
- Dystonic reaction.

History

- Determine nature and time of ingestion
- Determine co-ingestions, e.g. alcohol.

Source for further advice

TOXBASE: www.spib.axl.co.uk (requires password): the clinical toxicology database of the NPIS open to registered users only.

National telephone number (NPIS—National Poisons Information Service): 0870 600 6266.

Specific antidotes

- Anticholinergic agents: physostigmine
- Arsenic: dimercaprol
- Benzodiazepines: flumazenil
- Beta blockers: glucagon
- Calcium antagonists: calcium chloride or gluconate
- Cyanide: dicobalt edetate alone or sodium nitrite + sodium thiosulphate
- Digoxin: digoxin-specific antibody fragments (Digibind)
- Ethylene glycol: ethanol or 4-methylpyrazole
- Fluoride: calcium gluconate
- Iron: desferrioxamine
- Lead: dimercaprol or penicillamine
- Mercury: dimercaprol or penicillamine
- Methanol: ethanol or 4-methylpyrazole
- Opiates: naloxone
- Organophosphates: atropine
- Paracetamol: N-acetylcysteine; methionine
- Paraquat: Fuller's earth
- Thallium: Berlin Blue
- Warfarin: vitamin K or FFP.

Toxidromes (toxicological syndromes)

Antimuscarinic (anticholinergic) syndrome

- Tachycardia
- Dilated pupils (mydriasis)
- Dry, flushed, hot skin
- Dry mucosae
- Urinary retention
- Reduced bowel sounds: reduced peristalsis
- Mild elevation in body temperature
- Mild hypertension
- CNS: confusion, hallucinations, seizures, sedation, agitated delirium, myoclonic jerking and choreoathetoid movement
- Cardiac dysrhythmias.

Cholinergic (muscarinic) syndrome

- Excessive salivation
- Lacrimation
- Bronchorrhoea
- Wheezing
- Abdominal cramps: hyperperistalsis
- Urine and faecal incontinence
- Vomiting
- Sweating
- Miosis
- Bradycardia
- Muscle weakness and fasciculation
- PE
- Confusion or lethargy
- CNS depression
- Seizures.

Peripheral syndromes may be described as

- SLUDGE: salivation; lacrimation; diarrhoea; gastrointestinal motility, emesis
- BBB: bradycardia; bronchorrhoea; bronchospasm.

Sympathomimetic syndromes

- Tachycardia
- Hypertension; with severe hypertension, reflex bradycardia may occur
- Hyperthermia
- Sweating
- Dry mucosae
- Piloerection
- Mydriasis
- Hyper-reflexia
- Agitation
- Delirium

- Paranoid delusions
- Seizures
- Stroke
- Cardiac dysrhythmias.

Opioids

- Bradycardia
- CNS depression
- Reduced gastrointestinal motility
- Hypotension
- Miosis
- Respiratory depression.

Sedative–hypnotics

- Bradycardia
- CNS depression
- Hypotension
- Respiratory depression.

Benzodiazepines

- CNS depression
- Normal vital signs
- No respiratory depression in oral overdose without concomitant CNS depressants.

Sympatholytic syndrome

- Reduced BP
- Reduced pulse rate
- Low body temperature
- Small or pinpoint pupils
- Reduced peristalsis.

Beta blocker

Management of beta blocker toxicity

- Treat hypoglycaemia
- In the presence of bradycardia and hypotension:
  - IV fluids
  - Atropine
  - Beta agonists
  - Glucagon
  - Calcium
  - Vasopressors: dopamine; noradrenaline; dobutamine.

Glucagon 5–10mg IV (50–150mcg/kg in children), diluted in 10mL. saline as a bolus, followed by an infusion of 1–10mg/h depending on the response. Glucagon is only available in 1mg vials. It activates adenylate cyclase and increases myocardial cyclic AMP independently of beta receptors. Raising cyclic AMP levels has a positive inotropic and chrono-tropic effect. Vomiting is a useful indicator that an adequate dose of glucagon has been given and occasionally an anti-emetic may be required. Some patients do not respond and if vomiting has occurred without an effect on the blood pressure, further glucagon is unlikely to be of benefit.

- IV calcium
- Glucose–insulin–potassium regimen
- Cardiac pacing.

Cocaine

Presentations of cocaine toxicity

Cardiovascular
- VT or VF
- Heart block or asystole
- Unstable angina
- Myocardial infarction (usually non-Q wave)
- Severe hypertension
- Cardiomyopathy
- Aortic dissection.

Neurological
- Tremors; agitation
- Seizure or status epilepticus
- Excited delirium
- Coma
- Stroke: cerebral infarction
- Subarachnoid haemorrhage.

Psychiatric
- Euphoria
- Hallucinations
- Disorientation
- Acute toxic psychosis.

Pulmonary
- Bronchospasm
- Haemoptysis: alveolar haemorrhage
- Acute non-cardiogenic pulmonary oedema
- Hypersensitivity pneumonitis (crack lung)
- Pneumothorax, pneumomediastinum, pneumopericardium.

Systemic
- Rhabdomyolysis leading to myoglobinuric renal failure
- Hyperthermia
- Metabolic acidosis
- Gastrointestinal: bowel ischaemia; body packer syndrome; hepatitis
- Disseminated intravascular coagulation
- Obstetric and perinatal: spontaneous miscarriage, abruptio placentae, premature labour, neonatal cerebral infarction, neonatal seizures, neonatal myocardial infarction.

Management
- IV access
- ECG monitoring
- Diazepam 10mg IV slowly, for agitation, seizures, hyperadrenergic states
- Dantrolene 1mg/kg over 15min, repeated every 15min up to a maximum dose of 10mg/kg/24h, for hyperpyrexia
- IV calcium antagonists for ventricular tachycardia

- Consider CT head to rule out SAH in the presence of headache.
- Beta blockers are contraindicated as unopposed alpha-adrenergic activity may occur, leading to paradoxical increase in BP, and coronary artery vasoconstriction.
- Hypertension can be safely managed with either an alpha blocker such as phentolamine, or with vasodilators such as hydralazine, nitrates (GTN) and nitroprusside.
- Myocardial ischaemia should be initially treated with oxygen, aspirin and benzodiazepines. If there is continuing ischaemia, then vasodilators should be administered. Patients with persistent ST segment elevation should receive reperfusion with thrombolysis or PCI.
- Body packers should be treated with multidose activated charcoal and whole-bowel irrigation.

American Heart Association recommended treatment for cocaine-related myocardial ischaemia or infarction

First line agents
- Oxygen
- Aspirin
- Nitroglycerine
- Benzodiazepines.

Second-line agents
- Verapamil
- Phentolamine
- Thrombolytic agent or primary angioplasty.

Agent to be avoided
- Propranolol.

Digitalis

Digitalis toxicity

Digitalis is a therapeutic agent with a narrow therapeutic–toxic margin of action. Vigilance is needed to recognize and treat toxic complications.

ECG features

- Sino-atrial exit block or arrest
- AV block
- Atrial tachycardia with 2:1 AV block
- AF with slow and regular ventricular rate (regularization of AF)
- Non-paroxysmal junctional rhythm
- Frequent ventricular premature beats
- Ventricular bigeminy and trigeminy
- Fascicular tachycardia/bidirectional ventricular tachycardia
- VT.

Management of digitalis toxicity

- ECG monitoring
- Determine plasma potassium and maintain at 4mmol/L
- Discontinue digitalis and diuretics
- Monitor magnesium levels
- Monitor acid–base balance
- Observe until at least 6h post-ingestion
- Consider administration of repeat dose activated charcoal, especially if symptomatic
- Consider temporary pacemaker
- Fab fragments of antidigoxin antibodies: ventricular dysrhythmias; bradyarrhythmias with hypotension; hyperkalaemia >5.5mmol/L
- Avoid cardioversion.

Ecstasy

Ecstasy toxicity

Management

- Give oral activated charcoal 50g for an adult, 10–15g for a child, if within 1h of ingestion
- Observe for at least 4h if asymptomatic
- Monitor pulse, BP, cardiac rhythm and body temperature
- 12-lead ECG
- Measure U & E, creatinine, LFTs and CK
- If features of severe toxicity are present, monitor coagulation and arterial blood gases
- Diazepam 0.1–0.3mg/kg orally or IV to control anxiety and agitation. Control convulsions with diazepam 0.1–0.3mg/kg or lorazepam 4mg in an adult and 0.05mg/kg in a child
- Correct metabolic acidosis with sodium bicarbonate: 250mL of 1.26% contains 37.5mmol
- Treat symptomatic narrow complex tachycardias in an adult with beta blockers: esmolol or metoprolol
- If the systolic BP is >220 and diastolic >140mmHg in the absence of long-standing hypertension, give diazepam 0.1–0.3mg/kg in adults and children. Repeat doses may be necessary
- Correct hyperthermia with sedation and cooling. Dantrolene 1mg/kg by rapid IV injection to a maximum of 10mg/kg
- Treat liver failure by standard measures.

Paracetamol

Paracetamol overdose

Paracetamol is a common cause of deliberate self-poisoning in the UK, where it is the most common cause of acute liver failure. Paracetamol may be co-ingested with a variety of other toxins, and following national treatment guidelines is vitally important.

General information

- Time of ingestion: <1h; <8h; 8–15h; 15–24h; >24h; staggered; time unknown
- Amount ingested in milligrams
- Significant ingestion: >150mg/kg; >75mg/kg AND enhanced risk of liver damage
- Enhanced risk of liver damage
- Taking liver enzyme-inducing medications: carbamazepine; phenobarbitone; phenytoin; rifampicin; St John's wort
- High alcohol intake: >21U/week for a man; >14U/week for a woman
- At risk of glutathione ingestion: eating disorders; HIV infection; cystic fibrosis; malnutrition
- Known liver disease
- Co-ingestion.

Parvolex (N-acetylcysteine)

- 150mg/kg in 200mL 5% dextrose over 15min
- 50mg/kg in 500mL over 4h
- 100mg/kg in 1000mL: over 16h.

Levels in mmol/L		
Time of ingestion (h)	High risk	Normal risk
4	100	200
5	85	170
6	70	140
7	60	120
8	50	100
9	42.5	85
10	35	70
11	30	60
12	22.5	45
13	20	40
14	17.5	35
15	15	30

Toxic dose

- >150mg/kg or 12g
- >75mg/kg in high risk groups
- <1h: 50g charcoal orally
    Levels at 4h
- <4h: Levels at 4h
    Treat with *N*-acetylcysteine (NAC) based on levels
- 4–8h: Levels on arrival
    Treat with NAC as required
- 8–15h: Level on arrival
    Commence NAC if toxic dose ingested prior to obtaining result
- 15–24h: Levels on arrival + INR, LFT, U & E + venous blood gas
- >24h: Check INR, U&E, LFT, Venous blood gas (VBG)
    Commence NAC. Contact NPIS.

Staggered overdose: Start NAC and check INR, LFT, U & E, VBGs
Continue NAC at 150mg/kg/day.

Salicylate

Salicylate poisoning

Features

- Nausea and vomiting
- Epigastric pain
- Tinnitus
- Deafness
- Sweating
- Blurred vision
- Hyperpyrexia
- Dehydration
- Tachypnoea
- Non-cardiogenic pulmonary oedema
- Acute renal failure
- Mixed respiratory alkalosis and metabolic acidosis
- Hypokalaemia, hypernatraemia, hyponatraemia
- Hyperglycaemia; hypoglycaemia
- Hypoprothrombinaemia
- Confusion
- Delirium
- Coma.

Early management

Dose ingested

- >120mg/kg
  - Adult: give 50g activated charcoal
  - Child: give 1g/kg activated charcoal.

Consider charcoal even for late presenting patients; peak absorption may be delayed up to 12h post-ingestion especially with enteric coated tablets

- >500mg/kg
  - Adults only: consider gastric lavage followed by 50g activated charcoal, if patient presents within 1h.

Maintenance management

- Check salicylate levels 4h post-ingestion; then every 2–3h until peak concentration is achieved and levels are falling consistently
- If history is reliable for an ingestion >120mg/kg and tablets are enteric coated, consider measuring levels for minimum 12h post-ingestion even if no salicylate is detected initially
- Monitor and correct U & Es, arterial blood gases and pH, blood sugar, PT
- Rehydrate (oral or IV fluids) to correct dehydration. Moderate or severe cases may need CVP monitoring
- Repeat doses of activated charcoal: adult 25–50g; child 1g/kg every 4h until salicylate level has peaked and is consistently falling, to prevent delayed absorption.

Urine alkalinization
- Indications: moderate or severe toxicity
- Alkaline urine (pH 7.5–8.5 optimally) enhances salicylate elimination
- Forced alkaline diuresis is not recommended because of the risk of fluid overload
- Adults: 1L of 1.26% sodium bicarbonate (isotonic) + 40mmol KCl IV over 4h and/or 50mL IV bolus of 8.4% sodium bicarbonate, ideally via a central line
- Children: 1mL/kg 8.4% sodium bicarbonate + 20mmol KCl diluted in 0.5L dextrose saline infused at 2–3mL/kg/h
- Hypokalaemia prevents urinary excretion of alkali so must be corrected.
- Check urine pH hourly aiming for pH 7.5–8.5
- The rate of bicarbonate administration alone may need to be increased if pH remains <7.5
- Check U&E every 2–4h and keep K^+ between 4.0–4.5.

Indications for haemodlalysis
- Renal failure
- Congestive heart failure
- Non-cardiogenic pulmonary oedema
- Convulsions
- CNS effects not resolved by correction of acidosis
- Acid–base or electrolyte imbalance resistant to correction
- Persistently high salicylate concentrations unresponsive to urine alkalinization.

Additional criteria relating to severity
- Age >70 or <10yrs
- CNS features
- Hyperpyrexia
- Metabolic acidosis
- Pulmonary oedema
- Late presentation.

Aspirin risk assessment

Table 11.1 Salicylate risk assessment

Ingested dose (mg/kg body weight)	Estimated severity
<150	Toxicity not expected
150–300	Mild to moderate toxicity
300–500	Serious toxicity
>500	Potentially fatal

Table 11.2 Peak concentration interpretation

Adult	Child/elderly	Management
<350mg/L (2.52mmol/L)	<250mg/L (1.8mmol/L)	Mild clinical effects; further treatment unlikely to be necessary
<500 m/L (3.6mmol/L)	<350 mg/L (2.52mmol/L)	Mild clinical effects; continue maintenance management
500–700mg/L (3.6–5.04mmol/L)	350–600mg/L (2.52–4.32mmol/L)	Moderate clinical effects; continue maintenance management and institute urine alkalinisation
>700mg/L (5.04mmol/L)	>600mg/L (4.32mmol/L)	Severe clinical effects; haemodialysis recommended

Tricyclic antidepressant

Management
- Assess and treat ABC as appropriate
- Correct hypoxia
- ECG monitoring; monitor QRS duration: when <100m, significant toxicity is unlikely to occur; QRS duration >100m is associated with an increased risk of seizures; QRS duration>160m is associated with a high risk of ventricular dysrhythmias.
- IV access
- 50g charcoal if within 1h of ingestion
- Check U & E: look for low potassium
- Check arterial blood gases: look for metabolic and respiratory acidosis.
- Correct metabolic acidosis
    - Serum alkalinization with parenteral sodium bicarbonate boluses (1mmol/kg)
    - Target pH for alkalinization: 7.45–7.55.

The distribution of tricyclic antidepressants within the body largely depends on the degree of ionization of the drug. Low pH favours ionization of the drug, reducing lipid solubility and tissue affinity. Plasma binding is decreased by a low pH.

Lignocaine should be used to treat ventricular dysrhythmias if systemic alkalinization fails.

- DC cardioversion for tachyarrhythmias with haemodynamic compromise
- Treat seizures with diazepam or lorazepam; phenytoin is contraindicated
- Physostigmine is no longer recommended to treat anticholinergic manifestations as its use has been associated with seizures, vomiting, bradycardia, asystole and death
- Patients who display signs of toxicity should be monitored for a minimum of 12h
- With cardiac arrest, prolonged resuscitation may be successful.
- Indications for systemic alkalinization: 300mL of 1.26% sodium bicarbonate
pH <7.1
QRS >160msec
Cardiac arrhythmias
Hypotension.

Carbon monoxide

Exogenous sources

- Internal combustion engines: exhaust fumes (deliberate poisoning); catalytic converters do not prevent carbon monoxide poisoning completely
- Smoke inhalation
- Incomplete coal burning
- Burning of fossil fuels in oxygen-restricted environments or with poor exhaust outlets
- Badly installed ,poorly maintained or malfunctioning domestic combustion appliances using gas, oil or solid fuel, or the use of such appliances in inadequately ventilated areas
- Tobacco smoke
- Methylene chloride (dichloromethane), found in paint removers and other solvents.

Clues to the diagnosis of domestic carbon monoxide poisoning

- More than one person in the house affected, including pets
- Symptoms better when away from the house, e.g. on holiday, but recur on returning home
- Symptoms related to cooking; stove in use
- Symptoms worse in winter; heating in use.

Carboxyhaemoglobin levels

- Measured in a heparinized blood sample (arterial or venous)
- Useful biomarker of exposure to carbon monoxide
- Poor correlation between COHb levels and symptom severity
- Patients with identical COHb levels can show wide variations in clinical manifestations
- Symptomatic levels 30–50%
- Significant risk of tissue hypoxic injury 50–70%
- Death 0–75%

Criteria for admission for carbon monoxide poisoning

Indications

- Carboxyhaemoglobin >20% or >15% in the presence of cardiac or pulmonary disease
- Loss of consciousness at any time
- Neurological signs and symptoms, other than headache
- Myocardial ischaemia; cardiac arrhythmia
- Pregnancy
- Metabolic acidosis.

Treatment of carbon monoxide poisoning

- 100% oxygen by tight fitting mask with an inflated face-seal until carboxyhaemoglobin falls below 5%. On this regimen the half-life of carboxyhaemoglobin is 74min (compared with 320min breathing air)
- Complete bed rest
- Sedate if necessary

- Monitor blood gases and correct pH
- Monitor BP and give IV fluids if necessary
- Monitor ECG and ICP
- Control convulsions with diazepam
- Consider hyperbaric oxygen therapy: the half-life of carboxyhaemoglobin at 3 absolute atmospheres of oxygen is only 23 min
- Arrange checking of appliances and flues and measurement of CO concentration in the house before allowing anyone back.

Hyperbaric oxygen

Indications
- Neurological signs including a reduced level of consciousness
- History of unconsciousness at any stage without another explanation
- Carboxyhaemoglobin level >40%
- Pregnancy (very high affinity for foetal haemoglobin), with carboxyhaemoglobin level >15%
- Cardiac arrhythmia or ischaemia diagnosed by ECG
- Symptoms not resolving on normobaric oxygen over 4–6h.

Contraindications
- Asthma
- Cardiac arrhythmias that may need immediate correction
- Claustrophobia
- Theoretical benefits of hyperbaric oxygen
- Faster reduction in carboxyhaemoglobin levels. The half-life of carboxyhaemoglobin at 3 absolute atmospheres of oxygen is 23min
- Increased intracellular delivery of oxygen
- Impairment of platelet adhesion in the capillaries
- Improved mitochondrial function
- Reduced neutrophil activation and adherence, reducing lipid peroxidation.

Half-life of carbon monoxide
- In air: 4–6h
- In 100% oxygen: 40–80min
- In hyperbaric oxygen: 15–30min

Neurological examination should include
- Tests of fine movement and balance (finger–nose movement, Romberg's test, normal gait and heel–toe walking)
- Mini-Mental State examination
- Testing of short-term memory and ability to subtract 7, serially, from 100.

Gastrointestinal and gynaecological resuscitation

Caustic burns of the oesophagus

Features

- Oro-pharyngeal pain and mucosal burns
- Excessive salivation and drooling of saliva
- Refusal to eat and drink
- Dysphagia
- Airway obstruction, with stridor
- Subcutaneous emphysema in the neck with palpable crepitus
- Retrosternal and epigastric pain in the presence of full-thickness oesophageal injury
- Haematemesis.

Management

- Management of A, B, C
- The passage of a nasogastric tube is contraindicated
- Referral for early fibreoptic oesophagoscopy, which allows grading of severity and planning of ongoing management.

Barogenic rupture of oesophagus

Mackler's triad

- Vomiting or retching
- Lower thoracic pain
- Subcutaneous emphysema.

Upper gastrointestinal bleeding

Haematemesis and melaena signify upper gastrointestinal bleeding, arising proximal to the ligament of Treitz. The extent of revealed bleeding does not necessarily correlate with the actual loss of blood volume.

Initial assessment

- Estimated blood loss
- Alcohol abuse
- Medications: aspirin/NSAID/warfarin/hepatotoxin ingestion
- Pulse rate; BP (standing and lying)
- Skin: pallor; jaundice; spider naevi; telangiectasia; purpura; hyperpigmentation
- Signs of chronic liver disease and portal hypertension (suggests varices)
- Prior abdominal aortic aneurysm repair: suggests aorto-enteric fistula
- Abdominal mass; hepatosplenomegaly
- Co-morbidity
- Melaena: blood in gastrointestinal tract >14h
- Preceding retching and vomiting (Mallory–Weiss tear).

Causes of upper gastrointestinal bleeding

- Peptic ulceration
- Oesophagitis
- Mallory–Weiss tear of lower oesophagus
- Oesophageal varices
- Gastric erosions
- Tumours
- Swallowed blood from nasal bleeding
- Rare:
  - Aneurysms: aortic; splenic artery
  - Aorto-enteric fistula
  - Arterial malformations (Dieulafoy lesion)
  - Pancreatic tumours; chronic pancreatitis
  - Haemobilia: haemorrhage into a biliary duct
  - Hereditary haemorrhagic telangiectasia
  - Pseudoxanthoma elasticum.
  - Haemostatic disorders.

Coffee ground vomit

- Any dark liquid: bile; faeculent vomit
- Thin liquid with black bits: gastric stasis
- Thick, black, grainy liquid: true altered blood.

High risk gastrointestinal bleeding

- Age >60yrs
- Syncope
- Systolic BP <100mmHg
- Postural hypotension (orthostatic decrease of 20mmHg in systolic BP or postural increase in pulse rate of 20 beats/min)
- >4 units blood transfused in 12h

- Significant co-morbidity (cardiac, respiratory, renal, malignancy, neurological disease)
- Coagulopathy.

Investigations
- FBC
- Renal and liver function tests: disproportionate rise in urea over creatinine
- Group and cross-match
- Clotting screen
- 12-lead ECG.

Initial management
- High concentration inspired oxygen
- Two large bore upper limb IV lines
- Volume replacement: aim for pulse <100bpm; Systolic BP >100mmHg; urine output >30mL/h
- Urethral catheterization with hourly urine output monitoring for large volume bleed
- Correction of coagulopathy
- Packed cell transfusions for low HCt; maintain haemoglobin between 8 and 10g/dl
- Withdraw aspirin and NSAIDs
- IV proton pump inhibitor: omeprazole 80mg IV bolus followed by infusion at 8mg/h over 72h, with peptic ulcer bleed with bleeding stigmata; keeps gastric pH <6
- Referral for endoscopy, usually performed within 12h
- Surgical intervention may be required for continued bleeding.

Indications for CVP line
- Large volume bleed
- Co-existing renal/cardiac failure
- Persistent hypotension/tachycardia
- Suspected/proven varices.

Special measures for bleeding oesophageal varices
It is useful to remember that most alcoholics with gastrointestinal bleeding do not have chronic liver disease (or varices)
- Airway protection is indicated in the presence of severe uncontrolled bleeding, haemodynamic instability, severe encephalopathy and an SpO_2 <90%
- Cross-match 6 units of blood; conservative blood replacement
- CVP line
- Correct coagulopathy
- Terlipressin 2mg IV bolus followed by 1–2mg 4–6 hourly for up to 72h; or vasopressin 0.2–0.4U/min IV infusion for up to 72h, titrated to response up to maximum of 0.9U/min. The solution for infusion is prepared by dissolving 20U of vasopressin is dissolved in 100ml 5% dextrose, OR
- Octreotide 50–100mcg IV loading dose, followed by infusion at 25mcg/h to a maximum of 50mcg/h (500mcg in 50mL 0.9% saline at 5mL/h)

Rockall prognostic score. The higher the Rockall score, the greater the risk of rebleeding and death.

Age
<60	0
60–79	1
>80	2

Shock
Pulse <100bpm; Systolic BP >100mmHg	0
Pulse >100bpm; Systolic BP >100mmHg	1
Pulse >100bpm; Systolic BP <100mmHg	2

Co-morbidity
No major co-morbidity	0
Cardiac failure; ischaemic heart disease; any other co-morbidity	2
Renal failure; liver failure; disseminated malignancy	3

Endoscopic stigmata
None; dark spot seen	0
Blood in upper gastrointetinal tract; adherent clot; visible or spurting vessel	2

Diagnosis
Mallory–Weiss tear; no lesion seen and no stigmata of recent haemorrhage	0
All other diagnoses	1
Upper gastrointestinal tract malignancy	2

- Prophylactic antibiotics
- Flexible fibreoptic endoscopy at the earliest possible time
- Consider Sengstaken–Blakemore tube; prior airway protection ±
High risk lesions on endoscopy
- Active bleeding at the time of endoscopy
- Visible vessels in ulcer
- A sentinel clot over the ulcer
- Recurrent bleeding in hospital.

Sengstaken–Blakemore tube insertion
- Wear surgical scrubs and full protective clothing including face visor and mask
- Submerge balloons underwater and test inflation with air to identify any leaks
- The left lateral position is best if the patient is vomiting
- Deflate balloons and pass tube orally beyond 50cm.
- Inflate gastric balloon with 300mL. water/10% hypaque; ultrasonographic confirmation of placement is possible by recognizing echogenic bubbles after inflation with 50mL air initially

Rockall, TA, Logan, RF, Devlin, HB, *et al.* Risk assessment after acute upper gastrointestinal haemorrhage *Gut.* 1996; **38**: 316–321.

- Pull tube up until resistance is felt, owing to the gastric balloon impinging on the oesophago-gastric junction
- Gauze tape to secure tube to face or 500mL bag of fluid as traction
- A CXR can be taken to confirm tube position
- Check hourly that the tube has not slipped back down
- Gastric aspirate-free drainage. Flush with air or 20mL water every 30min
- Oesophageal aspirate—continuous suction or drainage
- Do not routinely use the oesophageal balloon
- The gastric balloon should be deflated 12 hourly
- When used, the oesophageal balloon is inflated to 30–40mmHg and deflated 6 hourly.

Components of Sengstaken–Blakemore tube

- Gastric balloon
- Oesophageal balloon
- Tube for gastric aspiration
- Tube for pharyngeal aspiration.

Acute liver failure

Features

- Jaundice
- Encephalopathy: altered level of consciousness; abnormal behaviour; liver flap
- Hyperdynamic circulation (high cardiac output; reduced systemic vascular resistance and mean arterial pressure)
- Coagulopathy
- Renal failure
- Gastric stress ulceration
- Metabolic acidosis
- Lung disease: acute respiratory distress syndrome; pulmonary arterio-venous shunting with hypoxaemia
- Cerebral oedema.

Causes

- Toxic: paracetamol overdose; *Amanita phalloides*
- Viral agents: hepatitis A, B, C, D, E
- Drug reaction
- Metabolic disorders: hepatolenticular degeneration; Reye's and Reye's-like syndromes.

Investigations

- Venous blood: FBC; U & E; LFT; clotting screen; hepatitis serology; paracetamol levels
- Arterial blood gases
- 12-lead ECG
- Ultrasound of liver and biliary tree
- Investigations may reveal hypoglycaemia, hyponatraemia, hypokalaemia, hypocalcaemia, hypomagnesaemia and renal failure.

Management

- A, B, C
- Monitor blood glucose and treat hypoglycaemia with 10–20% glucose infusion
- Treat coagulopathy: vitamin K
- Avoid blood product use if possible
- NAC infusion for paracetamol toxicity; can be used in other causes of acute liver failure although benefits are not proven
- Reduce gut nitrogen load: lactulose 20–30mL qds; $MgSO_4$ enemas
- Prophylactic H2 receptor antagonist
- No sedatives or opiates
- Mannitol for cerebral oedema: 1g/kg of 20% solution.

King's College Hospital criteria for liver transplantation

Paracetamol-induced acute liver failure

- Arterial pH <7.3 (irrespective of the grade of encephalopathy)

OR

- The presence of the following together:
  - PT >100s
  - Grade III/IV encephalopathy
  - Creatinine >300micromol/L

Non-paracetamol-induced acute liver failure
- The presence of three of the following
  - Age <10 or >40yrs
  - Aetiology of non-A, non-B, or drug/halothane-induced acute liver failure
  - Bilirubin >300micromol/L
  - Jaundice to encephalopathy time >7 days
  - PT >50s

OR

  - PT >100s

Acute pancreatitis

Causes
- Obstructive:
  - Gallstones
  - Pancreatic and ampullary tumours (periampullary carcinoma)
  - Afferent loop obstruction following gastric surgery
- Toxins:
  - Alcohol
  - Scorpion venom (ampullary spasm)
- Idiopathic
- Iatrogenic: post-endoscopic retrograde cholangio-pancreatography (ERCP); abdominal surgery

Rare causes
- Congenital pancreatic abnormalities: pancreas divisum
- Trauma: blunt (e.g. bicycle handlebar injury, seat belt injury), penetrating
- Post-renal transplant
- Drugs: thiazide diuretics, steroids, azathioprine
- Viral infections: mumps, Coxsackie B virus, cytomegalovirus, hepatitis A and B
- Hypercalcaemia: hyperparathyroidism
- Hyperlipidaemia
- Vascular
- Hypothermia.

Features
- Upper abdominal pain, may radiate to back or chest
- Nausea and vomiting
- Epigastric tenderness and guarding
- Abdominal distension
- Mild jaundice
- Low grade fever
- Hypovolaemic shock
- Signs of retroperitoneal haemorrhage
  - Grey Turner's sign: flank discolouration (ecchymosis)
  - Cullen's sign: periumbilical discolouration (ecchymosis)
  - Fox's sign: inguinal ligament ecchymosis
- Subcutaneous fat necrosis.

Investigations
- Serum amylase: ×4 normal (diagnostic): remember that amylase levels may not reach diagnostic levels in the presence of acute relapses superimposed on chronic pancreatitis with loss of exocrine cell mass; amylase level does not correlate with prognosis
- Urine amylase
- Serum lipase: ×2 normal
- FBC
- U & E

- Calcium
- Glucose
- Blood gases
- LFT
- CXR: raised hemidiaphragm; pleural effusion; atelectasis; pulmonary infiltrates
- Abdominal X-ray: sentinel loop; colon cut-off sign; obliteration of psoas shadows
- Early imaging to elucidate cause: ultrasound of the biliary tree
- CT usually done after day 3.

Management of acute pancreatitis
- Low threshold for referral for critical care admission
- Pulmonary support
- Arterial blood gas monitoring
- Oxygen (if hypoxaemic on room air)
- CPAP often helpful if pleural effusions present or acute lung injury developing
- Assisted ventilation with PEEP for worsening respiratory failure
- Fluid resuscitation:
  - IV colloid challenges, guided by CVP monitoring
  - Correct electrolyte imbalance
  - Blood transfusion
- Pain relief: titrated IV opioid analgesia
- Nasogastric tube placement
  - Enteral feeding possible especially via post-pyloric feeding tube
  - IV feeding if enteral route not possible
- Close monitoring of renal function
- Plasma calcium monitoring
- Plasma glucose monitoring; control of hyperglycaemia with insulin
- Antibiotic therapy: phlegmon; occluded bile duct
- Early ERCP and sphincterotomy: acute pancreatitis due to biliary obstruction with sepsis.

Severity markers
Ranson criteria
The presence of three or more criteria defines severe acute pancreatitis:

At presentation
- Age >55yrs
- WBC >16 × 10^9/L
- Blood glucose >10mmol/L (non-diabetic)
- Serum lactate dehydrogenase (LDH) >350U/L
- Serum aspartate transaminase >250U/L.

During first 48h
- HCt fall >10%
- Urea rise >10mmol/L
- Serum Ca <2.0mmol/L
- Base deficit >4mmol/L

- $PaO_2 < 8kPa$
- Serum albumin <32g/L
- Fluid requirement >6L.

Differential diagnosis of hyperamylasaemia
Intra-abdominal
- Perforated hollow viscus
- Mesenteric infarction
- Biliary obstruction
- Ruptured ectopic pregnancy.

Impaired renal clearance of amylase
- Renal failure
- Macroamylasaemia.

Early pregnancy complications

Collapsed miscarriage patient
- Two large bore upper limb IV lines
- Venous blood for FBC, group and save/cross-match; clotting screen
- Per speculum examination and removal of products of conception from the cervical os. The cervical shock syndrome represents a degree of shock disproportionate to the extent of blood loss, and is caused by cervical distension by the products of conception.
- Ergometrine if the cervical os is open
- Gynaecological referral.

Collapsed ectopic pregnancy
- Two large bore upper limb IV lines
- Venous blood for FBC, group and save/cross-match; clotting screen
- Urethral catheter for urine beta-human chorionic gonadotrophin (H) or venous blood beta-HCG
- Avoid vaginal examination; in stable patients one might expect to elicit cervical motion tenderness (cervical excitation), and a tender unilateral adnexal mass may be felt
- Urgent gynaecological referral
- Notify operating theatres.

> ### Risk factors for ectopic pregnancy
>
> - Previous ectopic pregnancy
> - Long history of infertility
> - Tubal surgery
> - Assisted conception techniques
> - Pelvic inflammatory disease
> - Intrauterine contraceptive device *in situ*
> - Progesterone-only oral contraceptive pill
> - Congenital abnormalities of the genital tract

Suggestive clinical features
- The triad of ≥2 weeks of amenorrhoea, irregular vaginal bleeding and lower abdominal pain
- Unilateral pain
- Vaginal bleeding
- Pain with defaecation; diarrhoea
- Pain on sexual intercourse
- Faintness; syncope
- Shoulder tip pain.

Sepsis

SIRS criteria

Systemic inflammatory response syndrome criteria for diagnosis

Two or more of the following:
- Temperature >38°C or <36°C
- Heart rate >90bpm
- Respiratory rate >20 breaths/min (or $PaCO_2$ <4.3 kPa (32mmHg))
- White cell count >12 000 cells/mm^3 or <4000 cells/mm^3 or >10% immature (band) forms.
- For every 1°C rise in body temperature, the heart rate increases by 10 bpm and the respiratory rate by four breaths per min.

Sepsis = SIRS + documented source of infection

Sepsis syndrome = sepsis + altered organ perfusion or evidence of dysfunction of one or more end-organs:
- Cardiovascular system: lactate >1.2mmol/L; SVR <800dynes/s/cm^3
- Respiratory: PaO_2/FiO_2 <30; PaO_2 <9.3kPa
- Renal: urine output <120mL over 4h

CNS: GCS <15 in absence of sedation or neurological lesion.

Septic shock = SIRS + hypotension refractory to volume replacement alone

Septic shock

Pathophysiology of septic shock

(a high-output, low-resistance state of hyperdynamic circulation)
- Tachycardia
- Arterial hypotension
- Reduced systemic vascular resistance: vasodilatation and venous pooling of blood, leading to refractory hypotension
- High cardiac output
- Reduced splanchnic blood flow leading to intestinal ischaemia
- Increased capillary endothelial permeability leading to a capillary leak state with third space losses
- Depressed myocardial contractility
- Low to normal pulmonary capillary wedge pressure
- Normal or raised mixed venous oxygen concentration.

Monitoring in septic shock
- ECG
- Non-invasive blood pressure
- Pulse oximetry
- Hourly urine output
- Arterial line should be considered.

Initial investigations in sepsis
- Venous blood: FBC; renal and liver function tests; inflammatory markers: CRP, pro-calcitonin, ESR/plasma viscosity; culture and sensitivity (two samples at least); coagulation screen.

Goal-directed approach to septic shock

This approach involves optimization of cardiac preload, afterload and contractility to balance oxygen delivery with oxygen demand. The resuscitation end-points in the first 6 hours (sepsis handle) include:

- Urine output >0.5mL/kg/h
- CVP 8–12mmHg
- MAP 65–90mmHg
- $ScvO_2$ (central venous oxygen saturation—superior vena cava or right atrium) >70% during emergency department resuscitation
- Arterial lactate concentration <3mmol/L
- Base deficit—5 or less
- pH 7.35 or above.

Interventions in goal-directed therapy for haemodynamic optimization

- Supplemental oxygen
- Endotracheal intubation and mechanical ventilation
- Central venous and arterial catheter placement
- Sedation, paralysis (if intubated) or both
- Low CVP: crystalloid; colloid
- Low/high MAP: vasopressors/vasodilators
- Low $ScvO_2$: red blood cell transfusion (to Hct of 30%); inotropic agents (dobutamine).

Antimicrobials in sepsis

- Second-generation cephalosporins
  - Cefuroxime 750mg–1.5g IV 8 hourly
- Third-generation cephalosporins
  - Cefotaxime 1–2g IV 12 hourly
  - Ceftriaxone 1–2g IV 12 hourly
  - Ceftazidime 1–2g IV 8 hourly
- Vancomycin 1g IV 12 hourly
- Teicoplanin 400mg 12 hourly
- Meropenem 2g IV 8 hourly
- Amoxycillin 1g IV 6 hourly
- Flucloxacillin 1g IV 6 hourly
- Metronidazole 500mg IV 8 hourly.

Remember the door to needle time!

American College of Chest Physician/Society of Critical Care Medicine Consensus Conference: definitions for sepsis and organ failure and guidelines for the use of innovative therapies in sepsis. *Critical Care Medicine*, 1992; **20**: 864–874.

Rivers EP. Early goal-directed therapy in the treatment of severe sepsis and septic shock. *New England Journal Medicine*, 2001; **345**: 1368–1377.

Dellinger RP, Carlet JM, Masur H, *et al.* Surviving Sepsis Campaign: Guidelines for management of severe sepsis and septic shock. *Intensive care medicine* 2004; **30**: 536–555.

The ill patient with fever and skin rash

Petechial or purpuric rash
- Bacterial: meningococcaemia; gonococcaemia
- Viral: viral haemorrhagic fevers; atypical measles; enteroviral infections.

Diffuse maculo-papular rash
- Bacterial: early meningococcemia; *mycoplasma*
- Viral: measles; acute HIV infection; infectious mononucleosis; hepatitis B
- Rickettsial.

Vesiculo-bullous rash
- Toxic epidermal necrolysis
- Disseminated herpes zoster
- Varicella
- Echthyma gangrenosum.

Diffuse erythematous rash
- Staphylococcal scalded skin syndrome
- Toxic shock syndrome
- Scarlet fever syndrome
- Kawasaki syndrome.

Toxic shock syndrome

Toxic shock syndrome is a multisystem inflammatory toxin-mediated disease associated with infection caused by either *Staphylococcus aureus* or group A beta-haemolytic *Streptococcus*. In children, particularly, it can complicate otherwise minor burns.

Diagnostic criteria

Major criteria

- Fever: temperature ≥38.7°C
- Rash: diffuse, macular erythroderma
- Mucosal membranes: hyperaemia, oropharyngeal or conjunctival
- Desquamation: 1–2wks after onset of illness (typically palms and soles)
- Hypotension: systolic BP ≤ fifth percentile by age (children under 16yrs of age) or systolic BP ≤90mmHg (adults), or orthostatic hypotension.

Minor criteria

Multisystem dysfunction—at least three:

- Chest: tachypnoea; tachycardia
- Gut: vomiting and/or diarrhoea at onset of illness
- Renal function: diminished urine output or raised plasma creatinine ≥ twice the upper limit of normal, or pyuria (≥5 leukocytes per high-power field) in the absence of urinary tract infection
- Hepatic: serum bilirubin or liver enzymes (AST/ALT) elevated ≥ twice the upper limit of normal
- CNS: confusion or irritability
- Haematologic: <100 × 10⁹/L platelets; >10.0 × 10⁹/L neutrophils.

Clinical settings

Menstrual TSS

- Tampon-associated
- Not tampon-associated.

Non-menstrual TSS

- TSS related to the female genitourinary tract. Associated with barrier contraception use (diaphragm, contraceptive sponges) occurring in the puerperium following non-obstetric gynaecological surgery associated with septic abortion
- TSS related to skin or soft tissue infections primary staphylococcal infections (folliculitis, cellulitis, carbuncle, muscle abscesses)
- Staphylococcal super-infections of pre-existing lesions (burns, insect bites, varicella zoster infections, surgical wounds)
- TSS related to respiratory tract infections: upper respiratory tract focus (sinusitis, pharyngitis, laryngotracheitis, odontogenic infection). Lower respiratory tract focus (staphylococcal pneumonia)
- TSS related to skeletal infections: osteomyelitis, septic arthritis.

Illnesses that may resemble TSS
- Severe group A streptococcal infections: scarlet fever, necrotizing fasciitis, toxic shock-like syndrome
- Kawasaki syndrome
- Staphylococcal scalded skin syndrome
- Rocky Mountain spotted fever (USA)
- Leptospirosis
- Meningococcaemia
- Gram-negative sepsis
- Exanthematous viral syndromes: measles, adenovirus infection, certain enteroviral infections, Dengue
- Severe allergic drug reactions.

A useful resource is the toxic shock syndrome information service at 24–28 Bloomsbury Way, London WC1A 2PX (Telephone: 020 7404 2120).

Management is for impending shock + antibiotics + immunoglobulin.

MARS BAR score for TSS

Mental state	Irritable/drowsy	2
	Hypertonic/floppy	5
Appearance	Shocked/sick	5
Renal output	<0.5mL/kg/h	2
Skin	Rash only	2
	Pyrexia >40°C	3
Blood	Heart rate >140	1
	Haemoglobin <9g/L	3
	Platelets	1
	WBC <6.0	5
	Hypocalcaemia	1
Alimentary	Diarrhoea	5
	Vomiting	2
	Abdominal distension	2
Respiratory	Tachypnoea	1
Total		40

Score	Action
0–9	No treatment
10–15	Suspect; probably treat
16–25	Highly suggestive
>25	Diagnostic

Necrotizing soft tissue infections

Classification
- Cellulitis: clostridial; non-clostridial. Involves superficial fascia and subcutaneous tissue
- Necrotizing fasciitis: monomicrobial (type II; group A *Streptococcus*); polymicrobial (type I; mixed aerobic and anaerobic). Involves deep fascia and involves progressive destruction of fat and fascia, while the skin may remain intact
- Myonecrosis: involves muscle.

Necrotizing fasciitis

Clinical findings
Early
- Pain
- Cellulitis, especially refractory to treatment
- Fever
- Tachycardia
- Swelling
- Induration
- Skin anaesthesia.

Late
- Severe pain out of proportion to local findings
- Oedema and tenderness beyond the limits of skin erythema
- Skin discoloration: purple or black
- Blistering
- Haemorrhagic bullae
- Palpable crepitus
- Discharge of 'dishwater' fluid.

With progression:
- Severe sepsis or SIRS
- Disseminated intravascular coagulation
- Acute renal failure from hypovolaemia and/or rhabdomyolysis
- Cardiovascular collapse
- Multiorgan failure.

Adjuncts to help diagnosis
Laboratory investigations
- Leukocytosis with left shift
- Metabolic acidosis
- Raised serum CK
- Altered coagulation profile
- Hypoalbuminaemia
- Abnormal renal function.

Plain radiography
- Soft tissue gas.

CT or MRI
- May delineate extent of disease
- Soft tissue gas.

Incisional exploration or biopsy (can be done at the bedside)
- Histological confirmation of diagnosis
- Tissue culture to identify pathogens and sensitivities.

Management
- Early recognition is the key to successful treatment
- IV antibiotics
- IV fluid resuscitation
- Packed cell transfusions
- Ventilatory support
- Aggressive early and complete surgical debridement; incisions to deep fascia; excision of all non-viable tissue
- Surgical re-exploration 24–48hrs later
- Repeated debridements may be necessary.

Malaria

With widespread long-distance travel to exotic locations for both business and pleasure, the possibility of contracting malaria has assumed increasing importance. A thorough travel history, including details of stay in malaria-endemic zones is mandatory for all acutely unwell patients, especially in the presence of unexplained illness. *Plasmodium falciparum* infection is specially noteworthy because of its propensity to cause micro-circulatory effects from schizogony in deep capillaries, in the brain, kidneys, liver and lungs.

Investigations
Venous blood
- FBC
- U & E; LFTs
- Clotting screen
- Thick and thin blood films for malarial parasites: at least three negative films at intervals.

Management of acute attack
- Chloroquine-sensitive benign malaria: oral chloroquine for 3 days
- Chloroquine-resistant malaria; falciparum malaria: oral quinine for 7 days then maloprim if quinine resistance suspected (tetracycline if maloprim-resistant)
- Severe disease: IV quinine infusion; intensive care as necessary.

Plasmodium falciparum malaria
WHO criteria for severe disease:
- Cerebral malaria
- Severe normocytic anaemia
- Hct <15% or haemoglobin <5g/dL in the presence of parasitaemia >10 000/μL
- Renal failure: urine output <400mL/24h in adults or 12mL/kg/24h in children failing to improve after rehydration
- Serum creatinine >265μmol/L(3.0mg/dL)
- Pulmonary oedema or ARDS
- Hypoglycaemia: whole blood glucose <2.2mmol/L (40mg/dL)
- Circulatory collapse (shock)
- Systolic BP <70mmHg in adult or <50mmHg in children aged 1–5yrs
- Spontaneous bleeding from gums, nose, gastrointestinal tract, etc. and/or substantial laboratory evidence of disseminated intravascular coagulation
- Repeated generalized convulsions
- Academia: arterial pH <7.25; plasma HCO_3 <15mmol/L
- Macroscopic haemoglobinuria (not drug-induced)
- Post-mortem confirmation of diagnosis on brain biopsy

Other manifestations
- Impaired consciousness, but arousable

- Prostration, extreme weakness
- Hyperparasitaemia
- Jaundice
- Hyperpyrexia (rectal temperature >40°C).

Quinine regimen
- Quinine dihydrochloride 20mg/kg in 200mL normal saline or 5% dextrose over 4h
- Then 10mg/kg over 4h, every 8h, until oral medication is started.

Adjunctive measures
- ABC
- Blood transfusion
- Treatment of hypoglycaemia
- Anticonvulsants
- Renal replacement therapy
- Exchange transfusion
- Discussion with specialist in infectious diseases.

Meningococcal septicaemia

Meningococcal septicaemia is a potentially lethal illness, with often non-specific clinical features in the early stages, leading to missed and delayed diagnoses. (See p. 446.)

Clinical features

- Fever
- Flu-like symptoms
- Diarrhoea
- Intense leg pain interfering with ambulation
- A vasculitic skin rash: rapidly evolving and progressing, and coalescing non-blanching red skin rash, usually appearing within 24h of onset of illness
- In many cases, in the initial phases a red blanching maculo-papular rash may be seen, mimicking a viral exanthema
- Cold hands and feet
- Digital infarction.

Management

Airway + breathing

- Oxygen therapy
- Early tracheal intubation and ventilation.

Circulation

- Large bore venous access
- Antibiotics: IV 2g cefotaxime or ceftriaxone
- Volume resuscitation
- Avoidance of lumbar puncture
- Inotropic/vasopressor support
- Physiological replacement corticosteroid therapy in the presence of refractory circulatory failure.

Priority investigations in suspected meningitis or meningococcal septicaemia

- Venous blood: FBC; U & E; glucose; LFTs; CRP; clotting profile; culture; EDTA blood for PCR; clotted blood
- Arterial blood gases.

Table 13.7 Glasgow meningococcal septicaemia prognostic score

Criterion	Score
Hypotension <75mmHg if <4yrs age <85mmHg if older	3
Rectal/skin temperature difference >3°C	3
Base deficit <8mmol/L (capillary blood sample)	1
GCS <8 or deterioration >3	3
Lack of meningism	2
Parental opinion that child's condition has become worse over past hour	1
Widespread ecchymoses or extending lesion on review	1
Maximum score = 15	

A score of 8 or above indicates a potentially fatal outcome.

Yung, AP, McDonald MI Early clinical clues to meningococcaemia, *Medical Journal of Australia*, 2003; **178**: 134–137.

Contact addresses

Advanced Life Support Group
ALSG Centre for Training and Development
29–31 Ellesmere Street
Swinton
Manchester M27 0LA
0161 794 1999
(APLS and PLS Courses)

ALERT Course Coordinator
Portsmouth Hospitals NHS Trust
Queen Alexandra Hospital
TEAMS Centre
QUAD Centre
Portsmouth PO6 3LY
020 9228 6000 X 5831
ALERT@port.ac.uk

BASICS HQ
Turret House
Turret Lane
Ipswich IP4 1DL
0870 1654499
www.basics.org.uk
(Pre-hospital emergency care courses)

College of Emergency Medicine
Churchill House
35 Red Lion Square
London WC1R 4SG
020 7404 1999
www.emergencymed.org.uk

European Resuscitation Council Secretariat
Universiteitsplein-1
PO Box 113
BE-2610 Antwerp
Belgium
www.erc.edu

Postgraduate Medical Education and Training Board
7th floor
Hercules House
Hercules Road
London SE1 7DU
0207 160 6100
www.pmetb.org.uk

Raven Department of Education
The Royal College of Surgeons of England
35–43 Lincoln's Inn Fields
London WC2A 3PE
0208 7869 6300
www.rcseng.ac.uk
(ATLS Courses)

Resuscitation Council (UK)
5th floor, Tavistock House North
Tavistock Square
London WC1H 9HR
020 7388 4678
www.resus.org.uk
(ALS, EPLS, ILS and NLS courses)

The Royal College of Anaesthesia
Churchill House
35 Red Lion Square
London WC1R 4SG
020 7092 1500
www.rcoa.ac.uk

Useful websites

BRITISH COMMITTEE FOR STANDARDS IN HAEMATOLOGY
www.bcshguidelines.com

BRITISH THORACIC SOCIETY
www.brit-thoracic.org.uk

BRITISH TRANSPLANTATION SOCIETY
www.bts.org.uk

DIFFICULT AIRWAY SOCIETY
www.das.uk.com

EMERGENCY MEDICINE UK
www.emergencymedicine.org.uk

EUROPEAN SOCIETY OF CARDIOLOGY
www.escardio.org

INTENSIVE CARE SOCIETY
www.ics.ac.uk

JRCALC
Joint Royal Colleges Ambulance Service Liaison Committee
www.jrcalc.org.uk

MENINGITIS RESEARCH FOUNDATION
www.meningitis.org.uk

NATIONAL PATIENT SAFETY AGENCY
www.npsa.nhs.uk

NATIONAL POISONS INFORMATION SERVICE
www.npis.org.uk

NCEPOD
National Confidential Enquiry into Patient Outcome and Death
www.ncepod.org.uk

NICE
National Institute for Health and Clinical Excellence
www.nice.org.uk

SIGN
Scottish Intercollegiate Guidelines Network
www.sign.ac.uk

Index